INNER HYGIENE

INNER HYGIENE

CONSTIPATION AND THE PURSUIT OF HEALTH IN MODERN SOCIETY

James C. Whorton

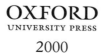

OXFORD
UNIVERSITY PRESS
2000

OXFORD
UNIVERSITY PRESS

Oxford   New York
Athens   Auckland   Bangkok   Bogotá   Buenos Aires   Calcutta
Cape Town   Chennai   Dar es Salaam   Delhi   Florence   Hong Kong   Istanbul
Karachi   Kuala Lumpur   Madrid   Melbourne   Mexico City   Mumbai
Nairobi   Paris   São Paulo   Singapore   Taipei   Tokyo   Toronto   Warsaw

and associated companies in
Berlin   Ibadan

Copyright © 2000 by Oxford University Press, Inc.

Published by Oxford University Press, Inc.
198 Madison Avenue, New York, New York 10016

Oxford is a registered trademark of Oxford University Press

Library of Congress Cataloging-in-Publication Data
Whorton, James C., 1942–
Inner hygiene : constipation and the pursuit of
health in modern society /
James C. Whorton.
p.   cm.   Includes index.
ISBN 0-19-513581-4
1. Constipation—History—19th century.
2. Constipation—History—20th century.
I. Title.
RC861.W39 2000   616.3'428'009034—dc21
99-16812

1 3 5 7 9 8 6 4 2

Printed in the United States of America
on acid-free paper

For Adrian

PREFACE

OH DEAR, man's bowels! What a trouble his bowels are! What an oversight of omniscience to have made man in such a way that he cannot get through life without being plagued by his bowels! . . . Surely prescience and omniscience might have constructed man's frame that poor mortality could have passed through the world without the fearful probability of having life cut short unless he attend everlastingly to his bowels. Oh dear, man's bowels! What a bother his bowels are!

John Smedley, 1872

FREEDOM of the bowels is the most precious, perhaps even the most essential, of all freedoms—one without which little can be accomplished. . . . As a consequence, obstinate constipation constitutes not merely a minor and temporary unpleasantness, . . . but to the contrary a true infirmity, *a pathological condition*, that one must defend against like the plague. . . . How could it be forgotten that—before having a brain, dear reader, before having a heart, dear lady reader—you have . . . a digestive tube open at both ends, an obstruction of which will promptly cause a turn toward disaster?

Émile Gautier, 1909

Why do Drs think that people have to have an eye Dr and throat dr and a foot Dr Prettie soon they will have to have a liver Dr heart Dr and a blood Dr and a skin Dr. The only thing to Dr is the bowels.

Mrs. Martha Rasmussen, 1932

On the 27th day of June in the year 1770, Monsieur Alphin, an army officer stationed in the provinces, suddenly fell feverish and weak. The local apothecary, an M. Blanchard, was summoned, and he immediately proposed the administration of an enema to "reopen and establish the bile flow." When Blanchard attempted to insert his instrument, however, he encountered "great hindrance and vexation," so, naturally, he spread the sick man's buttocks to search out the source of hindrance. He then discovered how truly profound vexation might be, for when he peered into his patient's fundament, the unsuspecting apothecary was greeted, "contrary to all usage and customs," by "AN EYE WHICH STARED HIM IN THE FACE" (this was a phenomenon, he noted, "that had NEVER before happened in the seven years he had been practicing"). Seven years of pharmacy practice will surely breed considerable aplomb toward the face of human deformity. But being scrutinized by a sphincter was more than even Blanchard could bear: considering "that his honor had been outraged," he left the scene at once. Alphin, meanwhile, passed away before a surgeon could arrive to remove the obstruction, leaving Blanchard, who had abandoned a patient in extremis, to face a charge of malpractice. In this instance, fortunately, the apothecary met with a satisfactory end, for the next day a trio of surgeons laid open Alphin's *anus mirabilis* and discovered an artificial eye lodged therein. After hearing servants testify that their master kept his glass eye in a glass of water when he slept, and deciding he must have swallowed it by mistake in the delirium of fever, the surgeons determined that though the case was surely "novel and extraordinary," all "errors and obstinacies are on the side of the deceased."[1]

A person who dies so ignobly, then gets blamed for his death to boot, mustn't be allowed to die in vain. Some redeeming moral should be sought in the tale of Alphin's eye, and in fact at least three can be found. One lesson is that turnabout is fair play. For centuries—millennia, even—the eyes of apothecaries and physicians had been directed toward their patients' bowels. The gut had been presumed to be the source of much disease, and debilitating purgatives and humiliating enemas had been routinely prescribed to flush foul matter from the intestines. It would be simple poetic justice for a patient's bowels to at last return the stare of medicine and provoke outrage in its practitioners.

A second moral is that an ounce of prevention is worth a pound of cure. If Alphin had paid any heed at all to what he was drinking, he would certainly have spared himself considerable discomfort and embarrassment, and conceivably might have escaped an untimely death. No less today do people dig their own graves prematurely, whether by inhaling tobacco smoke, eating fat-sodden junk foods, or acquiring the perfect tan. We can now statistically demonstrate numerous risk factors associated with cancers, cardiovascular disease, and other mortal ills, factors which are elective activities, and therefore, like Alphin's glass eye, avoidable insults. More and more, the profession of medicine turns to doctoring people's lifestyles in addition to their diseases, and preventive measures threaten to crowd out miracle drugs and high technology: "We got him onto an exercise bike," a *New Yorker* cartoon doctor consoles the grieving widow in his office, "but I'm afraid it was too late."[2] Furthermore, in exploring the connections between lifestyle and morbidity and mortality, we have come to recognize that many of our risky behaviors are relatively recent acquisitions, frivolous indulgences fostered by the industrialization and urbanization of Western society. As a consequence, developed nations are all but overwhelmed by "diseases of civilization," or, as they've recently been rechristened, "Western diseases."

Thus we arrive at a third interpretation of the Alphin saga: the more things change, the more they remain the same. The period of his death, the late 1700s, was one of fundamental change in medicine, of the emergence of an orientation that would give medical practice its modern shape. This changing orientation was largely a shifting of the clinical attention of the physician from the whole sick person to the specific pathologically compromised organ or tissue at the seat of the disease. By establishing new definitions and explanations of disease, this localizaton of pathology also fostered new methods of treatment, the growth of medical specialization, and the ever more complex instrumentation and technology that are earmarks of medicine in the late twentieth century. This revolutionary transformation nevertheless failed to tear physicians' attention away from the bowels. On the contrary, medical anxiety over intestinal impurity rose steadily higher through the nineteenth and into the early twentieth century. And though the uneasiness subsided somewhat for a half century beginning in the 1910s, it has returned in recent decades in the form of the dietary fiber hypothesis. Drawn from extensive epidemiological studies, this proposal links "Western diseases" as different as varicose veins and colon cancer to the inadequate fiber content of Western diet; low fiber intake, the reasoning runs, results in low fecal bulk and slow fecal movement, exposing the bowel to greater irritation from its contents as well as altering certain metabolic processes. With the dietary fiber hypothesis, ancient suspicions that fecal decay must trigger physical decay have been modernized and made scientifically respectable. *Plus ca change.* . . . By shifting his gaze to the local site of his bowels, Alphin was turning his eye to the future.

The two centuries since Alphin's passing have witnessed an enduring apprehension over the effects of constipation that has not only gripped medical professionals and the public but also motivated a diverse congregation of health reformers, medical entrepreneurs, and outright quacks to put forward an astonishing variety of preventives and remedies for the dread affliction. A veritable culture of constipaton has developed, a culture enlivened by examples of the most naive idealism and crass materialism, all the while drawing on the latest concepts in medical science. I became involved with the history of this culture while contemplating a book on the historical development of the concept of diseases of civilization. As I immersed myself in medical literature relating to that larger topic, I was struck by the recurring attention to constipation as the fundamental disease of civilization. I soon came to discover that however mundane a matter inactive bowels might at first seem, the modern history of constipation is a fascinating epic, at once an amusing off-color record of human misery, and an instructive account of the evolution of medical thought and its shaping of popular health beliefs and behavior. The original project was set aside in favor of a study of constipation's impact on modern health culture.

Modern preoccupation with bowel health might be described as a concern for "inner hygiene." This phrase, however, should connote a good bit more than simple cleanliness of the intestinal tract. Like so many ancient words, hygiene has undergone degeneration in modern times. The undergraduate who understands by the term anything other than washing of the body surface is a rare scholar today (why hygiene should now mean so little to so many will be addressed in a later chapter). To the ancient Greeks, hygiene meant health and all the things necessary for health. There was even a goddess of health—Hygeia—though it was understood that one worshipped Hygeia not by supplicating the goddess to confer health as a gift but by acting to build and preserve health for oneself through obedience to her clearly understandable rules of living. Hygiene meant above all a regimen, a systematic code of behavior with respect to diet, exercise and evacuation, sleep, and sex—all the habits (including cleanliness) that govern the well-being of the body. This regimen would continue as hygiene's meaning into the nineteenth century, and it would be accepted throughout that those little daily rituals were the great determinants of life-long health. Precisely by being so prosaic, however, so routine and taken for granted, as well as so gradual in their impact, practices of personal hygiene have generally been passed over by historians of medicine in favor of devastating outbreaks of pestilence and revolutionary scientific discoveries. Only recently has the intellectual and social history of hygiene been subjected to respectful study; scholarly analysis of the development of professional and popular health beliefs and practices has in fact grown into a thriving academic industry over the last two decades. Coverage of the subject nevertheless remains somewhat one-sided, for diligent inquiry has been made only into "outer hygiene," or the body's interactions with, and activities within, its surrounding environment: air, water, movement, and the assimilation of food and drink taken from without.[3]

Both medical and lay respect for the beneficent agents of the external world have been paralleled, however, by anxiety about the internal world. The body also surrounds an environment—the alimentary canal—that harbors materials that can seem every bit as threatening as outer agents seem helpful. Thus unless one attends to inner hygiene, the body becomes, by the metaphor Shaw used in *The Doctor's Dilemma*, a whited sepulchre, an outwardly clean edifice whose hidden core reeks with filth and decay. Yet the filth and its retention are ultimately the effects of various errors of diet, exercise, and other life activities. That means inner hygiene requires not merely the cleaning of the bowel of its obnoxious contents but more essentially the practice of all outer hygienic measures that prevent the accumulation and retention of intestinal filth. Medical historians have regularly taken note of this ancient preoccupation with the inner person, yet have found the subject either too puerile or too distasteful to merit much attention beyond asides about the violence of the cathartics and the indignities of the enemas that dominated prescientific medicine and self-care. A balanced understanding of the evolution of modern health consciousness requires a thorough exploration of the philosophies and practices of intestinal purity, a subject that, considering its prominence in medical and popular culture from antiquity to the present, is the most neglected element in the history of hygiene. From Louis XIV's faith in frequent enemas as the foundation of his personal well-being to Princess Diana's reported insistence on an annual allowance for the expenses of colonic irrigation as part of her divorce settlement, cleanliness of the bowels has been a ruling concern in the pursuit of health in modern times.[4]

The reader might well interject that the quest for inner purity is nevertheless only one element of modern health culture, and that focusing so narrowly on a single component of hygiene's history risks magnifying its significance to the point of distortion. It should be clear, then, that the intent of the chapters that follow is nothing more than to demonstrate that intestinal irregularity has always caused (as it does still) a good deal of uneasiness for physicians as well as the public, and has long been looked upon as a fundamental health problem stemming from the advance of civilization. This does not suggest, however endless the talk of constipation may seem at times, that fear of torpid bowels has dominated modern medical thought to the exclusion of all competing health concerns. That established, the reader must be reminded to guard as carefully against trivialization as against overmagnification, not least because intestinal lethargy is anything but a trivial matter to those who suffer it. No matter that it is often only a preoccupation instead of a genuine physical problem; preoccupations cause discomfort too. And when constipation truly does exist, it can produce considerable distress and inconvenience, and even (particularly among the elderly) incapacity. A blessed few may get through the experience unscathed, or even improved (lifelong constipate Martin Luther received his famous "revelation in the tower" while straining at stool); for the rest, the condition is a curse. "Who is more of a misanthrope," asked George V's personal physician, "than the subject of the loaded colon?" By engendering misanthropy, constipation, more than most afflictions, affects the victim's family and friends as well. "I have known . . . the happiness of a whole household to hang daily on the regularity of an old man's bowels," a turn-of-this-century English practitioner commented. "The gates of Cloacina open, the heavens smile and all goes smooth. 'Master's bowels have not acted today,' from the lips of the faithful butler and the house is shrouded in gloom."[5]

Constipation has ever been a source of gloom, and indeed has often been regarded as the most insidious ailment to which human flesh is heir. During the later 1700s, however, constipation began to be widely considered the most insidious ailment of *civilized* human flesh. Throughout the decades since, intestinal in-activity has been consistently attributed, through any number of arguments, to the unnatural modes of life fostered by urban, industrial civilization. To speak of civilization and the rise of constipation, therefore, is not to hyperbolize for the sake of humor. Rather, it acknowledges the true depth of modern society's absorption with intestinal hygiene.

One of the most striking of all records of constipation comes from the sixteenth century, from the coarse epics of Gargantua and Pantagruel. Rabelais was trained in medicine, so one might expect disablement and disease to play prominently in his fiction. His telling of the giants' adventures is as abundant in medical imagery as in medical incident. As the practical study of life and death, medicine, he understood, serves the novelist in a way few disciplines can, providing a powerful tool for exam-ining the timeless questions about human nature and the world. Rabelais used the human body, a modern admirer has commented, as "a pulsating, throbbing meta-phor for the whole of life." Thus when the unfolding plot called for Pantagruel to become ill, the ailment selected for him as the one best calculated to fell a colossus was constipation, bowels crammed with a "heap of ordure and filth," of "fecal mat-ter and corrupted humors . . . more stinking and infectious than ever was Mephi-tis."[6] For while constipation may not be the "whole of life," even to its sufferers, it has played an extraordinary role in human history. Pantagruel's complaint has been everyman's. Much more than just another of his creator's excursions into scatology, Pantagruel's prodigious attack of constipation stands as a parable of human intui-tions about health and disease, and as a marker for an extensive yet barely explored territory in the development and interactions of medical theory and therapy, self-medication and personal prophylaxis, health faddism and quackery, the commer-cialization of hygiene, and modern ambivalence about the blessings of civilization. This book will attempt to show how thoroughly concern for inner hygiene has per-meated Western health culture over the past 200 years.

It will not, however, be possible to consider every single strand of philoso-phy, prevention, and treatment of constipation. The amount of attention that both medical and lay writers have lavished on the costive bowel over the last centuries is enormous, and thorough exploration of all aspects of the topic would render the book unreadably long. I am therefore concentrating my discussion on the twen-tieth century. After two context-setting chapters on inner hygiene in the nineteenth century, six chapters will examine the period of roughly 1900 to 1940, when the threat of "autointoxication" (self-poisoning) from uneliminated waste motivated the public to partake in a remarkable assortment of anti-constipation measures. The two final chapters will follow that early-century fear of intestinal intoxica-tion through the close of the century.

Coverage will be narrowed as well by focusing on constipation anxiety as it was expressed in Great Britain and the United States. The British have long been

seen to be as preoccupied with their bowels as the French are with their livers—
"obsessed," an English physician has lately observed, "with the frequency, consistency, diameter, and appearance of their stools." At the same time, one of the
most frequently recurring declarations of American independence since the Revolution has been the perverse insistence that Uncle Sam's citizens are notably more
constipated than John Bull's. It has also been the case that this competition over
costiveness has been balanced by generous sharing between the two nations of ideas
and practices for escaping constipation.[7] Yet even after imposing these chronological and geographical constrictions, I have found it necessary to select only
certain themes, those that seem to be most significant and representative of constipation as a health concern of modern society.

In the end, no matter how hard one tries to dignify the subject, it remains
constipation. Preceding justifications notwithstanding, the topic may seem too
vulgar, or worse, too insignificant, to justify directing an historical eye at the anus.
In defense, I can only call on Dr. S——t, the pseudonymous author (no, it was not
Jonathan Swift, copromaniacal though he was) of an eighteenth-century tongue-
in-cheek treatise, *Human Ordure, Botanically Considered*. As the "First Essay, of
the kind, Ever Published in the World," it may strike readers, S——t feared, as tasteless or unimportant. Yet "there is no Man that ever was so humble as to observe
Human Ordure, but must confess there is a wonderful Variety in all Productions
of this Nature. . . . The World may say, perhaps I had very little to do, and that
so solemn and serious a Preface ill became so foul a Subject; but, let what will be
said, I can't help communicating my Sentiments, but will endeavour to wrap 'em
up in as cleanly a Manner, as the Dirtiness of the Theme will admit."[8]

Seattle, Wash.   J. C. W.
May 1999

ACKNOWLEDGMENTS

This book has taken a good deal longer to write than I ever would have guessed when I undertook the project (though given the nature of the subject matter, what else could have been expected?). Consequently, I have had more than the usual stretch of time to accumulate intellectual debts, and am indeed deeply in arrears to many people and institutions who assisted me in bringing the work to completion.

Research for the volume was supported in part by NIH Grant LM 05141. Financial assistance was received as well from the Sonnedecker Residency Program, American Institute of the History of Pharmacy. Finally, Albert Jonsen, my department chair at the University of Washington, encouraged my efforts with departmental travel funds (in addition, as Latin scholar, Al reviewed and gently corrected more than one of my attempts to render an antique passage into English).

Staff at a number of libraries and archival depositories provided invaluable aid in locating materials. I wish particularly to thank Colleen Weum, of the University of Washington Health Sciences Library, who was indefatiguable in the tracking down of whatever obscure works on colon function or bowel pathology I requested, and ever ready to help a novice find his way through the maze of Internet databases. Other members of the Health Sciences Library staff who smoothed my path were Hilary Carkeek, Mary Rainwater, Mary Van Court, and Kathleen Von Der Hofen. Special thanks go as well to Jan Todd, Curator of the Todd/McClean Physical Culture Collection at the University of Texas. Jan went far beyond the call of her duties in making my week in Austin productive.

I received kind help from staff at other institutions, including the National Library of Medicine, Bethesda, Maryland; National Museum of American History, Smithsonian Institution, Washington, D.C.; American Institute of the History of Pharmacy, University of Wisconsin, Madison, Wisconsin; the American Medical Association's Historical Health Fraud Collection in Chicago; The College of

Physicians of Philadelphia; the Edgar Cayce Foundation, Association for Research and Enlightenment, Virginia Beach, Virginia; Wellcome Institute for the History of Medicine, London; British Library, London; University of London Library; Royal Pharmaceutical Society, London; Gordon Museum, Guy's Hospital, London; St. Thomas's Operating Theatre Museum, London; Royal College of Physicians, Edinburgh; Special Collections Department, Edinburgh University Library; National Library of Scotland, Edinburgh; the Cheltenham [Gloucestershire] Art Gallery and Museum, and the Cheltenham Library; the Harrogate [Yorkshire] Library, and the Royal Bath Hospital, Harrogate. In Harrogate, Dr. Sheila Moore gave generously of her time in introducing me to research opportunities in that beautiful town.

I am especially grateful to the late Denis Burkitt and his wife Olive for sharing memories of the early development of dietary fiber theory, while simultaneously entertaining me at tea in their cottage in Bisley, Gloucestershire. I had an equally charming time at tea with Dorothy Chapple at her home in Sunbury-on-Thames, Middlesex, hearing her recollections of her grandfather, Sir William Arbuthnot Lane (a gentleman who figures large in this book). Tea was also taken with surgeon David Preston, of Louth, Lincolnshire, who gave up much of an afternoon to show me materials he had collected on Lane. William Helfand, of New York City, surrendered a morning directing me through his extraordinary collection of art works relating to the history of medicine and drugs (and has kindly granted permission to reproduce several items in this volume).

Others who assisted me in any of a number of ways include Michael Barfoot, Marilyn Barnard, Kim Beckwith, Susan Bowker, Andrew Brown, Bob Burke, Janet Caplan, James Carson, James Cassedy, Barbara Clarkson, Alisa Clein, David Cochran, George Constantine, Daniel Cox, J. H. Cummings, Ann Dally, J. J. Daws, Richard Engeman, John Eyler, Christina An Finkelstein, Norman Gevitz, Charles Greifenstein, William Haubrich, Kenneth Heaton, Lonny Hecker, Greg Higby, Adam Hornbuckle, Thomas Horrocks, Robert Joy, Suzanne Junod, Jimmy Lara, Barron Lerner, Harvey Levenstein, Sharon McGrayne, Lorene Mayo, Douglas Migden, Elaine Monsen, Richard Nelson, Melissa Oliver, John Parascandola, Roy Porter, Robin Price, John Quinn, Reimert Ravenholt, Nancy Rockafellar, Gail Sekas, Julia Sheppard, H. M. Sinclair, Dale Smith, Glenn Sonnedecker, Woody Sullivan, Michaela Sullivan-Fowler, John Swann, Cassandra Tate, Elaine Taylor, Hugh Trowell, Larry Vincent, Arnold Wald, Emily Wilkinson, Mary Ann Woodruff, and James Harvey Young.

Edith Barry, Jeffrey House, and Nancy Wolitzer of Oxford University Press were a pleasure to work with and very helpful with suggestions during the process of editing the manuscript.

Two dear friends have given freely of both intellectual and moral support. Jack Berryman, of the University of Washington, provided numerous leads to reading in the history of physical culture. Robert Nye, of Oregon State University, read and criticized parts of the manuscript, and was his usual fount of provocative ideas and constructive ridicule, offered through every medium from e-mail messages to conversations one spring week in what must have been half the village pubs of Gloucestershire.

I spared my wife Jackie any reading of the manuscript, but she certainly had to listen to enough anecdotes about the history of constipation, and usually at dinner. She was also frequently called into duty to vet my translations of French sources. For her forebearance, and for making nonworking hours so joyful, I am profoundly grateful.

Finally, I wish to thank my son Adrian, who has lived with this project longer than anyone but me, and, first as medical student, now as resident, has been expected to answer more than a few technical questions running the gamut from physiological mechanisms to surgical techniques; I'm proud to say he almost always had the answer. I am far prouder though, of the fine man he has made himself into.

CONTENTS

INNER HYGIENE

1

INNER HYGIENE IN THE NINETEENTH CENTURY: THE CONSEQUENCES OF CONSTIPATION

DAILY EVACUATION OF THE BOWELS is of the utmost importance to the maintenance of health. Without this the entire system will becomes [sic] deranged and corrupted
. . . a diseased stomach, bad breath, sallow complexion, enlarged and diseased liver, rush
of blood to the head, loss of memory, headache, heart disease, bleeding at the lungs, a thick,
coarse skin, loaded and contaminated blood and bile, falling of the womb, dyspepsia, piles,
hectic fever, consumption . . . are induced by neglect of this matter.

Harmon Root, 1856

Constipation (from the Latin *constipo*, to press or crowd together) is defined by *Dorland's Medical Dictionary* as "infrequent or difficult evacuation of the feces."[1] *Dorland's* is a standard source of medical definitions,
but if the story that follows is to be clear, the nonmedical reader needs
a more thorough explanation of constipation than that. The condition is the result
of a complex physiological process being disrupted by any of several interfering
factors, and both the process and the factors play leading roles in the evolution of
physicians' and lay persons' thinking about constipation.

One may as well begin with a consideration of feces. As the products of digestion that do not get absorbed into the circulation pass through the small intestine, they become mixed with bacteria resident in the digestive tract and with the
bile secreted by the liver for the digestion of fats; it is through bacterial action that
the various malodorous substances associated with bodily waste are produced,

1

while bile gives feces their characteristic color. Mucus, cells from the intestinal lining, and water become incorporated into the waste matter as well. Depending on the amount of fiber in the diet, the weight of a stool can vary from as little as an ounce to as much as a pound or more. Three-quarters of the weight of an ordinary stool is water, and more than half the dry weight of a movement consists of bacteria.[2]

Waste enters the large intestine at the *ileocecal junction*, where the ileum, the last segment of small intestine, connects to the cecum in the lower right abdomen (refer to Fig. 1-1, taken from a 1928 manual on constipation written by a physician for lay readers). The *cecum*, a pouch to whose nether end the appendix is attached, extends upward into the ascending colon, which ascends to the upper right abdomen before turning to the left at the hepatic flexure (i.e., a bend near the liver) to become the *transverse colon*. This latter section stretches across to the left side of the abdomen, then turns downward at the splenic flexure (near the spleen) to form the *descending colon*. In the lower left abdomen, the descending colon turns back to the right in a loop called the *sigmoid*, or *S-shaped*, *colon* (pelvic colon in the diagram). Finally, the sigmoid twists downward in the center of the body into the *rectum* (M), which terminates at the *anus* (L). The length of the colon, the distance from the ileocecal junction to the anus, is about 6 feet in the adult, and feces, moved along by contractile movements of the colon wall (peristalsis), require from 1 to 5 days to complete the passage (this *transit time*, as it is called, is dependent on the amount of indigestible bulk in the diet, and is typically longer in developed countries, where diets contain relatively low levels of fiber). Throughout the transit, water is absorbed from feces. Hence, if waste matter moves too rapidly, stools will be watery; if too slowly, they will be dry and hard, formed into so-called scybala. Normally, fecal material collects at the junction of the sigmoid colon and the rectum, until, through a nervous system reflex, some quantity of waste passes into the rectum, producing distention and the desire to defecate.

Frequency of defecation is highly variable. The great majority of people have an evacuation on a daily basis, but anywhere from 3 bowel movements a week to 21 is accepted as within the normal range (men generally have a somewhat greater frequency than women, and produce larger and softer stools). Physicians think of constipation as two or fewer movements per week, and/or the frequent necessity of straining to evacuate; painful defecation and the expulsion of scybala are common accompaniments. For patients, of course, the question of when one is constipated is open to far broader interpretation, being just about as subjective a judgment as the definition of pornography. Indeed, what the Supreme Court justice observed of pornography applies equally well here: people may not be able to define constipation with exactness, but they know it when they have it. "I know this," a British physician confided early this century, "that if my habit is not one of the most absolute daily regularity I am a worm and no man."[3]

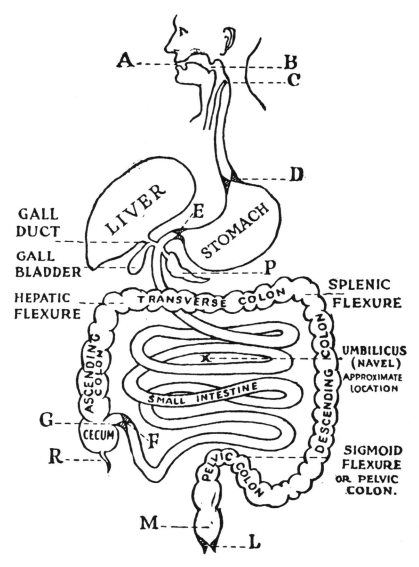

Figure 1-1. Diagram of the human intestinal tract [from William Stemmerman, *Intestinal Management for Longer, Happier Life*, p. 30].

Other signs of prolonged retention of feces include coating of the tongue, foulness of breath, loss of appetite, headache, and mental sluggishness (these follow apparently from mechanical pressure on the wall of the rectum). Nevertheless, there are exceptional individuals who go extended periods without emptying their bowels yet suffer no apparent injury or illness. A patient "who looked the picture of health" told a turn-of-this-century English physician that her bowels were perfectly regular; when asked to elaborate, she replied that they moved every 8 days. Many other doctors have recorded cases of healthy patients whose "regularity" was fortnightly, or monthly, or even more infrequent. There are also people who enjoy normal regularity, yet still retain considerable quantities of waste matter in the colon. A case in point is the nineteenth-century patient who suffered for 10 months with abdominal pain, even while having a daily evacuation. At the end of that time, he "passed with great pain sufficient faeces to fill seventeen chamber-pots"; after that, his pains disappeared for good.[4]

Constipation is sometimes caused by organic conditions, pathological changes beyond a person's control (an intestinal tumor, for example, or megacolon, an abnormally large intestine). The history of health culture, however, is the story of elective activities, of the particular things people have chosen to do that have positive or negative effects on their well-being, and it is poor choices in daily behavior that most frequently produce constipation. Today we are most conscious of the importance of including fiber in the diet, from whole grains, legumes, vegetables, and fruits. But we are also taught early in life the need to establish regularity by retiring to the toilet every morning after breakfast (the entrance of food into the stomach stimulates the intestines to move feces into the rectum). Unfortunately, the morning visit to the water closet is not always convenient, and though feces may voluntarily be held in the rectum until evacuation is feasible, if waste is retained too long, the desire to void will subside; if denial of the urge to empty is persistent, chronic constipation will result. The most frequently assigned cause of constipation historically has in fact been neglect to answer the daily call of nature (a medieval health guide stressed this necessity most pointedly, enjoining readers to "all alvine [intestinal] calls obey, Nor pause should e'en the King pass by that way").[5] Sedentariness is another common contributing factor in the establishment of constipation.

The mind matters too, as the functioning of the bowel is subject to the individual's emotional state; "the gastrointestinal tract," a twentieth-century physician has observed, "is the primary battleground for the conflicts between the psyche and the soma." An immediate challenge (the imminence of a public speaking engagement, the threat of physical assault) loosens the bowels and incites a need to evacuate. Chronic anxiety, with resultant feelings of depression or demoralization, suppresses intestinal activity and brings on constipation. As with seemingly every aspect of personal well-being in the late twentieth century, it appears that high self esteem is critical for good bowel health. A 1981 psychological analysis of "Personality Factors as Determinants of Stool Output" demonstrated that defecation occurs at its optimum level in "persons who are more socially outgoing, more energetic and optimistic, . . . and who describe themselves in favorable terms." It is tempting to hypothesize that constipation has necessarily increased with the emergence of modern civilization because of the accelerated rate of social change characteristic of the industrial world. Rapid change confronts people with uncertainty, inducing anxiety and a feeling of loss of control. Might society as a whole become anal retentive in the same way as the child who rebels against parental control by holding back the feces the parents are demanding of him? The argument has been made, but speculation about the impact of social progress on the demographics of bowel functioning will be left to those better versed in and more disposed toward Freudian theorizing.[6]

There is another psychological facet to constipation. Surveys of bowel habits in industrialized countries have determined that only 1% to 4% of the population have fewer than three movements a week—yet 20% to 30% consider themselves constipated. There is a "vast army of hypochondriacs," a British physician commented in the 1930s, "who are never happy unless their stools conform to an ideal which they have invented for themselves." Such people can be cured, he continued, only "by making them realise that faeces have no standard size, shape, consistence, or colour"; they need to be educated "to follow the example of the dog rather than the cat—and never look behind them." Whether imagined or real, constipation claims women as victims much more frequently than men. In a study conducted on more than a million Americans in the 1960s, for instance, 18.5% of the men questioned claimed to suffer from constipation (it was their sixth most common complaint); but among the women, 33.7% reported constipation, citing only headaches and fatigue as more common ailments (with both sexes, the incidence of constipation increased with age, to more than 50% among those 85 or older). This inflation of the incidence of constipation clearly stems from the widely held assumption (believed by more than 60% of the American public in a recent survey) that the colon has to be emptied every day if health is to be maintained: "a bowel movement a day keeps the doctor away" is the adage one medical writer has coined. And if a person takes that principle as medical gospel, even one unproductive day a week will cause concern. In another study, it was found that nearly half the subjects who identified themselves as constipated were in fact having more than five bowel movements a week. It seems ever to have been so. "No matter how perfectly well the person may be," an English physician wrote in the 1840s, everything "in the best order, no pain or ache present, no sense of fulness of the bowels: yet he is haunted" by the spectre of constipation. "All must go wrong, if all be not already wrong, unless his bowels are relieved: they were open yesterday, the day before, and for a year past, but not having been open on this precise day, the worst must happen. How hard, all but impossible, it is to drive into the understanding of patients that all this is error, every medical man of physiological education can say."[7]

Even if the worst might happen, the way to avoid it is obvious enough: alter the diet, take more exercise, attempt to reestablish nature's matutinal urgings. In recent decades, dietary change has taken over first place in the literature of constipation prevention, "dietary fiber" being recognized as nature's way of provoking peristalsis on a daily, even more frequent, basis. Fiber consists of the indigestible components of plant foods (celluloses, hemicelluloses, lignin), the material that moves unabsorbed into the large intestine. Since it attracts and retains large amounts of water, fiber assumes a much greater bulk than other food residues, thereby stimulating peristaltic contractions, being moved through the gut more rapidly, and prompting defecation more frequently. The softer texture of the wet fiber stool also allows for smoother passage of waste from the body. But all fiber is not equal. Though vegetables and fruits contribute varying amounts of cellulose to the fecal mass, bran, the shell of the wheat kernel, supplies significantly more. Consequently, whole wheat breads and cereals, products from which the bran has not been removed by processing, have come to be regarded as the most efficient, if not indispensable, means for assuring regular and complete bowel elimination: "Adding bran to our daily diets," one foe of constipation has recently written, "helps us to move our bowels as often as possible as easily as possible, and to pass stools as large as possible, so that when the procedure is over we'll feel as comfortable and satisfied as possible."[8]

But many people prefer the taste and texture of white bread and candied cereals, and the other steps toward maintaining regularity also require self-denial. So no matter how satisfying bran is supposed to be, the more popular option has been the easy solution—laxative drugs that purge the bowels without the constipated sufferer having to give it a thought. The alliterative suggestion of a twentieth-century British medical editor that "civilization, constipation, and cathartics carry a common denominator" hits the target dead center.[9] Civilization encourages constipation, and it also encourages a desire for quick and undemanding solutions to problems. Cathartics are the quick solution to constipation, so some introduction to laxative drugs is also needed if the chapters that follow are to be clear.

The bowel evacuant drugs in common use today are usually subdivided into the classes of laxatives, which produce soft, formed stools, and cathartics, which result in a more liquid evacuation. For most compounds, the distinction is a matter of dosage—small doses give laxative effects, larger ones cathartic results—so "laxative" and "cathartic" can be interchanged. (In former centuries, far more irritating compounds, the aptly named drastics, were prescribed; these agents induced profuse watery evacuations, accompanied by severe intestinal griping.) The terms purgative and aperient are also used to denote bowel-emptying drugs. In accord with popular usage, I will treat laxative, cathartic, purgative, and aperient as synonyms.

There are several categories of laxatives, determined by the mechanism by which evacuation is facilitated. Saline cathartics (Epsom salts, Glauber's salts) draw water into the intestine, increasing the bulk of fecal material. Stimulant or contact purgatives (senna, rhubarb, castor oil) operate through various pharmacological mechanisms to activate peristaltic waves in the intestinal wall. Bulk-forming laxatives (agar, psyllium) absorb and hold water, and there are still several other ways by which drugs produce aperient effects.[10]

But while laxatives do have a legitimate role to play in the maintenance of health, it is a limited one. They may be necessary to relieve acute constipation, to protect postsurgical patients from straining at stool, to accelerate the elimination of an ingested poison or of intestinal worms killed by drug treatment, and to clear the bowel for radiologic or colonoscopic examination. In each of these instances, however, laxatives are needed only for a short period, perhaps only a single administration. When the colon is subjected to repeated dosing with cathartic drugs, it soon becomes dependent on the artificial stimulus of the laxative compound and ceases to move of its own accord. The interpretation of the laxative user, though, is likely to be that the constipation is more entrenched than ever, and can be overcome only by continuing the drug stimulation. Furthermore, as the body does in response to most drugs, the colon steadily develops a tolerance for the laxative, requiring more and more of the drug in order to be stirred to activity; it's not uncommon for confirmed laxative users to take 20 or 30 pills daily over a period of years or decades. Such people become, in short, laxative addicts, dependent in mind as well as body on the relief afforded by cathartics, and often incapable of being weaned from their drug.[11]

The laxative addict's "cathartic colon" (the term used by physicians to denote the intestine damaged by purgative abuse) is a significant threat to health, productive of gastrointestinal disturbances, weakness and fatigue, and, in rare instances, death. Yet misuse of laxatives continues to be a serious public health problem: approximately 20% of the healthy population of industrialized countries still take cathartics regularly despite the profusion of medical warnings to avoid these drugs. Stretched over the centuries, that translates into many millions of people who have sought relief from constipation, whether real or imagined, through purgatives—only to induce more obstinate bowel dysfunction by destroying the natural action of the colon. The words of a mid-nineteenth-century English physician sum up this exasperating human preference for purgation over self-regulation admirably: "There is perhaps no disease so extremely common in this country as constipation of the bowels," he wrote, "no single disease which, in the aggregate, inflicts so large an amount of suffering on its inhabitants." Yet even though "all sorts of machines have been contrived in vain [and] all sorts of dietary plans have been laid down to no purpose—and the sufferers have been sent to every corner of the habitable globe in search of a remedy . . . equally to no purpose," people have imagined they could find relief in active cathartics, "until now . . . the daily use of pernicious drugs has become to thousands as necessary as their daily food."[12] This use of pernicious drugs, the machines contrived in vain, the dietary plans and desperate journeys to spas in every corner of the globe, and so many more attempts to counteract the constipating effects of modern civilization will be the themes of the pages that follow.

Sometime during the 1830s (a more precise date was not recorded), an otherwise healthy London woman began to experience periodic attacks of severe stomach-ache, "accompanied with most obstinate constipation." At first, the attacks were spaced at intervals a month or more apart, but gradually they became more frequent, eventually plaguing her daily. Eating brought on such paroxysms of pain that she began to restrict herself to a single daily meal of a dry biscuit with water or brandy, but even that caused extreme discomfort. Her bowels continued "at all times greatly constipated," despite heavy dosing with rhubarb, senna, castor oil, salts, and other purgatives. "She frequently had no evacuation for *six weeks*" at a stretch, and on occasion went 3 or 4 months with no relief. Indeed, when a movement did at last occur, it was a most perverse sort of relief, "her pains [of elimination] being more severe, if possible, than those of labour." The fecal matter brought forth "was enormous in quantity [and] formed into large round lumps . . . each certainly not less than a large foetal head." Urination became increasingly difficult and infrequent also, her joints and muscles lost flexibility, and she became incapable of opening her mouth. Progressive loss of weight and strength ensued, until "eventually the death she fervently prayed for closed a life embittered by a world of painful and unmitigated suffering."

Though the woman had consulted any number of physicians, none had been able to detect definite organic pathology. Nor could a probable diagnosis be made after her death, for she had stoutly resisted all suggestions of an autopsy. The fashionable Russell Square practitioner under whose care her ordeal had at last ended was thus uncertain what to assign as cause of death. Cancer was surely a possibility, though there had also been signs that made malignancy seem unlikely. "The many nervous symptoms," he proposed, pointed to disease of the brain and spinal cord, but there were reasons to doubt that diagnosis too. In the end, Dr. Williams headed his report simply, "the most remarkable case of constipation," and mailed it to a colleague for inclusion in his *Treatise on the Causes and Consequences of Habitual Constipation.* The implication of the unfortunate woman's illness, therefore, was that while overt pathological consequences might not be discernible, the underlying cause of disease could be clearly identified and situated in the body's core: "painful and unmitigated suffering" in virtually any form, even cancer and brain disease, might result from chronic inactivity of the bowels.[13]

The first step to be taken toward understanding humanity's enduring obsession with constipation is to appreciate the dreadful physical consequences that have always been presumed to arise from the costive intestine. The belief that retained feces can poison the body has, first of all, an unshakeable foundation in intuition. Reverence for cleanliness of all body parts, in fact, seems to be immortal. What religious ritual is more ancient than acts of cleansing to make people presentable to the gods? Holiness seems to require wholeness and freedom from blemish. Dirt defiles, and bodily evacuations in particular, whether mucus secretions, menstrual discharge, or feces, have been universally regarded as spiritual pollutants.[14]

For reasons of appearance, feel, and smell, they are also easily regarded as physical pollutants. It is impossible to insulate medicine from aesthetics, to resist supposing that what is ugly or unpleasant must also be injurious. And when attention is turned from the soul to the body, it is the bowel far more than any other part that arouses fear of dangerous pollution. The examples used in a work analyzing the history of dirt to illustrate the persistence of "irrational feelings of defilement . . . in the most sophisticated societies" make the point clearly: "Try serving soup in a chamber pot," author Terence McLaughlin suggests. No matter how well scrubbed, even disinfected the pot may have been after its previous use, the soup will go untouched. *That* kind of dirt, we all feel, can never be completely washed away. Who of us would react differently from the elderly woman "who was unlucky enough to drop her false teeth down the lavatory, where they were flushed into the sewer. When a search failed to find them, she heaved a sigh of relief. 'I would never have fancied them again,' she said."[15]

One can never fancy anything that has been touched even indirectly by the bowel, for the organ is a noisome sump in which is deposited filth whose texture and odor are the very definition of putrefaction, an obtrusively eloquent reminder of the eventual dissolution of death. Feces provide the analogy of choice for all things dirty, disagreeable, or useless: slums are cesspools of humanity, people with mistaken notions are full of crap, to a seventeenth-century Puritan the Anglican *Book of Common Prayer* was a "dungheap of popish abominations." Of all the mean dismissals of women as empty-headed prattlers, what makes the point so sharply as the old English proverb, "Many women, many words; many geese, many turds"? And if feces are foul in health, they can be even more vile in disease: an eighteenth-century Scottish lay term for the product of dysentery, "the green scour," is but one of many repellent phrases coined over the centuries to hint at the utter putridity of intestinal corruptions. Physicians who perform postmortems are unavoidably aware that the intestines are the first part of the cadaver to decompose. Pre-twentieth-century physicians, ignorant of the action of the millions of bacteria that colonize the colon, could interpret the sickening odor released when the abdomen was opened in no other terms than that the bowels must constitute the veritable throne room of all-conquering death. (Nor is the connection of fecal odor with death wholly fanciful; in recent years several fatalities have occurred among farm-workers overcome by hydrogen sulfide fumes while cleaning cow manure tanks.) The various parasitic worms so often found in the intestinal tract, as well as seen wriggling in stools from the living, buttress the conviction, calling to mind the worm-riddled corpse in its grave. The parallel has always been inescapable. In the 1989 novel *Love in the Time of Cholera* (itself an evocation of death within life), Garcia Marquez described nightfall in the Caribbean as "the oppressive moment of transition, [when] a storm of carnivorous mosquitoes rose out of the swamps, and a tender breath of human shit, warm and sad, stirred the certainty of death in the depths of one's soul."[16] Intuition and experience combine to virtually assure feces will be seen as fatal, and inner hygiene esteemed as an absolute essential of health.

Indeed, the oldest complete "book" extant is an Egyptian pharmaceutical papyrus (Papyrus Ebers) of the sixteenth century BC that offers as a basic expla-nation of disease the notion of a poisonous substance (rendered *whdw* by Egyptolo-gists) produced from undigested food in the intestines that overflows into the body proper and initiates putrefaction in the vital organs. In this respect, at least, medi-cal theory would not change drastically before the nineteenth century. Physicians of the 1700s, to illustrate, referred to the alimentary tract as the *primae viae*, or, as Latin usage declined in the eighteenth century, as the "first passages." The term connoted an avenue through the center of the body which, like any avenue, had to be kept clear, with traffic flowing. The purpose of a passage was to allow things to pass; any slowdown, let alone stoppage, was unnatural, and therefore danger-ous. Joseph Lieutaud, a highly placed doctor of the eighteenth century (he was personal physician to Louis XV), was one of the more articulate expositors of where fecal stagnation could lead. Like other physicians, he spoke ominously of the *sordes* (from the Latin *sordeo*, to be dirty), the residues of digestion in the *pri-mae viae* that should "be thoroughly carried off." If the sordes were not promptly removed, "the depraved juices, putrid matter, or depraved bile itself, lodged in the stomach and intestinal canal" might, he reasoned, be drawn into the blood through the "second passages," the lacteal vessels linking the intestines to the cir-culatory system. Lieutaud told of the "feculent blood" he found in victims of pu-trid fever, and described the elimination of corrupt matter through any of the body openings, not just the anus, as a "defecation." Even venesection, the bleeding then believed to be beneficial for just about all patients, would be harmful if not pre-ceded by a purging of the bowels, "because the emptied [by bleeding] vessels allow a more free *ingress* to the depraved remains of concoction." The first passages, then, constituted a physiological highway from mouth to anus that, in a state of constipation, was transformed into a pathological cul de sac (a "sewer," Lieutaud called it) from which the depraved remains of concoction could pass into the arterials of the blood vessels and overrun the system. Retained feces, in another physician's words, "must necessarily taint the fluids with a scorbutic acrimony, which may in time produce obstinate complaints."[17] All the clinical experience of the centuries had scarcely advanced understanding of the consequences of intestinal putrefaction beyond the concepts of the Papyrus Ebers; the constipated body still poisoned itself, whether with *whdw* or scorbutic acrimony.

The nineteenth-century public was subjected to even more dire warnings. London doctor Richard Reece, for example, opened his volume on constipation with the pronouncement that "there is no complaint more general or a more frequent precursor of disease, than costiveness. . . . It is often a predisposing, and not unfrequently an exciting, cause of the diseases that terminate the lives of more than one half of the human race. . . . [It is] more or less connected with all the diseases to which mankind is liable." One could hardly wonder, then, at his frightening additional observation "that subjects whose bowels have not been regularly relieved every or every other day, very rarely attain the age of forty." By an American physician's reckoning, constipation was the source of "three fourths of all the diseases . . . which torture the body, enfeeble the mind, and waste the life of civilized man." Medical and health literature teemed with case reports such as the one that opens this chapter, cases in which there was no demonstrable pathological alteration of tissue, but the patient had a history of costiveness, so . . . . death surely could be attributed to the slow but sure effects of habitual constipation. If a postmortem uncovered the presence of any significant amount of putrefying matter in the alimentary tract—the 60 pounds of "pudding-like material" found in the gut of a Frenchman who died suddenly in 1809, for instance—so much more certain was the diagnosis.[18]

The mechanism by which nineteenth-century doctors presumed costiveness to wreak such widespread havoc was essentially the same as that which eighteenth-century theorists had conjectured. "Excrementitial residue . . . retained in the bowel," according to one authoritative text, "becomes hard, knotty, dry, and friable: changes produced by the absorption of its fluids, which being necessarily conveyed into the blood, adulterate and corrupt it." Corruption could come by an indirect route, too, for hard and knotty residues would irritate first the intestine, then, by "sympathy," the stomach, thereby impairing digestion: "From impaired digestion, there must proceed impure chyle, from impure chyle impure blood; and if impaired digestion, produced and prolonged by habitual constipation, should endure, not for months only but for years, how can we wonder that the whole mass of the blood should become corrupt, or that the solids derived from that blood should be corrupt also?" A sampling of other texts uncovers statements such as the early-century warning that "the retained feces communicate a noxious quality to the [blood]"; the mid-century one that "the matter of alvine . . . excretions . . . cannot be long retained . . . without causing mischief" because it is "essentially pernicious"; and the late-century one that "the blood becomes poisoned by the retention and absorption of waste matters." Poisoned blood, yet another writer explained, means a thoroughly poisoned body, as "the horrible burden" is borne even to "the lip of beauty, which we kiss with so much devotion; [even] the very tear-drop of affection has mingled with it what ought to have been deposited in the privy a few hours before." "If what we eat today," he concluded, "does not pass from us to-morrow, it remains but to clog, and irritate, and inflame, and fester, and destroy, and rot every part with which it comes in contact."[19]

With everything festering and rotting, anything could happen. Lists of the consequences of constipation, to be found both in the texts used by medical professionals and the domestic handbooks consulted by the laity, indeed made good on Reece's assertion that the condition was "connected with all the diseases to which mankind is liable." The insidious course of destruction began slowly: "the person suffers from headache, from languor, from distention of the abdomen, . . . the breath is disagreeable, and the tongue furred, the state is not compatible with health, and should be corrected." But if not corrected, much worse than furring of the tongue could be expected to ensue; the heart disease, consumption, and other ailments cited in the quotation that opens this chapter comprised but a partial catalogue of constipation's supposed ravages. It was for good reason, then, that lay manuals such as *Letters to the People on Health and Happiness* stated bluntly that "there is no rule of health more important than this: *Take all proper methods to prevent constipation.*"[20]

Belief in systemic poisoning through fecal decay was reinforced in the nineteenth century by fear of another intestinal problem: flatulence. Intestinal gas had in fact long been supposed by some physicians to be a particularly effective medium for disseminating the depraved remains of concoction throughout the body (I will "send up fumes will make you worse," the abused intestines of a seventeenth-century Englishman threatened, and "in a word, I'le make your palate tast a tourd, And when you belch I'le turne the sent, To perfect smell of fundament"). By the nineteenth century, however, the threat could be defined with far greater clarity than "fumes." Analytical chemistry had developed to the point that it was possible to identify individual compounds even in gaseous mixtures. Hydrogen sulfide, in particular, was found to be commonly present in intestinal gas, and the compound was also determined to be a deadly poison when undiluted. It made sense, then, as readers of the *Library of Health* were informed as late as the 1840s, that "every degree of flatulence is disease," because hydrogen sulfide was "a poison so subtile as to penetrate . . . all the tissues of the body, . . . a most terrible poison." The danger was often overlooked, though, especially "among the laboring classes," who ignorantly thought of flatulence "as a sign of firm health," and supposed "that the power to eject the gas with violence, is one of the more certain indications of high health." For "multitudes," consequently, "the discharge of wind is as music to their ears." In actuality, it was poison to their bodies, and to their family and friends' bodies. "Him [sic] who loves his neighbor as himself," a nineteenth-century physician admonished (while presaging the next century's discovery of the dangers of secondhand smoke), must remember that "it is as much a crime to poison a neighbor with gas, as with a poison more tangible."[21]

Sparing one's neighbors, however, increased the risk to oneself. Benjamin Franklin, among others, fretted that "well-bred people" set themselves up for "future disease . . . often destructive of the constitution and sometimes of life itself" by holding in wind in social situations. Surely, he hoped, chemists could discover some substance that could be mixed with food to "render the natural discharges of wind from our bodies . . . inoffensive." And if flatulence could be detoxified, why could it not be deodorized as well? Could not science also improvise a way of "ex-pressing one's scent-iments," Franklin asked, that would make intestinal expulsions as "agreeable as perfumes," and thereby actually enhance social interactions through bowel exhalations? "The generous soul, who now endeavours to find out whether the friends he entertains like best claret or Burgundy, champagne or Madeira," he could foresee, "would then inquire also whether they chose musk or lily, rose or bergamot, and provide accordingly."[22]

In the meantime, intestinal gases had to be thought of as highly insalubrious. So great was the fear of fecal vapors, in fact, that even the fumes released from stools, material that had already been evacuated from the body, were regarded as dangerous. Thus the eighteenth-century's great authority on military medicine, John Pringle, attached much significance to the foul air released from "human excrements lying about the camp" as a cause of sickness in soldiers. Similarly, manuals written to guide nurses and other attendants to the sick almost invariably stressed the necessity of not allowing the patient's excrements to remain in the sickroom. On into the middle of the nineteenth century it is common to encounter such urgent advice as "the evacuations should be removed instantly from the room"; and "it is of immense importance in all acute disorders that the excretions of the patient should be immediately removed." Even Florence Nightingale, the nursing profession's sainted founder, insisted in her 1859 best-seller *Notes on Nursing* that "everything which the patient passes must be instantly removed away, as being more noxious than even the emanations from the sick [i.e., contagion]." It simply would not do to leave the chamber pot under the patient's bed until it had been filled or the time was more convenient. "Did you but think for one moment of the atmosphere under that bed," Nightingale reproved lazy nurses, and of "the saturation of the under side of the mattress with the warm evaporations, you would be startled and frightened too!"[23]

The frightfulness of fecal emanations was tightly bound, furthermore, to the most momentous of the nineteenth-century's medical advances, the institution of modern public health programs. Indeed, the early public health movement not only provided a seemingly scientific rationale for fear of flatus and feces but, by demonstrating the value of environmental sanitation for the prevention of disease, also heightened popular respect for the virtue of cleanliness and, by extension, of inner, intestinal sanitation.

Prevention of epidemic disease began to be conscientiously pursued during the 1840s and '50s through the sanitary reform movement, which attempted to eliminate the sources of mass illness by removing filth from the urban environment. Organic refuse was believed to poison the atmosphere with miasma (Greek for pollution), toxic vapors released from animal and vegetable material as it putrefied. The miasmatic theory was centuries old, traceable all the way back to Hippocrates, but it still had considerable rational appeal. The atmosphere was, after all, often the only obvious exposure all victims of an epidemic had in common, and miasma also explained why disease was so often the companion of economic deprivation and squalid environment. Miasmatic interpretations had been strengthened further by experience with the devastating invasions of bubonic plague and other acute infections that ravaged Europe time after time from the fourteenth century on. Although it was evident that a few of these diseases (smallpox, for example, and syphilis) were spread by person-to-person contact, in the majority of epidemics many people fell ill without having any direct exposure to the sick. The more subtle routes of transmission of microbes between infected and healthy persons—water, asymptomatic carriers, insects, and other animal vectors—were not known, and until these routes were discovered, an accomplishment of the second half of the nineteenth century, spread of sickness through the atmosphere was a perfectly satisfying explanation. In truth, in cases where insects carried infection, spread did occur through the atmosphere, but it was much more plausible to attribute malaria and yellow fever to miasma than to mosquitoes. Miasma, in short, ruled epidemiological thinking until the last quarter of the nineteenth century.[24]

This ancient theory achieved its peak of vigor during the middle decades of the 1800s, when it was adopted as the foundation for the modernization of public health measures. Prior to this, public health, the prevention of epidemics, had been a hit-or-miss, too-little and too-late affair. But the faith in the power of science to improve the human condition that had blossomed in the later eighteenth century inspired a new confidence that a population's health could be assured through environmental sanitation. If epidemics arose from miasma, and miasma originated in filth, then removal of filth from the environment should prevent epidemics. The need for environmental cleansing was dramatized further by the intensified urbanization associated with the Industrial Revolution. Organic refuse was directly correlated with population density, and as cities grew ever more packed, the garbage and waste that spawned miasma became ever more noticeable—and frightening. Indeed, the expected increase in disease (particularly tuberculosis, typhus, and cholera) did follow, and by the 1830s more than one study had reported a statistical correlation between levels of sickness and levels of filth. This spiraling disease threat was felt most acutely in Britain, the pacesetter in industrialization; so it was in Britain, in the 1840s, that environmental hygiene was first effectively translated from philosophy into practice under the banner of "sanitary reform."

The sanitary reform movement, directed by indefatigable civil servant Edwin Chadwick, was dedicated to the belief that disease could be virtually eradicated through such improvements as street paving and drainage, street cleaning and refuse removal, and above all, the construction of efficient sewer systems. Chadwick's epochal 1842 *Report on the Sanitary Condition of the Labouring Population of Great Britain*, an exhaustive survey of the wretched filth in which the British working classes lived, drew indisputable connections between the quantity of organic dirt in the environment and rates of morbidity and mortality. It educated the citizenry on the enormous toll in lives and public funds exacted by preventable disease, and gradually convinced the public that in the long run, prevention was far cheaper than cure.[25]

The resultant Public Health Act of 1848, the first piece of legislation directed at establishing a national system of disease prevention, inaugurated a grand environmental cleansing that brought about a significant lowering of the death rate (particularly from intestinal infections), despite being derived from an erroneous theory. Sanitary reform did do the right things (some of them, at least), if for the wrong reason, so no matter that toward the end of the century the venerable concept of miasma was put to rout by the upstart theory of pathogenic microorganisms. The early successes of sanitary reform had already made a profound and lasting impact on Western society's thinking about illness and prevention. Sanitary reform spread quickly from Britain to Europe and the United States, its universal endorsement by the medical profession and by the state impressing upon popular culture, as if it were a religious tenet, an unquestioning reverence for environmental cleanliness, a loathing and fear of every kind of filth. Miasma permeated Victorian consciousness as thoroughly as it did the city atmosphere, becoming the culture's byword for foulness and insidious evil. Holmes and Watson voiced the uneasiness of all their generation as they walked across the moor toward their appointment with the hound of the Baskervilles: "rank reeds and lush, slimy waterplants sent an odour of decay and a heavy miasmatic vapour onto our faces."[26] Rank odor, slimy decay—so deep was sanitary reform's imprint that, as will be seen, not even the overthrow of miasma theory by medical bacteriology could erase the certainty that putrefaction, wherever it occurred, foreshadowed death.

The overriding principle of sanitary reform philosophy, its most accessible lesson, was that bad odors are bad for health: "*all* smell is disease," Chadwick instructed a Parliamentary committee. To be sure, eighteenth-century medical writers had hinted at the same, almost always including the stink of city air as one of the major degenerative forces of civilization. "Fly the rank city," John Armstrong had enjoined Londoners in the mid-1700s; "shun its turbid air. . . . Sated with exhalations rank and fell." But smell assumed far greater odiousness as Chadwick and fellow sanitarians attacked it with the zeal of crusaders, making its suppression a matter of national pride, even honor. And though sanitary reformers turned their attention to every source of smell in the environment—garbage, standing water, carcasses, abbatoirs, overcrowded burial grounds—they sought out one offender above all others: human feces.[27]

To be sure, eighteenth-century authors had sometimes done the same: when Armstrong decried the rankness and fellness of city air, he at once laid it to "the spoil of dunghills." In the publications of the sanitary reform movement, however, the ill airs released from nature's necessities invariably outranked all other nasal assaults. The nationwide corps of sanitary inspectors who supplied much of the data and descriptions for Chadwick's celebrated *Report*, for instance, managed to find an astonishing number and variety of olfactory nuisances; in their minds, everything from pig sties to rotting potatoes contributed to preventable sickness and premature death. Yet no single source of smell was condemned so frequently and vehemently as "gases from reeking dunghills," "cesspools . . . foul and stinking," "emanations from . . . filthy ruinous privies," and "privies in the most disgusting state of filth . . . from which the most abominable odours are emitted." "There is hardly any source of disease more powerful as to its pernicious influence, or more general as to extent," Chadwick wrote, than these privies and dunghills. One of his dedicated local inspectors traced a dozen cases of fever in his Lancashire hometown to a clogged sewage drain, and even incriminated the wooden pole that had been used to force the drain open and then left to stand, smeared with ordure, between two closely adjacent houses.[28]

The same emphasis can be found in the work of sanitary reformers in other countries. When the Citizens Association of New York conducted a sanitary survey of their city in 1864 (a survey that was published in the *New York Times*), "a vast amount of disease and death" was attributed to "cesspool abominations"; "the contents of a privy" on Fifth Street were blamed for the deaths of "several children"; another privy was described as "worse than a Stygian pit," while of a third the survey stated that "it would seem impossible for human beings to create or endure such vileness."[29]

No one described the vileness of the urban atmosphere with such disturbing language as John Simon, the physician and public health officer who between 1848 and 1876 prepared annual reports on health for the Corporation of the City of London. Simon's well-publicized accounts, moreover, portrayed the city's filth in images unmistakably suggestive of constipation. Consider, for example, his discussion of the "extreme injury" resulting from cesspools. "It requires very little medical knowledge," Simon began his first report, "to understand that animals will scarcely thrive in an atmosphere of their own decomposing excrements." Yet "a very large proportion" of the human residents of London were confined within just such an atmosphere, the cesspits that received their waste being "actually within the four walls of the inhabited house; the latter reared over it, as a bell-glass over the beak of a retort, receiving and sucking up incessantly the unspeakable abomination of its volatile contents." If one thought about it, of course, the human body could readily be imagined as a house above a cesspit. That was how the author of a *Ladies Medical Companion* portrayed the constipated system, informing *ladies*, mind you, that if their inner cesspits ceased to drain efficiently, "the matter which should be discharged ferments, generates large quantities of foul air, which . . . stimulates to diseased action, as any other fumes introduced would certainly do." Any other fumes meant miasma, and flatulence was the body's own miasma: "You will readily admit this," the ladies were assured, "if you will advert to the difference in quality and quantity of the wind escaping from the bowels, when the contents are long retained."[30]

Alternatively, one might think of the intestinal tract as the body's sewer, but that hardly provided an escape. "Noxious gases are rapidly formed in the sewers," Simon explained in another report, from there to "escape . . . into the streets and houses"; if the noxious gas was constipation-induced flatulence, it escaped from the gut-sewer into the vital regions of the body. That this analogy had wide appeal is evidenced, among other ways, by its use in advertisements for home medicine chest purgatives. "The bowels are the common sewers of the body," one manufacturer reminded in issuing his warning that constipation "is the MOTHER OF ALL DISEASES." But there was still more to be said to suggest a correspondence between cesspits, sewers, and costive intestines. "The evil, before all others, to which I attach importance," Simon declared, was that of London's sewers all emptying into the Thames, a tidal river that was as likely to wash material back into the sewer outlet as to whisk it away. Much of the "excrementation of the metropolis . . . shall sooner or later be mingled in the stream of the river, there to be rolled backward and forward amid the population . . . . at low water, for many hours, this material shall be trickling over broad belts of spongy bank which then dry their contaminated mud in the sunshine, exhaling foetor and poison; . . . at high water, for many hours, it shall be retained or driven back within all low-level sewers and house-drains, soaking far and wide into the soil, or leaving putrescent deposit." Viewed from this perspective, it is the city that is constipated, its large intestine, the Thames, burdened by an ever-increasing mass of organic waste and

unable to void it. Likewise, the lesser intestines of the city, its sewers, are constipated as well. Kept from freely passing their contents onto the river, they too fill
with waste and become "chambers for an immense foecal evaporation." Obstructed
sewer, choked river, overloaded colon—they were all the same, "a gigantic poi-
son-bed," as Simon denounced the Thames. Sanitary reform thus may have made
people feel more comfortable with their cities, once streets were cleaned and sewers improved; but their colons were now more worrisome than ever, Simon having raised their consciousness of the danger of what he called "the slow rotteness
of unremoved excrement."[31]

Inner rotteness was made worrisome as well by the value nineteenth-century society attached to bodily purity, as opposed to environmental cleanliness.
For reasons beyond our present purposes, cleanliness of both body and clothing
came to be regarded as vital to health during the later 1700s and early 1800s. Specifically, the pores of the skin, it was believed, had to be kept open, free from waste
matter that was perspired by the body. Warnings that foul exhalates left on the
body's exterior surface would invade and poison the system, moreover, were forceful reminders that foul remnants left on the body's interior surface would do the
same. Indeed, theory indicated that when pores became clogged and trapped perspiration inside the body, waste matter would make its escape into the gut instead:
"it recoils in upon the bowels, and becomes, as it were spears, and darts." That
the two surfaces, skin and bowel, were consciously linked in eighteenth-century
considerations of cleanliness is also suggested by the development of the bidet.
Introduced in the 1720s, the "chair of cleanliness" was for some time a novelty.
Only from the 1750s onward did it gain common acceptance into first aristocratic,
then bourgeois, households on the continent. The bidet, however, was not originally restricted to those uses that today are so delicately described as "feminine
hygiene." The device was employed by men too, for its purpose was to provide
easier, more frequent cleaning of the perianal as well as pelvic region. That whole
area was judged to be unusually vulnerable, an area "where sweat, if left, produces
a disagreeable smell." And smell was a harbinger of disease. As another text went
on to point out, "apart from the unpleasant smell . . . part of these exhalations, and
of the substance of which they are formed, is taken up by the absorbent vessels
and carried into the circulation, . . . disposing the humours to putrefaction."[32]
Commentaries on the value of the bidet made the perineum seem just an extension of the colon, an external continuation of the body's inner skin. It was because
that inner skin was so especially filthy that a special piece of apparatus was needed
to cleanse its outer segment.

The bidet was just one example of the unprecedented significance that bodily
cleanliness was assuming in the theory, even practice, of daily hygiene by 1800.
The new status of washing as a health ritual was due primarily, however, to its

social mandate: cleanliness was more an expression of manners than of medicine. Making oneself clean so as to be presentable to others had been gaining appeal since the Renaissance, as part of what Elias has called *The Civilizing Process*, the process of society lowering its "threshold of repugnance" at objectionable appearance and behavior. Cleanliness was one of the qualities that conferred gentility. Purity of person and clothing made refinement visible, allowing the aristocrat and the sophisticate to clearly separate themselves from the masses. Gradually, cleanliness became a practical middle-class virtue too. Particularly during the later 1700s, with the advance of bourgeois respectability as the social norm, the ethos of neatness and order and control as the keys to worldly success made unsoiled skin and clothing appear a material statement of personal ambition and integrity; the business mentality entered a tidy body into the same moral column as tidy account books. Even handbooks of health backed up comments on the physical benefits of washing with moral encomiums: "Personal cleanliness is not only an amiable virtue," an American physician wrote in the early 1800s, "but a source of much comfort and satisfaction to all who pretend to the least degree of politeness and delicacy." Victorian disdain for, and determination to subdue, the brutish elements of human nature would soon make dirtiness an even more damning indicator of moral slackness. But already by the beginning of the nineteenth century, the implications of being coarse and vulgar, of being *uncivilized*, which neglect of personal cleanliness retains to the present, were embedded in the Anglo-American psyche. Dirtiness was a reason to feel shame.[33]

By being regarded as positive proof of rectitude and refinement, cleanliness exerted unique hygienic influence: as the Bushmans note, "cleanliness . . . was a moral ideal and thus a standard of judgment." Being clean was the one rule of healthful living whose violation was certain to meet with scorn from polite society. Heavy eaters, hard drinkers, and other lax livers got their share of condemnation too, but those blows were generally softened by society's unstated tolerance, if not envy, of the free and frolicking life of the *bon vivant*. Dirtiness had no redeeming qualities: neither healthful, nor pleasant, nor decent, it merited nothing but contempt. Hence as hygienic thought came to concentrate on the issue of how to adapt living habits to the rapidly changing and expanding world of urban civilization, cleanliness shone forth as the one accomodation that was already being made and that most brightly augured the hoped-for merger of healthful with civilized living. So complete was the cultural dominion of cleanliness that the concept steadily came to be used interchangeably with the broader concept of hygiene, until the word "hygiene" would as likely trigger thoughts of washing as it would the traditional associations of eating, exercising, or sleeping. The same transformation occurred with "sanitary." Derived from the Latin word for health, *sanitas*, it too implied all the non-naturals as late as the mid-1800s: "*Cleanliness* in towns," an American counterpart to sanitary reformer Chadwick wrote in 1850, "should constitute an indispensable part of sanitary" policy. At that point, environmental cleanliness was only *part* of sanitation, or health. The triumphs of the sanitary reform movement over the next quarter century, however, would make cleanliness and sanitation synonymous.[34]

The alteration of the meaning of personal hygiene was completed by the later-century elaboration of the germ theory, which made bathing a more urgent health practice than ever: "Cleanliness is the basis of hygiene," the author of *Les Monstres Invisibles* wrote in 1897, "because it consists of removing from us all dirt, and, in consequence, all microbes." The modern disease scourge, the invisible monsters of bacteria, seemed much more readily thwarted by soap and water than by moderation in food and drink. By 1890, New York City schoolteachers were training their pupils to reply to the question, "What must I do to be healthy?" with a litany quite different from the one students of a century earlier would have recited. "I must keep my skin clean," this new version of the hygiene catechism began. Wearing clean clothes followed, and only then did pure air and wholesome food, the traditional opening of the rules of hygiene, appear.[35] In the popular lexicon, at least, "hygiene" and "sanitation" entered the twentieth century with a considerably narrower meaning than they had held historically, reflective of the overriding significance cleanliness had acquired over the course of the nineteenth century. That change, of course, only made constipation more worrisome than ever; now it was unhygienic and insanitary not just because it was unhealthful, but also because it was unclean.

And since cleanliness was next to godliness, constipation might also be thought of as immoral. Indeed, the presumption that those of regular bowel habits enjoyed a condition of spiritual superiority was a final contributor to the establishment of inner hygiene as a cultural ideal, and the condemnation of costiveness as the scourge of civilization. However extreme that notion may sound today, it was a conclusion that was unavoidable if one accepted the worldview of many nineteenth-century writers on hygiene. For them, the whole philosophy of health was set within a theological framework that made the body every bit as precious in God's sight as the soul. The rules of body functioning, after all, the laws of physiology, were of God's making just as definitely as the commandments of morality, and thus had equal claim on the homage owed to the author of life. Women's health adviser Catharine Beecher (sister of Harriet Beecher Stowe) expressed what was a widely shared sentiment when she stated that the moral duties preached from the pulpit every Sunday "are no more important to the best interests of man than those 'laws of health' which are so widely disregarded. And yet they are as truly the 'laws of God' as any that were inscribed by his finger on tables of stone." If obedience to physiological law was, as a prominent American physician put it, "as much and as strictly a moral obligation, as is obedience to any command of the decalogue," then those who violated the rules of health were as certain to incur penalties as if they had stolen their neighbor's property or coveted his wife; lusting excessively in the flesh (as well as any other abuse of the body) was as risky as lusting in the heart. The penalty could be expected to occur gradually and through natural mechanisms instead of as a thunderbolt from on high. But in the end it would strike just as surely and lethally. "The folly and wickedness of our practical neglect of the great laws of human growth," Dr. Elizabeth Blackwell believed, "may be measured by the penalties of suffering, illness, and premature death." "Pain and decrepitude," by another hygienist's reckoning, were "the penalties of luxury and excess." By this interpretation, the practice of hygiene was an act of worship, "The Religion of Health," in Blackwell's words.[36]

At the same time, the abundant health enjoyed by those who did conscientiously abide by physiological law was interpreted as the Creator's reward for physical rectitude. Bodily health, furthermore, as the result of moral behavior, might be expected to generate still more morality. As one American physician told it, spiritual purity grew by giant leaps when people observed the "organic laws." "All at once is there given to them a supernatural energy," Elisha Bartlett sang; "benevolence and love run over, like gushing fountains of sweet waters. . . . Hope, on wings of celestial strength and beauty, stretches away her flight into the far depths of eternity, and lays hold on the future life." By being well, one became good and, just as important, was both strengthened and inspired to do good for others. The religion of health was to a considerable extent a social gospel, a physiological Methodism if you will. Combe's belief that "the laws of the human constitution" must serve as "the true basis on which our attempts to improve the condition of man ought to rest" was held by many in the ranks of health campaigners. "Extend your next walk," one exercise promoter suggested, "into a surburban locality. Enter a negro cabin; sit down in their midst; speak with them as a sister; . . . talk with them earnestly about their health; explain in a simple way the laws of ventilation; tell them how tobacco spoils their brains and lungs." Thus may the lowly be raised, and "you will . . . enjoy every walk, inspired by a truly Christian sentiment."[37] The feeling of Christian responsibility to save the bodies of others, and not just one's own hide, was a powerful force behind the marked increase in attention to personal hygiene in the 1800s.

In that cultural context, with health regarded both as moral duty and moral stimulant, the maintenance of bowel regularity could be accorded unprecedented significance. "As a Minister of Christ," a clergyman professed around mid-century, "I should be unfaithful to my trust, if I did not warn those who would . . . glorify God . . . that one great help towards physical or bodily, as well as mental purity, is [to pay] strict attention to the laws of Nature, which require imperatively regular daily expulsion of food we eat when converted into faeces."[38]

Inattention, like any other violation of hygienic law, would be punished; the punishment would be physical ("headache; flatulence; disordered stomach"), but it would also be spiritual. "The moral and mental evils [of neglecting the bowels] are still more distressing,—lowness of spirits; despondency, resulting in absolute assurance of having committed the unpardonable sin—sensuality; inability to apply the mind to any study; . . . utter hopelessness of success in any plan or undertaking,—all these, followed in some cases by insanity, are some of the evil consequences of confirmed constipation." But only some. There could be other, worse consequences in store. One American health writer, admittedly more of an alarmist than most, went so far as to propose that constipation, by producing congestion of the blood, which results in swollen vessels that press upon nerves and thus disturb mental functioning, could eventually lead to a "fearlessness of consequences" that would drive a person to "plunge headlong, and with utter recklessness, into any kind of wrong-doing which circumstances throw in his way—arson, robbery, murder, anything." An English surgeon argued the same possibility, noting that "the bloody miscreant Robespierre" was not only rumored to have been costive, but after his death, "his bowels were found one adherent mass!" It would be an interesting exercise, he recommended, "to consider . . . how far these morbid ailments influenced this monster in the bloody career in which he was engaged." Regularity wrought otherwise. Good bowel hygiene, the clergyman promised, "will lead to that evenness of temper, that cheerfulness of spirit, that firm assurance of hope that can alone make the sorrows of life tolerable, and may form some feeble foretaste of that never-ending happiness which is in store for God's people hereafter."[39]

Nevertheless, the spiritual rewards of intestinal cleanliness were never accorded the attention showered upon the physical benefits, and by the last quarter of the century, with the certainties of religion being increasingly called into question, assertions of a link between regularity and righteousness all but disappeared. One might suppose that with the onset of the great medical revolution of the germ theory during that same period, the link between constipation and general bodily corruption would have been shattered too. But in fact, the scientific breakthroughs of medical bacteriology only forged stronger connections between costive bowels and a host of more serious ailments. Thanks to the germ theory, constipation was transformed into an even greater menace: autointoxication.

To paraphrase Pudd'nhead Wilson, autointoxication was simply constipation with a college education, an age-old complaint elevated to new status by a more sophisticated name and a modern scientific theory. Autointoxication literally means self-poisoning, and though early twentieth-century physicians occasionally pointed to organs other than the colon as potential sites from which the body might poison itself, the term was generally understood to denote intoxication of the body by absorption of poisonous compounds from the large intestine.

It was the eighteenth-century notion of invasion of the bloodstream by depraved remnants of concoction dressed up in the stylish twentieth-century rationale of microbiology.

Autointoxication overshadowed the mere constipation of previous times because it involved germs. To be sure, microorganisms had been known for some time, since the introduction of primitive microscopes in the seventeenth century. But while a few physicians of the 1600s and 1700s had suggested germs might cause disease, their ideas were speculative and could not be taken too seriously until the 1860s and '70s, when the French chemist Louis Pasteur and the German physician Robert Koch devised laboratory methods to experimentally demonstrate causal relationships between particular species of microbes and individual diseases. Over the ensuing two decades, the causative agents of most of the major infectious diseases were discovered, and medicine (and the public) came to think of virtually all illness as due to germs: "the hostile microbe is in fact everywhere," a popular science writer warned in 1895, "within and without us, seeking, we might say, what it might devour."[40]

A linking of germs and illness to constipation followed almost inevitably, through reasoning about the phenomenon of putrefaction. Disease had been interpreted since ancient times as an internal putrefaction, a decomposition of body fluids or tissues (of which vomit, diarrhea, pus, and so on were evidence). Pasteur had essentially confirmed that interpretation by determining that putrefaction of animal and vegetable material outside the body was caused by the action of bacteria. The first practical application of the germ-putrefaction connection, carried out in the latter half of the 1860s, was Joseph Lister's introduction of antiseptic method into surgery; Lister employed a caustic chemical, carbolic acid, to suppress surgical wound infection because he thought of infection as a germ-induced putrefaction. Putrefaction, in short, held center stage in the developing germ theory. And what was constipation but the retention of a mass of putrefying matter in the core of the body, matter that microscopic studies revealed to be teeming with millions of bacteria.

It was simply a matter of a time before medical scientists would investigate the activities of intestinal bacteria. What they found was disturbing. Residues of protein in the large intestine, it became apparent by the mid-1880s, are broken down by microorganisms into a number of compounds (including the aptly named putrescine) that exhibit pronounced toxicity when injected into animals. There was, to be sure, no certainty that these substances were absorbed from the colon into the circulation, and even if they were absorbed, there was reason to suppose that the liver, the body's great detoxifying organ, might neutralize them. But by the same token, it was difficult to imagine that the compounds resisted absorption altogether, and though clearly any quantity taken into the blood did not pose an acute threat—people were not dropping in their tracks from putrescine poisoning, as laboratory dogs and rabbits did—there might nevertheless be enough to cause chronic deterioration of tissue. Who could say nay, as there was rampant confusion over such questions in this formative era of microbiology and biochemistry? It was, in fact, no great challenge to construct a plausible argument that people poisoned themselves through their bowels. The most vocal proponent of autoxication theory in the late nineteenth century, French physician Charles Bouchard, maintained that while intestinal toxins absorbed into the bloodstream never reached immediately lethal levels, because they were being continuously excreted by the kidneys as well as neutralized by the liver, they were never entirely eliminated either. Thus he could speak confidently of "stercoraemia" and "copraemia" (Latin and Greek derivatives, respectively, for fecalized blood), and remind colleagues that individuals differed greatly in susceptibility to various poisons and that aged or otherwise compromised kidneys and livers must allow the level of stercoraemia to rise. Constipation likewise would make blood more fecal, as the longer waste was retained, the more time the colon's bacteria had to work on it in toxin-generating ways. And if the blood were fecal enough for a long enough period, surely injury would result: "the daily production of the . . . substance in the intestine of a man," an American physician proposed, "and its absorption continued through weeks and possibly months may be of marked detriment to the health." Life was tricky; there were so many variables affecting whether people would slowly annihilate themselves with their own feces. In Bouchard's scheme of things, "man is . . . constantly living under the chance of being poisoned; he is always working toward his own destruction; he makes continual attempts at suicide by intoxication." Indeed, the very nomenclature of the new theory suggested that to live was to commit suicide by degrees. Not only was one of the putrefactive alkaloids produced in the bowel given the name "cadaverine," but the term coined as a categorical label for all the compounds was "ptomaines," derived from the Greek for corpse.[41]

Though it vexed Bouchard to see his ideas greeted with "incredulity and jesting," by the end of the century that initial reaction had given way to widespread acceptance. A physician writing in the *Journal of the American Medical Association* in 1893, for example, warned of "the morbid influence of habitual constipation," which generated "a mass of ptomaines to be seized by the active absorbents of [the intestine] and thrown back into the general circulation, poisoning tissues wherever they go and defying the liver, kidneys, or any other emunctory to cast them out." Autointoxication made a great deal of sense. Poisoning from the bowel had always had a powerful intuitive appeal, and now this age-old suspicion appeared to have the blessing of modern bacteriological science. Furthermore, it met a need that medicine has felt in every age; providing an explanation and a diagnosis for all those exasperating patients who insist they are sick, but are unable to present the physician with any clear organic pathology to prove it. Autointoxication, in other words, became its era's catchall diagnosis, the category into which cases of headache, indigestion, impotence, nervousness, insomnia, or any number of other functional disorders of indeterminate origin could be dumped. "The vapours" had served in that capacity in the eighteenth century (though more than one Georgian physician recognized vapours to be "so general and loose a Signification, that it is a common Subterfuge for meer Ignorance of the Nature of Distempers."). At the advent of autointoxication, the role was being played by neurasthenia, the nervous exhaustion believed since the 1860s to be epidemic among the professional, or brain-working, class in fast-paced, high-pressured modern urban society. (Why was the modern American, in particular, never quite well, always taking one medication or another tonic to brace himself up, a physician asked in the 1890s? Because of "his hurrying, restless, nerve-straining life, constant high pressure," his being "always ready to sacrifice the requirements of nature on the insatiable altars of business or pleasure." Because of neurasthenia.)[42] Constipation, of course, had commonly been regarded as a contributing factor to both the vapors and neurasthenia. But with autointoxication, constipation was the fundamental cause.

The appeal of the autointoxication diagnosis was enhanced, no doubt, by its similarity to an *environmental* health threat causing considerable uneasiness through the last quarter of the nineteenth century: sewer gas. The ancient notion of miasma as the cause of epidemic disease, as it turns out, did not immediately disappear with the adoption of bacterial explanations of infection. To the contrary, for a period, at least, the miasmatic theory had new life breathed into it by bacteriology. Miasma had always been understood as the gaseous product of putrefaction, so once it became apparent that putrefaction is the result of microbic activity, miasma could readily be reinterpreted as a product of germs. To be sure, it had to be acknowledged that one could no longer attribute malaria and cholera and fevers to foul odor—infections came from direct bacterial invasion. But it still could be supposed that nauseating miasma might be the source of various noninfectious ailments. Thus was miasma modernized.

Sewer gas was this updated version of miasma, sickening fumes that seeped into households through the very drains, ironically, that the sanitary reform movement had instituted to protect society from the old form of miasma. Sanitary reform had installed indoor water closets and constructed efficient sewer systems to rescue city dwellers from the malefic odors of the outhouse and dungheap. But the connection of the water closet to the sewer had left every house infiltrated by a network of pipes that over time became encrusted with fecal matter, matter that under the influence of germs decomposed into noxious gases. Over time, household drains corroded, cracks opened, leaks developed, and the vapors of the residents' own putrefied evacuations wafted upward into every room. As a Scottish doctor's 1882 "Psalm of Health" entreated,

> Tell me not in scornful numbers, Sanitation is a dream;
> Woe be to the man who slumbers, Thinking drains are what they seem.
> Drains are real, bad gas injurious, If the grave is not our goal;
> All past systems are but spurious; Carefully re-drain the whole.

"So far as the production of dangerous gas is concerned," New York City's leading sanitary engineer proclaimed as late as 1898, "the waste-pipe of the house itself, smeared from top to bottom with the foulest organic matter, putrefying often under the worst condtions, . . . is at least a brave rival of the worst street sewer." On further reflection, he saw it as more than a rival, as indeed "the worst enemy of those who live in modern houses." So common were such dire pronouncements up to the beginning of this century, that even stoic New Englanders, a public health authority joked, "feared [sewer gas] perhaps more than they did the Evil One."[43]

The chronological coincidence between the dread of this evil gas and the discovery of ptomaines enabled the same environmental analogy of sewer gas to autointoxication that miasma had to flatulence earlier in the century. The alimentary tract, especially the colon, was the body's drainage system, and the compounds generated by microbial action in the colon had a highly unpleasant odor; how else could one think of autointoxication, except as sewer gas in vivo? An American health educator's reaction to Bouchard, for example, was to propose that ptomaines invaded the body in the form of vapor: "by the reabsorption of the gases thus generated," he advised, there resulted "slow poisoning" and "invalidism whose cause is often undreamed of." "Perfect sewerage," he summed up, "is the price of health, in our bodies no less than in our houses, and any deviation from this is sure to bring its penalty." As late as the 1930s, people were still being warned that, "one cannot live over a cesspit in good health. How much more difficult to remain well if we carry our cesspit about inside us—especially when, as so often happens, the cesspit is unpleasantly full!" (Laxative manufacturers were quick to see, and exploit, the analogy too. The 1893 promotional booklet *Constipation and Beecham's Pills* described the gut as the body's sewer, and explained how "the sewage rots and generates poisonous liquids and gases [which] produce a kind of sewer-gas poisoning.")[44]

By the early 1900s, sewer gas had gone the way of miasma, a visceral hunch about the danger of bad odors that had been discredited by medical science. Autointoxication was hardly dependent on sewer gas for its survival, though. Through ways that will be related over several chapters, autointoxication enjoyed a golden age from 1900 into the 1930s; all the nineteenth century's uneasiness over the consequences of constipation, it turns out, were but a prelude to the fears that would haunt the early twentieth. Before the age of autointoxication can be profitably explored, however, two additional elements of the nineteenth-century's handling of constipation have to be considered. The next chapter will examine how Victorian society related bowel function to the changing habits of life fostered by urbanization, and sought to achieve intestinal health through reformed lifestyle or, that failing (as so often it did), with drugs.

2

INNER HYGIENE IN THE NINETEENTH CENTURY: CAUSES AND CURES OF CONSTIPATION

BE A REAL MAN—A LIVE MAN—Don't be satisfied to be a lump of inert, half-dead, rapidly decaying flesh. That's just exactly what the man is who suffers from neglected constipation. . . . It cannot be put too strong—a man in that condition is simply a mass of poisoned, rotting flesh. He is an unclean thing. Constipation poisons every atom in the human structure. It poisons the body with the filthiest poisons imaginable—the poisonous effluvium of foul refuse that should be excreted, but that is left in the clogged bowels to breed the foul poisons of contagion. Be clean—be clean inside as well as outside.

Advertisement for Dr. Pierce's Pleasant Purgative Pellets, late nineteenth century

one orders a vomit and t'other a purge
And with violent heat their remedies urge
Of the poor patient how hard is the lot,
For one way or other he must go to pot.

George Hamilton, 1806

On November 14, 1635, the most storied character in the long history of hygiene died in London. Thomas Parr—"Old Parr, the old, old, very old man"—lived for 152 years in the Shropshire hamlet of his nativity, and lived in robust health. As recently as his 130th year he had been engaged "lustily in every kind of agricultural labour," and apparently had still been lustfully engaged as well: at age 105, it was recorded, he had been ordered to do penance for fathering a bastard, and 17 years later had taken a new

29

wife, who afterwards testified that not "until about twelve years back [age 140] had he ceased to embrace her frequently."[1]

In the spring of 1635, rumors of the old, old man reached the ears of the Earl of Arundel, while the lord was visiting his estate near Shrewsbury. Deciding to display this "piece of antiquity" at court, the Earl had Parr transported to the capital, where, in September, he was presented to Charles I. Still as quick of wit as body, he answered the king's inquiry as to his religion by saying, "he held it safest to be of the religion of the king or queen that was in being, for he knew that he came raw into the world, and accounted it no point of wisdom to be broiled out of it." Parr spoke as a prophet, for he soon exited this world, still raw, suddenly passing away only 2 months after arriving in London. An autopsy was performed the next day by the city's foremost physician, William Harvey, discoverer of the circulatory flow of the blood. "All the internal parts," Harvey found, "appeared so healthy, that had nothing happened to interfere with the old man's habits of life, he might have escaped paying the debt due to nature for some little time longer." External parts suggested the same reservoir of vitality, the testes, "sound and large," attesting to the patriarch's prodigious virility.[2]

Parr's claims of age, unfortunately, were substantiated by nothing more than his own word and village gossip. These were still enough to gain him burial in Westminster Abbey (south transept), but hardly sufficient to withstand critical examination ("there is no doubt that Thomas Parr was a very old man," a Victorian cynic allowed; "an exceptionally old man; probably a hundred; possibly a year or two more"). That he was most likely an impostor, or at least an exaggerator, is not the point, however. What matters is the presumed cause of Parr's death, whatever his age. Harvey determined that something had "happened to interfere with the old man's habits." His sexual escapades excepted, Parr had followed an abstemious course before coming to London, living in pure country air, on simple country fare. But in the city, he was suddenly "set at a table loaded with variety of viands, and tempted not only to eat more than wont, but to partake of strong drink." Inevitably under such a change, "all the natural organs would become deranged."[3] Apparently Old Parr's intestines had not yet been made deranged by gluttony and strong drink, but constipation surely would have resulted had he continued on such a regimen much longer. Such was the fundamental understanding of costiveness in Parr's day, and it continued into the nineteenth century: constipation was caused by improper habits of life, and improper habits were for the most part caused by urban civilization.

The purpose of Harvey's delineation of the alterations in the old man's mode of living once he moved to London was to document the conclusion that "the cause of death seemed fairly referrible to a sudden change in the non-naturals." *Non-naturals* was the somewhat confusing term that had been used for centuries to categorize the various components of behavior and environment that one had to regulate so as to live in accord with nature. In the classic formulation, they comprised air, food and drink, sleep and watch, motion and rest, evacuation and repletion, and passions of the mind. Derived from everyday experience and common sense, the non-naturals simply recognized that people needed a wholesome atmosphere to breathe, adequate food, sleep, and exercise, regular elimination of waste, and emotional equanimity. That was the meaning of the word *hygiene* in the nineteenth century: adherence to the doctrine of the non-naturals.[4]

As suggested by the juxtaposition of opposites (motion and rest, evacuation and repletion), non-natural philosophy aimed at balance. All life's activities were to be exercised in moderation, at a level of neither too much nor too little, if health were to be enjoyed. So indisputable was this simple but wise philosophy that, even though the term "non-naturals" would fade away during the Victorian age, its content survives to the present. The only significant changes in traditional hygiene in modern times are not alterations, but refinements, fine-tuning accomplished by such new sciences as biochemistry, physiology, and epidemiology. The much-publicized seven rules of health recently determined by epidemiological studies relating life span to living habits merely confirm that the non-naturals were the right way all along: "Regular meals [breakfast every day, no between-meal snacks], adequate sleep, near average weight, physical activity, and avoidance of smoking and excessive drinking [are] all positively related to health" and longevity, re-searchers at UCLA's School of Public Health concluded in 1973.[5] Of course they are, nineteenth-century physicians would respond, and don't forget "passions of the mind" (stress management).

Parr lived by such rules for more than a century and a half—then something, Harvey observed, "happened to interfere with the old man's habits of life." What happened was that the pollutions and excesses of city life displaced the purity and simplicity—the naturalness (the non-naturalness)—of traditional country life. "We live in an artificial state," Harvard surgery professor John Collins Warren wrote in 1845, "a state that continually thwarts the course of the native disposi-tion of the animal economy."[6] That state, of course, was civilization. Even as early as the 1840s, a reader's reflex to Warren's statement would be "of course," for by then people had been conditioned for the better part of a century to think of civi-lized life as an artificial mode of existence that runs counter to the best interests of the human animal economy. Had Alphin's story been generally known, it might have assumed the status of a fable: this modern man died because he substituted the artificial—a glass eye—for the natural. Indeed, since approximately the time of Alphin's death, the last third of the eighteenth century, Europeans and Ameri-cans had been made intently aware of the widening gulf between their manner of living and that of their presumably more hardy forebears. Rousseau and the in-fatuation with noble savagery that he had stirred up contributed to this, to be sure. But all the literature of health, the professionally composed and the lay-authored alike, also pointed to estrangement from primitive regimen as the source of many of humankind's ills. Lamentations over the fall of humankind from the grace of physical perfection and despair at ever seeing humanity restored to primitive vitality were virtually obligatory prefaces to any text on hygiene or even pathology in the late eighteenth and early nineteenth centuries.

In truth, the pairing of village against metropolis, primitive against modern, pristine against corrupted, was ancient and had become commonplace by the end of the Middle Ages, as European society had grown steadily more urbanized, commercial, and prosperous. "Diseases of civilization" was well established as an idea, if not as a phrase, by the time Parr fell victim to one. Up to that time, however, succumbing to civilization was still regarded as a voluntary act; old Parr had been lured to the city, not forced to move to it. By the end of the following century, the city had so expanded in size and industrialism was exerting such economic pressures on the traditional way of life that premature death by civilization was taking on the appearance of inescapable fate. How much longer could people hope to live like Parr, "within bounds of nature's laws,"[7] when nature's bounds were being relentlessly pushed toward obliteration? Romanticism's exaltation of the primitive and the natural sharpened this anxiety about the unavoidable degenerative influence of civilization to a fine point.

Indeed, it was a generally unquestioned assumption that the pace of human self-destruction was actually quickening. Decline had been going on since the days of Methusaleh, it was admitted, but most people had still maintained a passable degree of health until the last century, or even the last generation. Such were the melancholy reflections of Benjamin Waterhouse, lecturing Harvard medical students at the beginning of the nineteenth century. He could personally recall students who had been robust and energetic, Waterhouse told his pupils. "But does this charming picture any longer exist? Is it not faded and fading, like a flower, that has passed its bloom; and which is about to wither on its stalk? . . . . *Whence this* deterioration?" he asked.[8] Civilization.

But all was not angst and resignation to sickliness and early death. While it was true, Warren continued, that "civilization . . . has . . . raised obstacles to the development of the physical powers, [it] has [also] copiously supplied the means of intellectual improvement."[9] Here readers were being led to see that while civilization could be viewed as synonymous with sickness, one might with equal reason think of illness as an anachronism in an age of such copious intellectual improvement. One of the distinguishing marks of Western culture since the Enlightenment is precisely this ambivalence about the relationship of health to civilization. Anxiety over the perpetual undermining of health by the effete manners of urban society has been inextricably bound up with optimism that extraordinary levels of health (today's "wellness") might be made available to all by civilized society's development of biological science, and the application of that scientific knowledge to daily life. Full health has thus been at once a cherished ideal and an exasperating chimera: the goal ought to be so near, given the achievements of the biological sciences, yet it has remained so far—thanks to the unnatural stresses of civilization.

The source of all that deterioration was not always civilization, however. Just as often it was identified more precisely as "luxury," the era's favored term for the softening self-indulgences associated with city life. "The sad effects of luxury are these," it had been written; "we drink our poison, and we eat disease." Excessive and overrich food and drink did, in fact, usually head the critic's list of urban society's luxurious gratifications. They were invariably followed, however, by equally distraught notations on the odious impurity of city air, the debilitating sedentariness of city "workers," and the psyche-shattering excitements of city business, politics, and entertainments. All were denounced as evils from which the traditional rural life was free. Whether shopkeeper or sybarite, the poor city dweller hadn't a chance, and to prove the point he was hauled forth, time and again, to have his stature measured against that of the farmer (and invariably to the former's humiliation). "Compare," one physician jeered, "the whistling plough-boy with the calculating stockbroker; the shepherd on the mountains with the merchant in the city; the village magistrate with the prime minister." Compare, others urged, the "slim soft-fibred man-milliner" to "the firm and brawny ploughman," the "delicate lady" to the "nut-brown country girl." Even the "sickly sallow . . . city child" was made to cringe before "the florid complexion and sound health of the country youth."[10] In all these cases, the book could be judged by its cover, the inner workings of the body—its health—being perfectly matched to its outward appearance.

The inner workings of the stockbroker or the merchant were particularly deficient in the intestines. No single harmful effect of civilization was warned about more frequently than constipation. Such was the message of several book-length expositions on the subject, including John Burne's 1840 *Treatise on the Causes and Consequences of Habitual Constipation*, and Richard Reece's 1826 *A Practical Dissertation on the Means of Obviating and Treating the Varieties of Costiveness, Which Occur at Different Periods of Life, and in Cases of Predispositions to Various Constitutional Maladies, in Peculiar Temperaments of Body, in Disorders of the Lungs, Stomach, Liver, Rectum, etc., and During Pregnancy*. The danger of constipation was the point of a London physician's opening chapter in *The Influence of Civic Life . . . on Human Health*: crammed intestines, James Johnson argued, "characterize nine-tenths of the diseases of civilized life." It was the gem of wisdom revealed by another London practitioner in his *Directions for Invigorating and Prolonging Life*: the prevention of constipation, according to this self-proclaimed "invalid's oracle," "is the fundamental basis of health and long life." It was the gist of the advice given costive old men by famed Edinburgh physician James Hamilton, Senior, the early century's acknowledged authority on matters of health

and the bowels. Correction of civilized living habits, he told valetudinarians, was
the first step to be taken by those hoping to regain regularity. "Forsake the haunts
and habits of fashionable life," Hamilton begged them; "quit the crowded city,
alluring amusements, and various occupations carried on in airless, or even in
tainted rooms; . . . shun luxurious tables, indolence, and late hours; . . . retrace
the steps by which [you have] deviated from simple nature, and . . . court the country, pure air, and simple diet."[11]

Hamilton pretty much said it all. The haunts of fashionable life were facto-
ries and offices by day, tenements and theaters by night—all places of muscular
idleness that sapped the intestines of their tone and vigor. That physical exertion
strengthened the abdominal organs to better perform the evacuative function had
long been an article of medical faith. The belief is evident, for example, in the facetious proposal in the mid-1600s for an excremental Olympics of sorts to be held
at Epsom, a spa notorious for the strength of its purgative mineral waters: "He
that gains the glory here," the Olympics organizer announced, "must scumber
furthest, shite most clear." And to rally competitors to their best effort, he reminded
them of the example set by their more muscular (less civilized) forebears:

> And for to make us emulate,
> The good old Father doth relate
> The vigour of our Ancestors,
> Whose shiting far exceeded ours.[12]

The connection between regular exercise and regular elimination was also
clearly appreciated by Dr. S—t, the compiler of that eighteenth-century treatise
on *Human Ordure*. Attempting to do for stools what Linnaeus and other scientists
were doing for plants and animals, the "Dr." classified human dejecta into five
categories, according to morphology, and gave each a descriptive Latin name.
Classification number 1, Merda Turbinata (cone-shaped dung), was the output of
health. Its shape, "like a boy's top reversed," showed it had made an assertive exit
from the body. Undoubtedly "the Product of well concocted Aliment," it was
"always generated in a robust strong Body," and gave "sure Indications of a firm
well ton'd set of Intestines." These noble specimens, "always of a firm Consistency," were "to be met with mostly in Plow'd Fields, High Roads, and sometimes in Meadows." To be sure, one might encounter "faint Icons" of the species
in suburbs—if farmers or other heavy laborers resided there. Even these would
be left behind once the city was entered, though, and one was surrounded by the
slothful. There one was almost sure to encounter only specimens from classification number 5, the "Button-formed" excreta, which occurred either as individual
small, round balls, or as "conglomerate" buttons, "joined so close and compact
together . . . like an ear of Indian wheat." Such pellets were certainly not the dejecta of well-formed, active bodies. The writer had observed them, rather, "to

flourish mostly among Colleges, Schools, and most Places of publick Education, as well as in and about Prisons, Jails, and all Places of Confinement."[13]

Nineteenth-century health literature sustained the theme. Thus *The Cyclopaedia of Practical Medicine* informed readers in the 1840s that "debility of the fibre of the muscular coat of the intestines" had generally been found "in those who led a sedentary life." Clerks and clergymen, students and seamstresses, any whose jobs involved physical inactivity (which was true of most of the new occupations of city life) were virtually doomed to suffer constipation. And doomed was hardly too strong a word. Only too typical was the case of the bookseller who suffered from costiveness most of his life, until at age 40, "finding himself grow weaker . . . as the . . . constipation continued, he gradually became exhausted, and died." Autopsy confirmed what his doctor had suspected: "the colon throughout its whole extent was enlarged, and its muscular fibres were thin and pale. . . . The muscular fibres, even near to the anus, were remarkably thin and pale." It was a medical truism that, "among business, professional, and studious men, . . . no condition is more common than that of constipation."[14]

The habits of fashionable life comprised first of all those "luxurious tables" scorned by Hamilton, particularly tables lacking in the bulkier, unfashionable foods that kept farmworkers' intestines active. Medical and popular health literature through the entire nineteenth century harped unceasingly on the binding effects of the common diet of meats, gravies, and pastries, all eaten in too great quantity and too much haste. "Put all these things" that civilized society stuffs down its gullet, an English physician suggested, "into a bowl instead of the stomach, and contemplate the noxious, fermenting mess. Isn't it enough to kill an ostrich?"[15]

Undoubtedly it was, especially if the ostrich were perpetually in a hurry. The speed with which people overate, in America particularly ("I never saw a Yankee that didn't bolt his food whole like a boa constrictor") was encouraged by the too rapid pace of life away from the table. The hurry to attend to business, the constant rush, the ceaseless pressure of affairs and the clock, created a level of morbid nervous excitement not felt by workers down on the farm. "The anxiety of mind . . . arising out of an advanced state of civilization," one medical authority wrote, "has a great influence . . . in rendering torpid the peristaltic action of the intestines. Look at the multitude of anxious faces one meets daily in the streets. Think for a moment on the contentions, competitions, and responsibilities that men have to encounter, and we shall not be surprised at the load of anxiety that oppresses the greater part. This anxiety depresses the energy of the nervous system . . . and the peristaltic action of the intestinal canal grows slow and retards the excretions." Amen said other medicos. When James Johnson proposed a comparison of the plough-boy with the stock-broker and the shepherd with the city merchant, he specified comparing "the state of their minds, and the state of their digestive organs," and assured "you will find a corresponding contrast in both." He might have stopped there, but knowing that not all readers would be able to examine their fellows' digestive organs, he explained that in the mentally agitated city dwellers one would find "the alimentary canal completely torpid," its contents running "into all kinds of decomposition and fermentation."[16]

An even more serious effect of the overscheduled life was that harried people so often failed to make room on the schedule for their daily intestinal obligations. This, doctors were almost unanimously agreed, was the chief reason for so much costiveness in civilized nations. "Of all the causes which originate and establish habitual constipation," Burne argued in his *Treatise*, "there is none certainly so general as inattention to the calls of nature." In some cases, inattention was due merely to indolence, to simple unwillingness to make the effort to visit "the residence of Mrs. Jones" (as the English sometimes called their toilets; "the coffee house" was another genteel appellation) "unless urged by an imperative necessity which they cannot resist." In other cases, inattention had a purely practical basis—an inconvenient location of the closet, perhaps; or inclement weather when the closet was outdoors.[17]

Bowel neglect might also stem from misordered priorities. Civilized folk felt great reluctance to withdraw, however briefly, from business or social activities for fear of missing a big sale or juicy gossip. Most commonly stressed by commentators, however, was what Burne called "a misplaced sense of delicacy." Itself a refinement of civilized society, delicacy often made a person hesitate to leave a group not for fear of what he might miss but because of the certainty he would be missed; surely everyone would guess he had gone to pay a visit to Mrs. Jones (guessing might not even be required, since Mrs. Jones so frequently resided outside and "access . . . often runs in front of the sitting-room windows"). Victorian ladies were believed to be particularly sensitive in this regard, so treatises on hygiene regularly included a section on the importance of providing women with a secluded water closet. "They who would secure the health of their families," one such discussion advised, "ought, when seeking a change of residence, . . . to make every inquiry about the situs of the closet, and to see that it be so placed that it may be made use of without the risk of being seen." A good arrangement, it was suggested, was to have the toilet on the far side of a vestibule in which coats, boots, and umbrellas were kept, so that ladies could "be seen going to or coming from it without any knowledge being given of the object for which they resorted thither."[18]

Predictably, embarrassment over attending to so basic a body function was more pronounced in Britain and America than on the Continent. There was the story of the most proper English gentleman who, while traveling in France, was mortified when he opened the unbolted door of a *cabinet d'aisance* and discovered it occupied by a lady. He hastily retreated to his room, but shortly another lady knocked on his door and informed him, "'*Monsieur! la place est libre!*' The Englishman blushed for an instant," but quickly realized the moral of the incident and shrugged, "*Eh bien*! If Madame feels no delicacy in this matter, why should I?" Such flexibility was the exception, it seems, for physicians and other health writers complained all century long about the prevalence of this foolish modesty in polite society, and the fearsome toll in suffering and death it exacted: "Little do such persons know the misery and ill health they entail upon themselves when they allow such habits [of delicacy] to grow upon them." But just as important was not to interrupt the effort once embarrassment had been overcome and Mrs. Jones called upon, "because if baffled," an American hygienist warned, "the spell is at once broken, the charm dissolved, . . . preparatory to interminable ills." In sum, one could do no greater good for oneself than to heed nature's urging daily. "The great practical lesson that I wish to inculcate," a British physician exclaimed, "to be engraven, as on a plate of steel, on the memory of children, and youth, young men and women, the mature and the gray-headed: Allow nothing short of fire or endangered life to induce you to resist, for one single moment, nature's alvine call."[19]

Interminable ills could stem from still other civilized habits conducive to constipation: late sleeping, soft beds, overheated rooms, too much clothing, protracted periods of study ("the exercise of the encephalic portion of the nervous system detracting from the energy of the abdominal portion"), and just about any other things "which divert the secretions to the surface of the body." Even the stance that civilized people assumed for the act of defecation could be faulted, the squatting posture of peasants in the field being "more conducive . . . than the more easy [read luxurious] position of a sitter upon the perforated board."[20] Clearly anyone who hoped to avoid constipation had to order her or his life very carefully.

Fortunately, there was no lack of guidance on how to achieve that order. The Enlightenment's faith in the power of science and education to improve the human condition had fueled an extraordinary burst of activity in the publication of handbooks of hygiene for the lay person. Such works were virtually flowing from the presses by the later 1700s. To be sure, health manuals had been available since the Middle Ages, and had increased in number with the advent of printing. Such titles as *The Haven of Health*, *The Castell of Helth*, and *Bulwarke of Defence* made hygiene seem a certain refuge in a hostile and dangerous world as early as the sixteenth century. What had been a gradual buildup through the 1500s and 1600s, however, became a torrent during the 1700s under the impulse of Enlightenment confidence that health was truly attainable for all. An early nineteenth-century survey of health promotion works of "note and merit" reported 54 volumes published during the seventeenth century, and 211, nearly four times as many, for the eighteenth.[21]

That momentum carried into the nineteenth century. Continuing optimism about the attainability of health and the power of science and education, dismay

over the debilitating effects of urban life, and the spread of public literacy assured
an ever-expanding market for handbooks of health throughout the 1800s. Physicians comprised the largest group of authors of these works on hygiene (or on
"physiology" or "physical education," as such texts were commonly titled by the
1820s). Many of their books were intended for consumption by fellow professionals; but just as many were popularized distillations of the substance of medical texts.
Many physicians felt dutybound to become popularizers, in light of the remarkable progress they saw taking place in physiological science. Historically subject
to "the most extravagant errors," physiology had newly come of age, doctors
maintained, and was now accurately surveying all "the mazy labyrinths of this
mysterious machine . . . in all their windings," pinpointing all "the lurking places"
of bad health. "We are privileged," nineteenth-century physicians believed, "to
live in a more propitious age," and with privilege came responsibility.[22] Ordinary
people deserved to have maps of the body's mazy labyrinths too. These popular
treatments of physical education were issued in great quantity by lay writers also
(educators, clergymen, women concerned about the special hygienic challenges
confronting their sex), writers who, like physician-authors, produced works for
schoolchildren as well as for adults (instruction in hygiene became a standard part
of the school curriculum in both Britain and America from mid-century onward).

   This enormous interest in physiology simplified can also be explained, perhaps, as a response to cultural demands that went beyond individuals' hopes for
physical security. By clarifying how the diverse specialized parts of the body
machine can smoothly integrate their functions so as to accomplish work and produce new material goods (body tissue), physiology provided a model for the operation of the new industrial order. "Health literature," Martha Verbrugge has
written of mid-nineteenth century American culture, "was a translation of middle-
class ideology into physiological terms. Moderation, self-control and persistence
were standard themes in the prescriptive rhetoric of the period. Codifiers of middle-
class norms declared that self-governance would enable people to endure social
change."[23] As a model of industrialism, therefore, physiology not only validated
the efficacy of the new system of production but also provided assurance that the
rapid and disturbing transformations sweeping through society could be kept under
control and the process made predictable; in a subliminal way, physiology shored
up people's hopes for economic security too, and calmed their fears of social tur-
moil. The physiology of the digestive tract had particular appeal in this regard,
illustrating as it did the utilization of raw material, the generation of power, and
the efficient elimination of waste. Regarded from that angle, constipation was grit
in the gears, a jamming of the body factory's machinery. The unrestricted operations of a laissez-faire system were as much to be desired in the animal economy
of the bowels as in the marketplace.

The onslaught of Victorian respectability during this very same period, on the other hand, was inhibiting frank discussion of body parts and functions. Presentations of sexual hygiene in particular were being clothed in opaque euphemisms by the 1830s, and one would expect the same veil to be drawn over the intestinal tract. That it was not, at least not nearly so tightly, indicates the significance colon hygiene was believed to have for overall health. "So important is the due and timely evacuation of the faeces," even one of the more straight-laced physiology popularizers recognized, "so injurious their retention in the bowels, . . . that no motive of delicacy would justify the construction of a code of health, which should omit to notice this subject."[24] So notice it hygienists did, repeatedly and as candidly as good taste would allow.

Notice first had to be taken of defecatory frequency, what constituted "due and timely evacuation." "Constipation is a term of relative import," an American expert explained. "It may be laid down as a general rule, that a daily evacuation of the bowels is indispensably necessary" ("some very hearty eaters may better have two"), but that was only a generalization. Also part of the medical definition of constipation was the specification that the feces be "retained longer in the intestines than is customary with the individual." Individuals' physiological schedules did vary considerably. For most, once a day was the natural rhythm, but for others nature preferred two days, and there were a few who lived in health with "a natural stool but once or twice a week." Doctors pointed out that rare specimens might go weeks, months, even as long as "upwards of eight years" without an intestinal evacuation (the last was a French woman who compensated, apparently, by having "copious greasy sweats"), and not be harmed. "These cases, however, are extraordinary, and should not affect the rule, that the bowels should be opened every day." What mattered, the index by which people determined if they were the rule or the exception, was the quality of the evacuation: "a healthy condition of the bowels demands . . . that each discharge be free, easy, and copious, . . . and without pain, straining, or irritation." Texture was a critical measure too. Less than a diurnal schedule was no cause for concern so long as the stools, once they appeared, "are of the consistence of mush, as the cook passes it into the dish for the table, . . . or of New Orleans molasses, when the thermometer is about twenty of Fahrenheit." It was when feces were "inspissated so as to render their evacuation tedious and imperfect" that one had to worry. But for the great majority, a daily movement was the ideal, and consequently, physicians frequently complained, people jumped to the conclusion that they had been struck with constipation whenever they passed a day without a movement, whether the eventual dejecta were inspissated and tediously expelled or not.[25]

That settled, hygiene handbooks turned to instruction in alleviating or avoiding constipation through correct living habits, emphasis being placed upon three of the non-naturals above the others. First came diet, the replacement of luxury at table with plenty of fruits, vegetables, and other bulk-producing foods. Whole-grain bread was recommended with particular enthusiasm now that white bread was coming into high fashion. Wheat flour had been bolted, or passed through strainers to remove the coarser particles of bran, for centuries, and the resultant lighter-colored flour had always been seen as more desirable, even accorded a touch of luxury status. In the early nineteenth century, however, the demand for lighter bread increased remarkably as the growing middle class determined they should ape even the staff of life of the upper crust. The lower classes demanded white bread too, though the loaves they could afford were whitened artificially, with various adulterants. "Bread is often spoiled to please the eye," one physician complained, but "the poorer sort will eat no other." Medical authorities recognized that bread "made of the whitest flour is apt to render [the bowels] costive," and recommended unbolted flour for bulk. Bran was also believed to stimulate the colon to regular action by an irritating effect; its "scales," an English dietary expert explained, "exert a mechanical action upon the intestines, and . . . excite them into action." The suggestion of "scales," projecting an image of rough-edged particles scraping the intestinal wall and inciting it to movement, was representative of scientific opinion throughout the nineteenth century: bran was "roughage" as well as bulk, and "rarely fails in procuring regular and natural stools."[26]

The benefits of brown bread were extolled still more insistently by the nineteenth-century's most notorious health reformer, Sylvester Graham. A minister of religion turned temperance crusader, Graham in the 1830s moved beyond the condemnation of Demon rum to renounce all manner of health-destroying indulgences. The Grahamite, or popular health reform movement enjoyed a heyday of only two decades or so, and converted at most a few thousand health abusers to active observance of its program of physiological rectitude (these mostly in the Northeast and Midwest). But Grahamite literature was profuse and widely circulated, and virtually all literate Americans were aware of the movement's teachings.[27]

The stated rationale for Graham's renunciations of coffee, spices, flesh food, corsets, tight pants, soft mattresses, etc. was that all were dangerous forms of overstimulation of body tissue. In truth, the stimulation that so worried the former preacher was the sensual kind. His outlook might be thought of as the antithesis of our own century's "Playboy philosophy": "if it feels good," Graham might have said, "don't do it!" There was, of course, a theological logic at work behind this analysis of health. Sensual stimulation leads to immoral behavior, and it is inconceivable God would allow any activity to be bad for the soul without also making it bad for the body. The result was a philosophy of hygiene that differed markedly from the non-naturals tradition. The latter had a quantitative orientation; just about any food, drink, or activity was consistent with health so long as it was not

such bad constitutions that no physician could save them, and the other six had such good ones that all the physicians in the world could not kill them."[39] It's human nature to suppose one belongs to the latter group until experience proves otherwise, and then to try to save oneself by relying more on medicine than manly resolution. For many, once the self-control demanded by hygiene was considered, an ounce of cure looked better than any amount of prevention.

Of the myriad constipation cures available, the simplest and most direct was "the sailor's remedy," "which is to push a piece of hard soap, shaped as the little finger, and hold it there until the evacuation comes on. A similar cut piece of wood, with a soaped or greased rag around it, will answer, as also the oiled finger." Suppositories of hardened honey or molasses candy, or the handle of a spoon were sometimes recommended as the "convenient instrument," but most often it was simply the oiled finger one was told to use to "actually pick to pieces the indurated fecal plug."[40]

To most people's way of thinking, however, there was a far more convenient instrument at hand than the finger. Why had the creator put so many purgative drugs on earth, both plants and minerals, if not to spare God's children the distasteful experience of the sailor's remedy, and the discomforting exactions of exercise and dietary restraint and an every-morning visit to the necessary house? Dosing with cathartics seemed the easy way out, and thus was the one generally taken. In truth, the administration of drugs to expel corruption from the bowels had been the most basic form of therapy employed by physicians for millenia. In the seventeenth and eighteenth centuries, physicians had in fact become notorious for the violence with which they flushed patients' intestines, using botanical preparations such as colocynth, gamboge, and elaterium (its name derived from the Greek word for "to squirt," signifying "the forcible manner in which it ejects the contents of the bowels") that have since been banished from the pharmacopoeia as much too active. It was perhaps elaterium that a seventeenth-century poet had in mind when he recounted "Mr. Smith's taking a Purge." "I powder took" one morning, Mr. Smith explained, and

> Long had it not in stomack been
> But from each part came powdring in
> Of uncouth gear such pregnant store
> That gutt 'gan grumble, nock runne ore.

(The nock, or notch, referred to the cleft between the buttocks).

> Downwards in a rage they drew
> To ramble, and bid nock adieu:
> But when they came to portal nastie
> Bumme was so straite, and they so hastie,
> That many a worthy pellet must

Into one Booming shott bee thrust,
At rumbling noyse the mastive growles
The frighted mice forsake their holes,
And Souldiers to my window come
Invited thither by my drum. . . .
Oh dismall Dose! oh cursed geere!
Will all my body runne out here?[41]

Numerous lesser, but still potent enough, cathartics were commonly utilized as well to remove excrement before it slowly poisoned the body, including jalap, scammony, Chinese rhubarb, aloes, senna, cassia, castor oil (all plant products), and Epsom and other mineral salts. Collectively, all such drugs were known as *physick*. But already by Mr. Smith's day, the 1600s, the dismal doses of physick dispensed by physicians were being challenged by the first wave of patent medicines (that was the common name given them, though since few were ever actually patented by any government, it is more accurate to call them proprietary medicines, which were nostrums manufactured by individual proprietors who generally had not received any medical training). Proprietary remedies were compounded from many of the same drugs prescribed by doctors, but recipes were trade secrets, and the products were advertised directly to the public as preparations very different from and far superior to the pharmaceuticals used by the profession. They were, in short, quackery, ineffective (and sometimes dangerous) concoctions fraudulently pressed upon consumers with extravagant therapeutic claims. Forerunners of today's over-the-counter medications, patent medicines constituted the first great step in the modern commercialization of health and hygiene.[42]

The British led the way in the production of patent medicines: by the mid-1700s, consumers could take their choice of Anderson's Pills, Stoughton's Elixir, Dr. James's Fever Powder, Dr. Hooper's Female Pills, Dr. Bateman's Pectoral Drops, Turlington's Balsam of Life, Daffy's Elixir Salutis, and still other highly touted compounds. By that time, the best-selling English brands were also available in the American colonies, too underindustrialized yet to manufacture their own medicinals. American production of patent nostrums would nevertheless get started before 1800, and actually overtake English output within a few decades. There were already enough products vying for public support in the eighteenth century, however, to force manufacturers to advertise aggressively if they hoped to make a go of it. Proprietary medicine producers, in fact, were the pioneers in developing the methods of exaggeration, deception, and psychological manipulation that have made the advertising industry the silliest, yet most pervasive and profitable, form of quackery in modern times. The first trail they blazed was that of newspaper advertising. Newspapers increased markedly in number during the eighteenth and nineteenth centuries, in response to expanding public literacy. Quacks immediately recognized papers as a medium for distributing their message much more widely, while publishers saw the patent medicine business as a huge source of revenue. It was love at first sight, and the affair has continued to the present.

But for patent medicine ads to work, they had to appeal to people's beliefs and intuitions about how disease originated and might be cured. Hence it is no surprise to find purging of the bowels as a common element in the patent medicine man's pitch to consumers. As far back as the late 1600s, for example, a London charlatan hawking his wares in the street was heard to describe his peppercorn-size pills as a "Diminutive Phanpharmica so Powerful . . . and of such Excellent Vertues, that if you have Twenty Distempers lurking in the Mass of Blood, it shall give you just Twenty Stools, and every time it Operates it carries off a Distemper." Half a century later, with patent medicine promotion relying primarily on newspaper advertising instead of street spiels and handbills, by far the most frequently advertised patent preparation in the newspapers of Bath (a spa that was the hypochondriac's heaven) was Scots Pills, a combination of aloes and jalap. In second place was Daffy's Elixir (senna), while two more purgative remedies (Dr. Bostock's Purging Cordial Elixir and Dr. Radcliffe's Famous Purging Elixir) helped to round out the top ten. Still another half century later, a poem about a quack by name of Doctor Drug'em joked that his pills had the power to "empty Pockets well as scour the Guts." When the poet looked for a way to characterize charlatanic medicine, in other words, he saw purgation as the standard readers would recognize.[43]

Conflict between professional and proprietary cathartics only intensified during the nineteenth century. As markets expanded and the stakes increased, the extravagance of patent medicine advertising grew ever more outrageous and pervasive. The symbiotic advertising relationship between proprietaries and newspapers was sustained, of course, becoming even more rewarding as public literacy and the number of newspapers continued to grow (in the United States, for example, papers grew in number from 200 to 4000 during the first half of the nineteenth century). But by mid-century, blurbs in the daily journals were being reinforced by all manner of other promotional methods. Medicine makers pushed product names and claims upon the public through posters and signs applied to windows, walls, fences, boulders, and any other prominent objects that didn't move; through mass mailings equivalent to the dreaded "Resident" mail of today; and through a host of publications running the gamut from pamphlets, song books, calendars, and cookbooks to pulp novels, almanacs, and home medical guides. Paper weights, porcelain plates, and untold other domestic appurtenances were emblazoned with patent medicine trademarks. And during the second half of the century, entertainment, in the form of the traveling medicine show and its troupe of singers, comedians, crack shots, and magicians, became the medium of choice of the most successful American entrepreneurs. Although expensive to mount, medicine shows attracted large crowds and put them in the mood to part with their money, in the end returning the startup investment many times over.[44]

Of the thousands of brands of patent medicines brought to market in Britain and America in the nineteenth century, more employed purgatives to produce a noticeable and presumably salutary effect than any other active drug (Fig. 2-1). The purgative employed, moreover, was most likely to be of botanical origin. This reliance on vegetable aperients played off of public dissatisfaction with the medical profession's wholesale adoption of a new cathartic, the mineral drug calomel. Through the first half of the century in particular, calomel (mercurous chloride) was the drug physicians prescribed most frequently of all, outstripping even opium. But this "Sampson of the Materia Medica," as its devotees reverently called it, could be as devastating to the patient as to her disease. Chronic mercury poisoning, with profuse salivation, ulceration of the mouth and gums, loss of teeth, and in advanced cases destruction of the jawbone, was a too common result of calomel treatment; Samson was actually Delilah in disguise, weakening her victims by pulling their teeth instead of cutting their hair.[45]

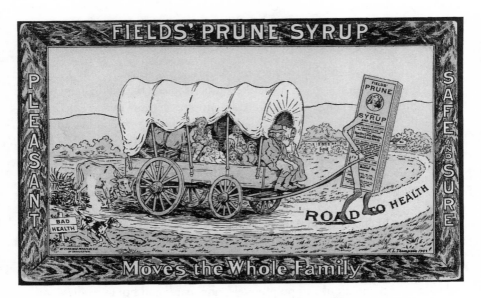

Figure 2-1. Advertisement for a laxative that moved the entire family along the road to health [The William H. Helfand Collection, New York].

The profession's critics, including some physicians, focused on calomel as the symbol of doctors' tendency to harm rather than heal. Virtually all practitioners "on both sides of the Atlantic," a medical man complained in the 1820s, "appear to be infected with purging mania, and the various classes of medical students let loose upon the world, following explicitly the dictates of their masters, commence their careers with equally unsparing hands." Unless calomel "be exhausted," he worried, "there is little hope for ourselves and our posterity. They, too, will be purged out of the world, as their fathers have been before them." The public had the same fear, and patent medicine manufacturers exploited it to the hilt. "Calomel is the great bug-bear—the raw head and bloody bones," a physician grumbled, "that has been used by designing knaves . . . to frighten. . . . Quacks . . . have raised a hue and cry against all minerals, and in the hope of throwing ridicule upon the profession they term us 'Mineral Doctors.' They cry *mad dog*, and set upon the chase."[46]

Those quacks, the nostrum peddlers, essentially styled themselves vegetable doctors, recognizing that profits were to be made by persuading people that herbal remedies were gentler yet no less active than mineral ones (never mind the fact that virtually all the purgatives other than calomel that physicians prescribed were of vegetable origin). "At the present day," one medical onlooker commented, "there is a great fondness for vegetable medicines. Anything having the prefix of vegetable to it goes down with the multitude." One who went down with multitudes was James Morison, a Scottish pill maker whose first attempt, about 1816, was a mixture of aloes and oatmeal. To his credit, Morison soon realized that so provincial a recipe would have limited appeal, and by 1825 was marketing a product that replaced the oatmeal with jalap, colocynth, gamboge, rhubarb, and/or senna. The exact formula is in dispute, but all ingredients were of botanical origin, thus justifying at least part of the product's grandiose name: Hygeian Vegetable Universal Medicine. The appellation Universal was justified by Morison's pharmacological rationale, carefully spelled out in advertisements that explained how all disease stems from impurities in the blood, and how it was the "quality and virtue" of his pills "to give that impulse to the blood, so as to make it bring all its impurities to the bowels to be purged off." Purgation was commonly equated with blood purification in proprietary ads, but few promoted the equation so successfully as Morison. His official motto, *Uno ictu*, at one blow, stated succinctly, if perhaps crudely, that all sickness could be overcome with a bludgeoning of the bowels. Under the simpler name of Morison's Pills, his remedy continued to be one of the most popular patent medicines for several decades after the discoverer's death in 1840. Heeding Morison's axiom that the "bowels cannot be purged too much," and that they should "have no dread of overdoses," customers swallowed his pills by the dozens, and more: one devotee testified under oath to having taken

20,000 over a 2-year period. No wonder a satirical song ("Morison's Pills," it was called) could propose that traditional purgatives be discarded and this more vigorously acting new product be taken in their stead:

> Give way ye slow-workers—ye jalaps and squills
> To 'Perpetual Motions' and Morison's Pills.[47]

If Morison further conditioned the British public to revere inner hygiene, the American public had its own horde of purgative salesmen to learn from, and none more commanding than Benjamin Brandreth. A native of Liverpool, Brandreth immigrated to (and at once opened shop in) New York City in 1835; within 5 years he had made his Vegetable Universal Pills one of the largest-selling preparations in his new country. Brandreth's adoption of a product name so similar to Morison's was part of his calculations, but it should not be construed as plagiarism—or at least not as unmitigated plagiarism. It exemplifies again the sales appeal of botanical over mineral preparations (Brandreth's Pills, "Entirely Vegetable and Innocent," "cure without hurting your teeth or gums"), and of the idea that purgation could be a panacea. How could one improve on Vegetable Universal as a name for such products? And for that matter, how could one improve on Morison's formula, except by simplifying it to three of his most potent ingredients: aloes, colocynth, and gamboge? Having borrowed so freely from name and composition, Brandreth must have felt no qualms about appropriating Morison's advertising line as well. Did Morison's Pills sweep impurities from the blood into the bowel, and thence flush them from the body? Brandreth's Pills "Puryfies [sic] the Blood" too, ads blared; their maker had determined that "life was in the blood; that by whatever name diseases were distinguished, impurity of the blood was the source of all."[48]

"To see a man or woman who never purchased a box of Brandreth's Pills," wrote an MD bemoaning the "national disease," "would be equivalent to seeing the fifth wheel of a coach. No such phenomenon exists." It was at least certain there was no man or woman in the country who never saw an ad for Brandreth's Pills. American society was figuratively papered over with Brandreth handbills and pamphlets (nor were they scarce in Britain). And they were as frightening as they were frequent. "Corruption gets the ascendancy" in many people; such unfortunates "carry in their bowels and blood a load of old, depraved humors," or else "corrupt humors"; then "there is an absorption into the circulation, of gases and gummy substances," "of poisonous vapors or matters," hence the sick, all of them, are in need of medicine that will not only clear the bowels, but make its way "through the whole system" as well, there to break up and expel "slime, mucus [and] congested poisonous matters." "Purgation," the public was told over and over, is "the magnet, the guide, the star of safety"; "Purgation is the Corner-stone of all Curatives." It was the cornerstone of preventives too. A New Jersey woman explained why her nine children always looked so healthy: "we raise them on Brandreth's Pills"; her husband chimed in with the assurance that the same "desired effect" was produced by the medication when he gave it "to [his] oxen, horses, pigs, fowls, cats, dogs . . . ." The Brandreth Calendar for 1880 (free calendars were a popular advertising medium) proposed that there was "no reason why the age of man should not rival that of the patriarchs" if people would just take Brandreth's pills whenever they fell sick. Apparently the ad that proclaimed Vegetable Universal Pills to be "second only to Christianity in the benefits it is capable of conferring upon mankind" was just a modest statement of truth (though not everyone was satisfied that the medication drove death away; a rival product, Parson's Purgative Pills, parodied Brandreth's Pills as Deathbrand's Pills).[49] Patent medicine purgatives not only cured constipation, their advertisements mightily reinforced the public's perception that constipation was the root cause of nearly all other disease.

The point was driven home as well through a second major advertising theme of proprietary purgative manufacturers: victory over constipation, they maintained, required stimulation of the liver, and cathartics provided just such stimulation. It was for this reason that Harter as well as Carter manufactured Little Liver Pills, Ingham marketed Vegetable Liver Cural Pills, Warner put out Log Cabin Liver Pills, and Malena sold Stomach-Liver Pills: "Don't Die with the slow but sure-killing disease, Constipation. . . . But Live" with Malena (Fig. 2-2). As the makers of McLean's Liver and Kidney Balm put it, "A High Liver with a Torpid Liver, never makes a Long Liver" (one manufacturer even hinted that eternal life could be had from his pills, promoting them "as a Factor in Spiritual Awakening," since "it is difficult to convert a man or woman whose liver is out of order" [50]).

But no one sold liver pills like Englishman Thomas Beecham. Rolled out at the rate of nine million every day, Beecham's Pills were the most heavily advertised product of any kind in the British Isles during the last third of the nineteenth century. They were perhaps the most advertised product in the world as well. According to a popular story, an English explorer hacking his way through the very darkest part of Africa, certain he was penetrating territory never before trod by Europeans, came upon a tree with an advertisement painted on it—for Beecham's Pills. Were the story true, the ad doubtless would have been one more proclamation of the remedy's restorative effects on the liver. A Beecham promotion with a different African theme depicted a half dozen "dusky natives" cavorting about a large box of pills that had washed up on their shore from a shipwreck. The natives had lately been in desperate need. Digestive tracts and livers had been thrown completely out of kilter by barbaric dietary practices, by

> The missionary, roast, that disagreed—
> The leathery hymnbook that would not digest—
> The tracts that lay like nightmare on the chest!

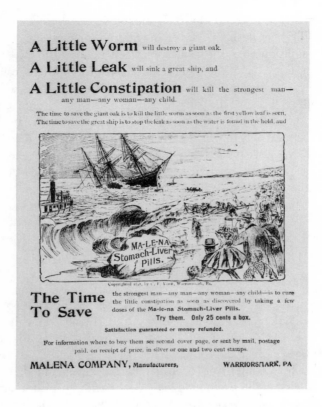

Figure 2-2. Advertisement for Ma-Le-Na, a popular laxative product of the late nineteenth century, warning of the dangers of constipation. [Warshaw Collection, Archives Center, National Museum of American History, box 25, file 5].

But just when hope seemed gone,

> . . . the savage breast with rapture thrills—
> For lo!—a mighty case of Beecham's Pills!
> Ah, priceless boon,—ah, treasure more than wealth!
> The banisher of pain, the key to health! . . . .
> So, eagerly, they set to with a will,
> And every darky took his utmost fill!

The saga played out at some length, but in the climax, a temple was raised to the great white benefactor:

> And, now, they worship Beecham as the giver
> Of Pills that purified a people's liver!

(The pills continue to serve as the salvation of entire nations. When Paul Theroux circumnavigated England by rail, less than 20 years ago, he discovered Beecham's to be the answer to the country's chronic unemployment problem. A comedian in a village in Norfolk requested of his audience, "Hands up, all those who aren't working." Nearly a dozen people raised their hands, but "the comedian was already laughing. 'Have some Beecham's Pills,' he said. 'They'll get you "working" again.'")[51]

But in fact, patent medicine purgatives did not keep people working efficiently. It was well established by the nineteenth century that the use of purgatives on a regular basis would depress bowel function and make the organ reliant on the artificial stimulus of ever-increasing quantities of drugs. "I never knew anyone get into the habit of taking medicine for keeping the body open," a Scottish physician stated, "who could leave it off. . . . Every dose makes way for another, till at length they become as necessary as daily bread." And the burgeoning of the proprietary medicine industry only promised worse to come. "Such, indeed, has been the mad rage for the purchase of *patent drastic pills*," an Englishman wrote in the 1830s, that "the necessity for a daily repetition . . . has been increased by every repeated dose, until the bowels are rendered callous to all remedies, and the case at last terminates in irremediable or fatal disease." He then added a facetious testimonial:

> Your pills can ne'er be praised enough,
> Although you charge so dear,
> They've killed my aunt, though dev'lish tough,
> And I'm her only heir.[52]

Like the aunt, people seemed to think they could abuse themselves with excess, then undo the abuse with cleansing drugs, *An Exposure of the Causes of the Present Deteriorated Condition of Health* commented. But they can't: the good liver "goes on alternately with his *peppers* and his *pills*; he thinks that *calomel* will beat out his *cayenne* and *curries*; and with his darling *poison* in the one hand, and darling antidote in the other," steadily descends into infirmity. It was, moreover, a bumpy ride downward, as the weakening effects of purgative dehydration forced the hapless addict to make use of tonic or stimulant drugs; but of course he was soon constipated again, and so on, "one dose [creating] a necessity for another, till the poor patient wants physic almost as much as he wants food." The health of the physic habitue thus "will be supported . . . like a shuttlecock between two battledores, by the alternate impulse of senna and sherry, of calomel and coffee, of jalap and gentian . . . to be continued as long as feather and cork resist the tendency which it has to knock them to pieces." Sooner or later, even the hardiest constitution would be broken apart: "terrible intestinal disease is induced by this dosing with purgatives"; "disease of the lower bowel has been produced, and death has at last been the consequence"; and "under the combined influence of improper habits and aperient drugs, the invalid is apt to go from bad to worse . . . til seized by acute, violent, and perhaps fatal disease."[53]

These first two chapters have surveyed a number of preoccupations and problems connected with constipation in the nineteenth century. All would continue into the twentieth. In fact, all would assume greater prominence than ever once autointoxication emerged as an even more daunting threat than simple constipation had ever been.

3

CUTTING OUT THE KINKS: SURGICAL TREATMENT

IF YOU WOULD KNOW WHY domestic friction exists, why children are bad, why boys run away from home, why girls seem sometimes possessed of the evil one, why business relations become intolerable, why workmen cannot get along together, why there is dissension in the church, why perfectly sane and sober folks suddenly develop the most outrageous cantankerousness, the cause is not in original sin nor the influence of psychic currents; it is more likely to be found in the vicious company of militant bacilli in the colon. . . . A great deal of what we call Sin is due to what the physician calls stasis.

Frank Crane, 1916

IF THE ORDINARY MAN OR WOMAN were confronted for the first time with the offensive contents of a constipated large bowel, and were told that the body he or she thinks so much about, decks out in fine raiment, and fears to part from more than he fears anything else in the world was the casket of such a jewel, the shock and disgust might almost prove fatal. Lifelong association with these things has bred the contempt of familiarity, the oblivion of the painfully obvious. Sir Arbuthnot Lane's rapier thrust through this armor of complacent forgetfulness lets a flood of light into the dirty corners of our human dustbins.

F. A. Hornibrook, 1934

Edith Eastlake was a sickly child. Throughout her growing-up years in the English coast town of Brighton, she was plagued with coughing, sore throats—and constipation. From the age of 15, painful menstruation was added to her woes, along with headaches and tonsillitis, and her "constipation seemed to increase." She left school at 18 and spent a year and a half confined to home, submitting to a variety of both orthodox and homeopathic remedies. Periodically she improved enough to work a few months as a teacher, then as a secretary, but by 1906, now in her late twenties, she seemed to have fallen into a permanent state of "very unwell. Severe headaches and constipation worried me very much." Though she engaged yet another doctor, and his drugs, Miss Eastlake continued to decline, until in 1908 there was nothing to be done but to move into a rest home.[1]

The rest was no help. Over the next 2 years, her weight dropped well below 100 pounds and she ceased to menstruate; her "constipation was very acute," her abdominal discomfort "almost unbearable." Unable to sleep without the assistance of morphine, "my life was a veritable hell on earth." Then, at the eleventh hour, in February, 1911, a friend advised her to consult the renowned London surgeon William Arbuthnot Lane. "It is almost impossible to describe my miserable condition when I saw Sir Arbuthnot," she confided some years later (for the record, Lane was not Sir at the time of this first visit; he was baroneted in 1913, in part for his successful operation on a member of the royal family). "Practically all life and hope had gone out of me, I hardly cared whether I lived. . . . However, Sir Arbuthnot's intense sympathy, goodness, and great understanding heart filled me with a new hope."[2]

Lane's surgical prowess helped a bit, too. Although a first abdominal operation, done in March of 1911, brought only brief improvement, then relapse, follow-up surgery resulted in "the miracle of miracles." Miss Eastlake immediately began to gain weight (she had sunk as low as 62 pounds), soon resumed menstruating, and no longer suffered from constipation. Before the end of her first postsurgical year she was able to return to work, and even to undertake matrimony. A decade later, she remained vigorous (at 150 pounds), and attributed it all to Lane: "To Sir Arbuthnot's skill I owe everything; Life, Health, Happiness, and even my husband. . . . My feelings and gratitude are too deep for words, and I just long to let the world know what he can do if his aid is sought."[3]

There were many who sought Sir Arbuthnot's aid, and seemingly many of those came away with health and happiness, if not always a spouse. Sir William Arbuthnot Lane was—on this all his medical contemporaries agreed—the "greatest modern interpreter" of autointoxication. And autointoxication, or constipation elevated to new heights by the scientific glamor of the germ theory, was apparently the most widespread illness of the developed world in the early years of this century. It was, in one physician's accounting, "one of the gravest physical disorders of civilized man, one that has truly been called the 'mother of diseases'." By others' reckoning, it "inflicts upon mankind vastly more misery, suffering and deaths than any of the great dramatic 'killing diseases' such as cancer, tuberculosis, heart disease, etc."; "civilized nations have become a prey to [autointoxication]. It is an insidious danger making steady inroads into health and stamina"; autointoxication "affects the rich and the poor, the idle and the industrious, the brain-worker and the manual labourer. . . . It causes numberless varieties of aches and pains, and produces endless forms of discomfort." Or, in Lane's own words— typically concise and cocksure—autointoxication "is the cause of all the chronic diseases of civilization, I have no doubt."[4]

Autointoxication enjoyed its age of greatest vigor in the years from 1900 to 1920. Even though by the end of that period the medical profession was beginning to abandon the theory, the public mind had become fixated on bowel health as never before. A London practitioner commenting in 1913 summed up what had happened since the beginning of the century. "Encouraged by us doctors," he wrote, "hundreds of thousands of human beings have grafted into themselves the idea that they were born into the world for the main purpose of getting a daily evacuation of their bowels, for should they fail in this they will be poisoned by the absorption of the noxious products that are, they suppose, grown in this their kitchen garden." He spread the blame around to doctors in general, but surely he knew (and indeed, elsewhere said so) that Arbuthnot Lane was the doctor above all others who fostered the image of the gut as a garden of deadly weeds. Lane led the way, furthermore, in implementing the most drastic of all the many measures that were instituted to offset the onslaught of autointoxication: surgery.[5]

Lane was effectively destined for a surgical career, a grandfather and a great-grandfather having both been doctors, and his father a military surgeon. Born in 1856 at an army post in the north of Scotland, Lane was taken to South Africa before he was a month old when his father's regiment was sent to fight in the first Kaffir War. Over the next several years, his family moved to Malta, to Nova Scotia, on to Dublin, and finally back to Scotland, where the young boy's schooling fostered an interest in anatomy and medicine. The interest came to fruition in 1873, when, at the age of 16, Lane moved with his family to London, and enrolled as a student at Guy's Hospital. He would spend his entire career there, as things worked out, and become one of the most illustrious of a long list of distinguished surgeons attached to the hospital over the centuries. He was a much-beloved figure as well, by all accounts as gentlemanly, gracious, and kind-hearted as Edith Eastlake remembered him. "To the world he was Sir Arbuthnot Lane, Bart.," one biographer begins, "but to us [students and colleagues] he was 'Willie,' and 'Willie' he will always be." But Willie was also possessed of extraordinary self-confidence, a trust in the certainty of his observations and reasoning that sometimes led him to hasty generalizations and dogmatic statements to which he held steadfast in defiance of evidence and argument to the contrary. "I wish I were as sure of anything," a highly placed American physician quipped, as Lane "is of everything." Nowhere was this proclivity for dogmatism more solidly demonstrated than in his crusade against autointoxication: "Upon that rock," his American critic observed, "Sir Arbuthnot has built his church."[6]

Lane was drawn early to the repair of fractures, and from the start made truly pioneering contributions to orthopedic surgery. That area of work naturally involved an interest in the mechanical structure and functioning of the body, an interest he pursued through careful dissections of bodies in the hospital's autopsy room. Through these dissections, Lane came to realize that repeated physical

stresses, such as the hauling of heavy loads, would induce changes in the muscu-
loskeletal structure. A man who worked as a coal heaver, for example, would
gradually develop a compressed spinal column and restricted movement of the
chest as a result of carrying heavy bags of coal over his shoulders. The upper ver-
tebrae of a bootmaker would also change, though somewhat differently, in response
to the peculiar position he assumed at the last. Lane actually came to pride himself
on his ability to identify a deceased laborer's line of work by the structural adaptations detectable in his skeleton.[7]

As Lane pondered nature's adaptive capacity, he came to see that there was
one form of labor in which everyone engaged, and by which everyone must be
deformed: hauling around the intestinal tract. The human digestive system, he
reasoned, had originated in four-footed ancestors. Thus when we evolved into
Homo erectus, the colon (along with other internal organs) became subject to an
altered gravitational pull, a mechanical stress. Under gravity's relentless tug, the
colon soon began to droop, a process that the body countered by forming mem-
branous bands or adhesions along the lines of greatest strain. Eventually the bands
would come to grip the sagging organ so tightly as to contract it in places and form
unnatural "kinks," as Lane termed them. The first kink to appear usually was at
the juncture of the descending colon and the sigmoid colon, just above the rectum; for this, Lane coined (and recited ad nauseum) the phrase "the first and last
kink" to describe the bend that developed earliest in life (the first) near the end
(the last) of the digestive tract. But of course the first was only the beginning. As
life progressed, gravity saw to it that more kinks formed in other areas of the
intestines (Fig. 3-1).[8]

Once kinked by gravity, the intestine would then begin to kink itself even farther. Band-narrowed passageways impeded the advance of feces, inclining the person toward constipation, which, however mild at first, increased the weight of the
colon, provoking the body to adapt with stronger bands, thereby tighter kinks. These
brought about a higher degree of constipation, making the bowel even more subject
to gravity's deforming influence, and so it went. It might go a second way. In people
of low vital power and weak abdominal musculature, the body was too feeble to
generate kink formation. Instead, the bowel was allowed to sag unopposed, to drop
into the pelvic floor and become twisted, or kinked, on its own. The end result was
the same—"an insuperable barrier to the passage" of feces. By early childhood, every
civilized person was trapped in a vicious downward spiral of tightening of the intestine and retention of waste matter in the body. (In his younger adult years, Lane
himself "suffered severely from constipation," because of limited physical activity,
he believed; how much his personal distress inclined him to suppose constipation to
be everyone's problem can only be guessed.)[9]

Every "civilized" person is specified because Lane's analysis suggested that
"savage races" should suffer much less intestinal deformation than culturally ad-

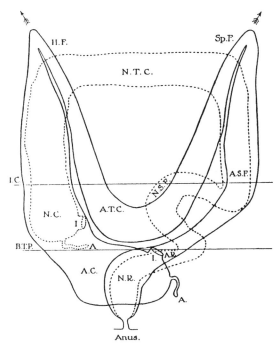

Figure 3-1. Arbuthnot Lane's somewhat mysterious diagram of the kinks of the colon [from Arbuthnot Lane, *The Operative Treatment of Chronic Constipation*, p. 16].

vanced populations. Precivilized modes of life, he pointed out, provided periodic relief from gravitational force. First, "savages" spend a good bit of their day in a squatting position, a posture in which the intestines are pushed up and supported by pressure from the thighs. They squat particularly for the purpose of emptying their bowels, adopting without thought nature's intended position for the act of defecation: "the forcible apposition of the thigh and abdomen empties the caecum and transverse colon [and] drags the rectum upwards and straightens it, so that the passage of faeces through it is very materially facilitated" (in truth, squatting does straighten the rectum and ease evacuation). Second, the prone position used for rest and sleep, which normally displaces the viscera upward, was largely neu-tralized in civilization by the use of soft mattresses, which allowed "the heavy buttocks and thighs [to] sink deeply into the bed," and so inclined the body enough to let the bowels sag toward the pelvis. Even when they slept, it seems, advanced races became constipated, and all because of their higher civilization.[10]

Lane devised a mechanical–anatomical analysis of intestinal kinking that was considerably more refined than the preceding paragraph might suggest. Its details needn't detain us, however, for it was, as it turned out, only theory. Anatomical reasoning suggested kinks should be present in people who had lived long enough, and autopsy found them, but further study by other anatomists determined that the kinks that so worried Lane were normal variations; most human beings have one or two kink-like sections somewhere in their digestive tract, and, as one critic put it, "a kink to you and me is no kink to it [the colon]." Some antagonists were much less diplomatic, objecting, so Lane reported, "that the kinks did not exist in the patient's body, but were present only in my brain." He persisted in his belief that kinking was a pathological alteration ("the first and last kink, is by far the most important evolutionary structure in the human body, . . . one that is productive of the most disastrous consequences to the health and happiness of the community"), but what worried him ultimately was the chemical transformations that occurred because of the kinks. Kinks, he maintained, caused "chronic intestinal stasis," and that resulted in autointoxication. "By chronic intestinal stasis," Lane explained, "I mean that the passage of the contents of the intestinal canal is delayed sufficiently long to result in the production . . . of an excess of toxic material, and in the absorption into the circulation of a greater quantity of poisonous products than the organs which convert and excrete them are able to deal with." Such "noxious substances," he elaborated, "produce degenerative changes in every single tissue of the body," indeed "produce disastrous results" if given enough time. Chronic stasis was not, however, exactly the same thing as constipation. The latter meant infrequent and labored bowel movements (stasis, to be sure), but the most regular people would suffer from stasis too if their daily evacuations were not thorough. The colon's contents must be "systematically completely removed," a Lane supporter instructed; otherwise there would be "an ever-increasing residue left behind." If only a fraction of each day's waste stayed trapped by the colon's kinks, feces would accumulate (even as far back as the small intestine) and putrefy and poison the unsuspecting victims no matter how unconstipated they were: "In other words, it is necessary to be sure that the patient is not passing to-day what he ought to have got rid of a week, or perhaps a month ago."[11]

That suggestion of a steady buildup of waste in the body reflects Lane's belief that most of the toxins taken into the circulation were absorbed from the small intestine, where the feces existed in a more liquid form and so were more easily acted upon by microorganisms. The role of the large intestine was more mechanical than chemical; the kinked colon, at any rate, was essentially a dam that so slowed the flow of waste it eventually backed up into the small intestine. The awful implications of the damming up of waste matter were conveyed by Lane in the most stark and compelling imagery. The human digestive tract, he reminded, was the biological equivalent of the household drainage system. The stomach was the body's toilet bowl, the duodenum the toilet trap, the small intestine the drainpipe, "and the large bowel the cesspool." No homeowner would put up with a clogged

drainage scheme that allowed "the discharge of offensive and perhaps poisonous gases" from fouled plumbing into his quarters (here the specter of sewer
gas appears, as late as 1926). He would look for the source of this "escape of foul
gases," he would "have the cesspool cleared of the material stagnating in it, or he
would have the house drain freed from the grease which was reducing its caliber
and obstructing the passage of material through it" (toilet drains could get kinked
too). Lane employed the analogy repeatedly, time and again describing the intestines as "the sewage system of the human body," demanding that people pay
attention to "the paramount importance of effective intestinal drainage," illustrating his books with diagrams of the alimentary tract laid out as a sanitary engineering
network, even generalizing direly that "death implies defective drainage."[12]

From 1903 onward, chronic intestinal stasis became Lane's medical preoccupation, if not obsession. Of the more than 400 articles he published on a wide
range of medical topics over his long career, fully one-fifth dealt with the causes,
effects, and cures of intestinal stasis (there was an inordinate amount of repetition
in these articles, though their redundancy might be seen as another measure of
Lane's obsession with the subject). The effects of stasis, which Lane believed he
observed in hundreds of patients through the years, were as numerous as they
were sad. There were the headaches, menstrual difficulties, and weight loss Edith
Eastlake experienced, but the long list also included complaints as varied as
abdominal pain, sallow or "dirty" complexion, breathlessness on exertion, pain
in the muscles and joints, cold hands and feet, facial tics, kidney disease, heart disease, baldness, and offensive perspiration ("a nasty graveyard odor" is how Lane
described the stasis victim's sweat to acquaintances). Such difficulties, furthermore,
were only the direct results of static bowels. Autointoxication also operated indirectly, its depressing effect on the body's resistance laying the sufferer open to every
opportunistic infection from pyorrhea to pulmonary tuberculosis. All these symptoms taken together, Lane concluded, "were merely a few obvious, typical" damages of the total that could be attributed to intestinal stasis. (Lane somehow became
convinced through clinical experience that red-haired people were much more
resistant to autointoxication than were others; "these favoured people," an ardent
follower of Lane described them, "with festooned colons, long loaded and undis-
charged, [who] nevertheless manage to show matchless complexions, exalted sexual
activities, great athletic enterprise, and an alertness of mentality which shames the
clean-bowelled brunette.")[13]

The worst of autointoxication's damages was cancer, which Lane supposed
could develop in any organ or tissue continually bathed in fecally contaminated
blood. At a time when understanding of the etiology of cancer was far murkier
than now, Lane stated without pausing that cancers have three causes. One is "trau-
matism," a state of injury or inflammation due either to acute damage or chronic
irritation, which, if not allowed to heal, degenerates into a cancerous lesion. Stasis-

generated poisons in the bowel, concentrated around kinks, of course, were chronic irritants, slowly traumatizing the organ, and were the chief reason for the high incidence of colon cancer in civilized nations. In addition, toxins absorbed from the intestine inhibited the healing of traumatic sites anywhere else in the body, thus contributing indirectly to cancer. The second cause of cancer was also intestinal poisons, for all body tissues required fully nourishing blood to maintain their vitality. If deprived of nourishment by poisons from the bowel (autointoxication both diluted the blood and suppressed an organ's ability to assimilate nutrients), tissue inevitably degenerated "in proportion to the degree of the fouling of its supply of nutrition." This process was particularly evident in the female reproductive system, comprising organs in which "function ceases at a comparatively early age." The uterus, ovaries, and breasts did not extract as much nutrition from the blood after menopause, Lane proposed, because they didn't require it for functional activity; consequently there was less nourishment to offset the effects of intestinal poisons.[14]

The third cause was "x," so-designated by Lane because "it is at present unknown to us." It might be a germ, he speculated, it might be something else, but whatever it was, x surely "cannot obtain a foothold in the tissues" unless they have already been weakened by "the traumatic and degenerative factors" of autointoxication. "*Cancer never attacks a healthy organ or tissue*," Lane repeatedly stated. So in the final telling, intestinal stasis was all three causes of cancer. "In every case in which I have had an opportunity of verifying it," he wrote toward the end of his long career, "I have found that the cancer patient was suffering from chronic intestinal stasis and that the . . . cancer was an indirect consequence of this condition." In every case! All this misery and wretched death from that infernal first and last kink? If so, one could hardly dispute Lane's assertion that the kink "spells the failure of civilization and is a veritable Pandora's box."[15]

As if every form of cancer weren't enough devastation, the ravages of stasis also included mental and emotional problems, some so severe as the melancholy that drove an occasional victim to suicide ("one hopeless person blew his brains out while we were arranging for his admission into a home"), the irascibility that drove others to violence ("it [intestinal stasis] is a more frequent cause of serious crime than is generally imagined," Lane intimated), even the psychic trauma that affected so many soldiers in World War I ("in all cases of shell-shock which came under my observation during the war the sufferer was invariably toxic"). For the most part, the psychological effects of stasis were milder than suicide or shell shock. They were, as it turns out, the very constellation of symptoms that previously had been regarded as the effects of neurasthenia, the nervous weakness or nervous exhaustion that physicians and the public alike had believed to be rampant during the last third of the nineteenth century. Neurasthenics, too, had been subject to anxiety and depression, insomnia and fatigue, headaches and sexual dysfunction;

in point of fact, many still were, for neurasthenia remained a frequent diagnosis well into the twentieth century. But by the 1910s, a British or American physician was as likely to tell a weary and anxious patient he had intestinal stasis or intestinal toxemia as to label him a neurasthenic. An English surgeon speaking in 1913 ticked off a long list of miseries associated with autointoxication, then asked his audience, "do not these symptoms correspond exactly with the symptoms of neurasthenia?" So convinced was he that nervous exhaustion was simply one (albeit it large) category of self-poisoning, that he treated more than 130 cases of neurasthenia with anti-autointoxication measures. The fact that most had improved under his care was proof positive, he submitted, of "my belief that chronic intestinal toxaemia is at the root of almost every case of neurasthenic trouble." His view was seconded by a practitioner whose specialty was the treatment of mental illness resulting from nervous exhaustion, and who had more than once "seen a prodigious evacuation of the bowels at the hands of the physician terminate a case of insanity." Lane concurred, stating matter-of-factly that "the mental condition which is brought about by auto-intoxication" was one that "medical men are very fond of calling . . . neurasthenia."[16] Thus did the old catchall diagnosis give way to the new.

Lane arrived at a diagnosis of chronic stasis for a patient on the basis of her presenting some (one hopes not all) of the symptoms noted above, backed by an X-ray examination demonstrating the presence of kinks and slow movement of a barium meal through the gut. Treatment of the condition depended on the severity of the case. In the early stages, damage could be undone with so simple a measure as a dose of paraffin oil (now called mineral oil; the oil operates as a laxative by retarding loss of water from the stools, hence keeping them bulky). It was with paraffin oil that Lane cured his own constipation, finding that "a sufficient quantity" taken before each meal greased the kinks of his intestines and allowed waste to slide through so easily that he could count on a postprandial movement every time: "I immediately improved in health, comfort and happiness." Understandably, Lane continued the practice to the end of his life, and urged it on his children and grandchildren (a granddaughter joked to me that she got married in part to get away from home and the daily dose of paraffin her father, a Lane disciple, made her take). Lane also imposed the regimen upon servants, a pet parrot, and a "little monkey that outlived all the years of possible longevity" thanks, presumably, to its daily oil (once when Lane was the guest of honor at a surgeons' banquet in the United States, the host placed a small champagne bottle of paraffin oil at each place). The highly viscous oil did produce frequent and large movements often accompanied by more than ordinary flatulence, and was prone to leak from the anus and soil the user's clothes ("an indignant lady" once returned to the physician who had prescribed paraffin for her "with a burning fire on her lips and a dressmaker's bill in her hand"). To Lane, however, that was still preferable to excoriating the intestine with the harsh cathartics traditionally used to empty the organ. Thus he prescribed paraffin in every case, even when more invasive measures also had to be resorted to. In memoirs composed 45 years after swallowing his first spoonful of paraffin, Lane still believed he could "safely assert that no remedy has rendered so much good to the human race as paraffin." Lane was an ardent advocate of the Curtis belt, too, a sort of truss for the abdomen that provided support for any sagging portions of bowel and kept them from further kinking. The belts were recommended for children particularly, for nipping a problem in the bud was clearly the best form of prevention. "Most children themselves recognize its value," a Lane compatriot maintained, "and refuse to be without it once they have learned to put it on properly, and even face the ridicule of their schoolfellows rather than give it up."[17]

In advanced cases of stasis, however, there was only one solution for a surgeon: cut out the kinks that cause it. To Lane, it seemed best to not only cut out any kinks that had already developed but to eliminate as well anything that might develop a kink in the future. By the beginning of this century, he was regularly performing what he called the "short-circuit operation," the bypassing of the large intestine from the point where it's joined by the small intestine (a common site of kinking, he believed) all the way to the sigmoid flexure, the S-shaped stretch of colon just above the rectum. Indeed, so eager was Lane to perform ileosygmoidostomy (connection of the ileum, or small intestine, to the sigmoid) for all manner of conditions, he quickly became notorious for it; even his students resorted to parody, mounting a skit about a surgeon who used "a sterilized trowel [to] short circuit the bowel," and who "sharpens his knives and . . . waits for the time," when short circuits "won't be a surgical crime."[18]

That short-circuit was the first operation done on Edith Eastlake. But, it will be recalled, she needed a second operation, and so did many others among Lane's patients, early improvement often being followed by a return of symptoms within a year or two. Although the short-circuit allowed waste matter to quickly move past nearly the full length of the colon, feces could, once having arrived in the sigmoid, be regurgitated upwards into the descending colon. Over time, considerable quantities of waste could accumulate in the colon, being dammed ever farther back toward the ileum, effectively undoing the bypass and reinitiating autointoxication. That was Lane's interpretation, anyway, and the way to fix the problem, clearly, was to perform colectomy, to completely remove the colon from the body.[19]

Colectomy was a much more complicated and risky procedure than ileosigmoidostomy, so Lane preferred to give the short circuit a try first. That was the approach he took to Eastlake's problems, but she required the second operation, and in her case, remember, colectomy proved to be a miracle of miracles. So it was for many others, Lane believed, and as he became convinced that total colectomy gave permanent results, he gradually abandoned the short-circuit procedure in favor of extirpation of the colon at the outset. He continued to perform ileo-sigmoidostomies on those who were too sick or weak for the more demanding colectomy, knowing that the latter operation could always be done after the patient had gained strength and vitality from the less-taxing procedure. Whichever surgery they received, patients had to continue the thrice-daily paraffin oil regimen afterwards too; paraffin was even more vital for them than for the uncolectomized, since the small bit of intestine they had left "is not of a calibre sufficient to accomodate the products of 24 hours' digestion, and to ensure perfect drainage it must be evacuated two or three times a day."[20]

Much more likely than not, the recipient of a Lane colectomy was female. In 1915, another English surgeon who had attained the title of Sir described "the victim of what we may call 'Lane's disease'" (a patient that "is now easily recognized") as "generally a woman." She was probably, in fact, a "lean, cadaverous, flat-chested" woman whose hands are "cold and clammy," whose skin "bears many crops of pimples," and whose body odor "is apt to be distressingly noticeable." Because her "abdominal muscles . . . are flabby and flaccid, and all the viscera which they should hold up are fallen in greater or less degree," she suffers "flatulence, and inveterate and incoercible constipation." Finally (and not surprisingly), a case of Lane's disease is "morose, querulous, and often suspicious," and just as often exhibits "a complete absence of the joy of life." Rarely does every last one of those attributes occur in an individual patient, the surgeon acknowledged, "but so many of them may coexist as to enable a distinct type of patient to be recognized." That type was female and, more likely than not, unmarried.[21]

Women are in fact affected by constipation more frequently than men. That was recognized by pre-twentieth-century physicians, who, even though they lacked the statistical documentation available today, were nonetheless certain from clinical experience that women were much more prone to costiveness. A nineteenth-century doctor who believed constipation to be the most common of all ailments, for example, specified that such was the case "especially among females." "This is the most prevalent morbid condition of all women in civilized society," a New Jersey physician maintained, while Austin Flint, one of the American profession's pedagogical leaders during the mid-1800s, stated that "most [girls] become affected with habitual constipation, and suffer from it all their lives." Yet another practitioner considered "most" an underestimate and insisted that irregularity was "universal" among the fair sex, or at least so nearly so that all doctors should adopt the practice he followed with female patients of always determining the state of their bowels before proceeding to other diagnostic possibilities. Similarly, cases of female constipation were often described in terms comparable to those used by Lane for his women patients. Among the many patients a nineteenth-century Scottish physician cured with purgatives, for example, were women who developed costiveness around the onset of puberty, then soon began to suffer abdominal pain, headaches, labored respiration, loss of weight and muscle tone, cessation of the menses, and "nervous symptoms . . . a peevish and recluse turn of mind, which makes the unhappy sufferer shun society, and court darkness and solitude."[22]

In the nineteenth century, however, surgery was not an option for female constipates searching for relief. Abdominal surgery became safe only after aseptic technique was perfected in the last two decades of the century, though even then, so extensive a procedure as removal of most or all of the colon involved a significant risk. Lane nevertheless performed hundreds of short-circuits and colectomies, and most were done on women. To be sure, patient records for all his intestinal operations are not available; all we have are three reports—two written by Lane, and one by Harold Chapple, Lane's assistant and eventually his son-in-law. Yet these papers detail 106 cases of chronic intestinal stasis treated with surgery, and indications are that they are representative of Lane's overall intestinal patient population: 89 of the cases were women. What could account for so skewed a distribution, for 84% of all severely constipated people being female? There was the supposed greater hesitation of women to attend to nature's call when with company (women have a "squeamishsness about being seen going to the toilet while in public places," an authority on the subject wrote in 1909, "no matter how strong the desire to empty the bowel may be"), and their relative physical inactivity.[23] But fundamentally, Lane believed, it was because females were far more likely to be kinked. Intestinal kinking, remember, came about in two ways: in the strong, constricting bands of tissue developed to support the bowel against the pull of gravity; in the weak, the undefended intestines were simply allowed to droop—and bend. Women were weak, or at least many more were than men, ideals of femininity discouraging them from any exertions more strenuous than playing the piano or conjugating irregular French verbs. Their untoned abdominal musculature thus offered no resistance to the sagging of the digestive tract.

In addition, the corsets favored by so many women positively pushed the viscera down into the pelvis. Tight lacing had been a commonly assigned cause of constipation in the nineteenth century, a representative critic objecting that by the pressure of the corset, "the colon is constricted, foecal matter accumulates in it, and life is destroyed as the result. Thousands thus perish every year." Lane's contempt for the corset was no less. "The English corset is disastrous," he protested, and at times he became so exercised about the device as to call it "by far the most important factor" in the production of intestinal stasis. For nineteenth-century physicians, corset pressure had directly retarded the movement of feces. For Lane, the corset encouraged kinking—"it exerts a constricting encircling pressure . . . and exaggerates the tendency to downward displacement"—which then inhibited the passage of waste. But this was only the beginning of a malignant downward spiral. Nature had endowed women with more body fat, which "plays a far larger share in supporting important organs and structures than it does in the male." Since loss of fat was one of the early consequences of stasis, the woman with falling (kinked) intestines would erode her intestinal support system, letting her bowels sink farther and kink more, thereby worsening her stasis and destroying more body fat, so that her intestines would fall deeper yet. [24]

The overriding importance of kinks in Lane's thinking is manifest in his interpretation of the relation of pregnancy to constipation. Nineteenth-century physicians looked upon the gravid uterus as nature's corset, a source of pressure pushing the bowel closed. Lane thought instead of the weight gained by pregnant women, "fat [which] pillows up the several organs," i.e., counteracts the drooping of the intestines (the growing fetus too would push upward against the bowel, so that "the kinking is as a general rule undone"). In that way, he hypothesized, "a toxic, thin, miserable girl may be converted into a plump, clean, happy one by a pregnancy. It would seem almost justifiable," Lane then mused, for "an unmarried girl [with stasis] to resort to a pregnancy rather than to operative interferences" ("almost" justifiable, for he had to concede that "in our present state of civilisation" there were "distinct and obvious objections" to such a recommendation). Still, possible objections didn't stop him from wondering if Brigham Young's commitment to polygamy involved an appreciation "of the influence of intestinal stasis on women, and the benefit which these people derive from matrimony." Even if unintentional, the Mormons' saving of so many women from autointoxication helped make Young "one of the greatest of the many great men of whom America can boast." [25]

The health-promoting power of pregnancy was not just an appealing theory; clinical experience validated it. Of the three articles mentioned above that reported on cases of treatment of autointoxication with surgery, two specified the marital status of every woman patient. Of the 57 women listed, 44—more than three-quarters—were identified as single or spinster. But whether married or not, female victims of intestinal stasis suffered distinctly female problems. Not only were their reproductive organs being continually irrigated with fouled blood but, Lane maintained through an elaborate anatomical argument, the straining at stool instigated by stasis placed peculiar forces on those organs and weakened them—there could even occur "kinking of the uterus." Protege Chapple asserted in 1914 that "it is no longer possible for us to consider many gynaecological conditions as separate diseases"; they had "masqueraded for so long in various disguises [but] now must fall in line with the many other abdominal conditions whose primary cause is intestinal stasis." He was, of course, echoing Lane, who had assigned autointoxication so large a role in the generation of female diseases "that the gynaecologist may also be regarded as a product of intestinal stasis. If women were not imperfectly drained," he speculated, "the gynaecologist would not have been evolved." [26]

Breast cancer might not have evolved either. Lane's clinical observations convinced him that autointoxication in women produced certain characteristic degenerative changes in breast tissue, "so much so that [the breast] may be regarded as the barometer of the degree of poisoning." The first stage of poisoning was induration, or hardening of the breast, succeeded by the appearance of nodules, then cysts. That these changes were due to stasis seemed evident from the fact that a patient's breasts soon returned to normal if she had her colon removed: "Take the breast while it is indurated and nobbly, . . . eliminate the supply of toxins, and a soft healthy organ results." Another, somewhat less traumatic option was increased sexual activity. Though Lane did not have an explanation for the phenomenon, he had frequently observed that "degenerative conditions do not arise in the breasts of women having regular sexual intercourse, however toxic they may be"; if for any reason intercourse ceased to be regular, induration and nodules quickly appeared (if she had stasis). The moral was obvious enough: "one who suffers sufficiently from imperfect drainage will of necessity undergo changes of varying severity in her sexual organs if she remains a virgin." The most severe change was, of course, cancer of the breast, which "appears with remarkable frequency."[27]

What usually brought women to Lane, though, was not fear of cancer, but pain and bloating in the abdomen, the pain "sufficient to make the sufferer lead the life of a chronic invalid." Some combination of headaches, weight loss, constipation, disturbed menstrual function, ovarian cysts, infertility, and other manifestations of autointoxication commonly figured in as well. Indeed, so unmanageable had autointoxication made these women's lives that they demanded surgical help even when Lane advised against it. "She was urged not to incur the risk of the operation," Lane reported of one woman, "which in her toxic condition was a very serious one." But her reply was "that if it were not done she would terminate her existence." So much for the predictions of colleagues that "patients would never submit to such a serious operation as removal of the large bowel." They were overlooking the fact that to the typical stasis invalid, "life has no attraction," "the world seems always chill and gloomy to them." Obtaining consent was thus not, in fact, a problem. Lane actually claimed that not a single patient "expressed to me the slightest anxiety, . . . but has most willingly grasped the opportunity of parting with his other troubles at all costs and at the earliest opportunity."[28]

Lane does not, however, seem to have needed much inducement in most cases. So long as medical measures such as laxatives and enemas had been tried first, and the patient was strong enough to undergo surgery, he was only too ready to perform it. To be sure, things did not always turn out as hoped—case reports occasionally end with such notations as "several days after . . . acute peritonitis set in, and she died," or "she suffered severely from shock. Vomiting commenced . . . and continued till her death three days later." Far more common , however, were endings such as "most pleased with the result of this operation," and "declares she has not felt so well for ten years" (only about 6.5% of the patients in the three articles mentioned previously died). Those actually were modest appraisals, much less sweeping than the claims Lane often made when promoting the surgical solution to professional peers. Symptoms that had plagued patients for years quickly disappeared after either short-circuiting or colectomy, he maintained, at times sounding not unlike a miracle healer. A woman "who had been confined to bed for many months," too weak to walk and so mentally lethargic "that she was regarded by many as an imbecile," was transformed into both an "active" and an "intelligent woman within a few weeks" of her colectomy. Another woman experienced such intense headaches that she was diagnosed by a neurologist as having a malignant tumor and urged to undergo brain surgery. Instead, she consulted Lane, decided a short-circuit suited her more, and her "headache disappeared at once" after the operation, with no later evidence of cancer. In sum, "the poor, wretched, stupid, feeble woman, who is rendered ugly and unattractive by her . . . general appearance of irritable old age, with her cold, clammy hands, with the aches and pains in her legs, loins, and arms, becomes in a few days a bright eyed woman, sweet smelling, active mentally and physically. Each week and each month shows a steady improvement and she gradually recovers her youth."[29]

Lane's operations restored youth not just to organs but to temperament and physical appearance as well. Stasis soured the disposition as thoroughly as it poisoned the tissues—note the preceeding quotation emphasizes an appearance of *irritable* old age; "bad temper" occurs in an unquoted part of the paragraph. The language of disagreeability and unruliness runs through all Lane's descriptions of the effects of stasis on women (not that he makes constipated males sound any more charming). A man was better off living "with a drunken woman rather than a toxic one," he is reported to have said; "a drunken person is occasionally merry, but a toxic one never!" On another occasion, Lane remarked that he had recently treated a man who had cut his own throat. An attendant with a facetious streak asked, "Did you want to do a short-circuit on that case, sir?" Lane's quick reply: "not on the man, only on his wife. If she had a short-circuit she would probably be better tempered, and he wouldn't want to cut his throat." (The man perhaps needed the advice of the palm-reader who was consulted by the constipated patient of another London doctor: "after looking at her hand [the palmist] said, 'If I were your husband I would take a stick to you!'")[30]

That surgery tamed the shrew was evidenced by the fact that "several of these cases [of autointoxicated women] have married after the operation," Lane reported, adding he was "certain that no one would have married them previous to the operation." Their preoperative lack of appeal was not entirely a matter of unpleasant disposition, however. The autointoxicated were not physically attractive either. More than one nineteenth-century hygienist had suggested a correlation between inner filth and outer ugliness, though the more common theme before

Lane was that while a female constipate might be as lovely as the most regular woman, her beauty was only superficial: immediately beneath her skin lurked unspeakable foulness, blood tainted with "the essence of a material, which a few hours before was too despicable to be touched, to be named, to be looked at, to be thought of, and yet now circulates in the very dimpled cheeks, and simpering tongue, and lisping lips."[31]

With the advent of autointoxication, however, inner nastiness was commonly presumed to seep through to the surface: "Toxins . . . springing from the intestinal cesspool," a London physician explained, "prowl about the tissues seeking what they may convert from the beautiful and useful into the ugly, the painful, and degenerate." In the even more vivid language of an American medical writer,

> It was an image good to see, with spirits high and full of glee,
> And robust health endowed;
> Its face was loveliness untold, Its lines were cast in beauty's mold;
> At its own shrine it bowed.
> With perfect form in each respect, It proudly stood with head erect
> And skin surpassing fair;
> Surveyed itself from foot to head, And then complacently it said:
> "Naught can with me compare."
> When lo the face began to pale, The body looked too thin and frail,
> The cheek had lost its glow;
> The tongue a tale of woe did tell, With nerves impaired its spirits fell;
> The fire of life burned low.
> In the intestinal canal, Waste matter lay, and sad to tell,
> Was left from day to day;
> And while it was neglected there, It undermined that structure fair,
> And caused it to decay.[32]

By Lane's analysis, the same stasis-induced loss of fat that allowed a woman's colon to droop left her exterior to sag too. Wrinkles appeared and bones protruded, "most distressing and conspicuous features. The buttocks also become flat and flaccid, instead of firm and round," he lamented; "the breasts also waste and flop downwards, and the whole form and contour of the woman alters conspicuously in the most objectionable manner." Beauty, in other words, was bowel deep. "Beauty starts from the stomach," a Lane supporter wrote, "and ends at the epidermis."[33] But all could be set to rights again, to firmness and roundness, by restoring a woman's drainage scheme.

No wonder, then, that Lane's patients worshiped him. "I shall be grateful to you all my life," one woman told him by post, while another, writing more than a decade after her colectomy, swore "I can't ever forget you, for if it wasn't for you I shouldn't be alive and well and happy now! . . . . I have been a different person ever since."[34] But were such women the norm? Many of Lane's contemporaries insisted they were rare exceptions, that for the great majority of patients, men as well as women, the experience of being "a different person" was short-lived, and that in more than a few cases the patient herself was short-lived. The efficacy and safety of Lane's operation as the therapy for Lane's disease was in fact a hotly contested issue in the medical world of the 1910s.

Debate was complicated by the fact that for pure operative skill Lane was held in higher esteem than perhaps anyone in the profession. "Lane was the most perfect surgical workman I have ever watched," an English colleague effused (an opinion subscribed to by many among surgery's elite); "no matter how difficult the operation, in his hands it appeared easy." Even colectomy looked easy in Lane's hands. "To those who . . . have watched Lane perform a total extirpation of the colon," prominent New Orleans surgeon Rudolph Matas enthused, "his very small operative mortality was not at all surprising. One could not see Lane perform this exacting and technic-testing operation, without feeling that he had seen something done as well as it could possibly be done." In Matas's opinion, Lane was "a real virtuoso," a man possessing "incomparable perfection" as "an abdominal technician."[35]

The virtuoso himself maintained that "the removal of the large bowel is not accompanied with any special danger to life." That, of course, was easy enough for Lane to say, but others bore him out. To offer one example, a New York surgeon who visited London five times between 1907 and 1913 watched Lane operate during every trip ("witnessed his masterly technique"), then followed the progress of the patients over several months. Not only did he find "many former human derelicts . . . made over into useful and happy people," but also determined that out of 52 ileosigmoidostomies and 54 colectomies performed by Lane during a 4-year period, only nine patients had died. "The mortality in operations for cases of intestinal stasis," he concluded, "is astonishingly low" (happily for us, a mortality of almost 9% would be considered astonishingly high today). Judging from other reports, the speed of recovery was astonishing too. Consider the patient with palsy and such mental confusion that "he was unable to do two things at once, e.g., blow his nose while walking." He was diagnosed as a case of stasis, and "Sir Arbuthnot Lane operated. . . . Improvement set in at once. Before the wound was healed the complexion had improved and the mind had cleared up 'as though a veil had been lifted'; . . . his whole aspect and outlook changed from gloom to brightness," and his palsy was cured. This case, described a year and a half after surgery, "has every appearance of permanency."[36]

On the other hand, consider George B., an American who sought Lane out only after enduring a full decade of relying on enemas to empty his bowels. Lane extracted the man's colon, along with 56 pounds of semi-liquid feces, but a week later, George B. died from peritonitis (inflammation of the abdominal lining; the unfortunate man's colon, incidentally, is on display in the pathology museum at

Guy's Hospital, exhibit A477). To Lane's credit, he acknowledged that, "I have lost more than one patient in this way." He did not actually consider these losses his fault, though, but rather blamed them on the advanced state of autointoxication such patients had reached by the time he was consulted. "Considerable risk of infection," Lane maintained, existed only with "patients who are supremely toxic," and those who were "feeble," with low "resisting power to organisms."[37]

Nevertheless, "statements of great mortality" from Lane's colectomies circulated through the British and American medical communities. Nor was rumor any kinder to the survivors. Another American physician, a gastroenterologist, singled out Lane as an example par excellence of "decerebrate medicine," backing the charge with a friend's report that he had once visited Lane's clinic and "watched him present to the audience a number of colon-less patients who [sic], he said, he had cured of this and that." But when the friend succeeded in getting into the room where patients were waiting to be shown off as cures, and asked how they were doing, the patients "said they were utterly miserable and unable to work, but the surgeon gave them a little money each week to come and be demonstrated, and 'they much needed this help.'" On occasion, supposedly cured patients admitted their misery directly to Lane. A Tooting woman wrote him in 1921 to let him know that despite a short-circuit operation in March 1913, followed by a colectomy 11 months later, "I am still having mucus colitis [likely a mistaken self-diagnosis, since she no longer had a colon], and it keeps me very thin." She was plagued by "bleeding piles" as well, "but I could not have another operation. . . . I feel afraid to see you. I have got such a coward lately." Nevertheless, she requested his advice on nonsurgical remedies, and hoped "you will not mind my writing. I have such faith in you. . . . Awaiting your reply/I am yours faithfully."[38]

Hettie Bacon's letter is a capsule characterization of the mix of misgivings and faith that Lane's surgical and medical brethren felt about his theory and treatments. He was too extraordinary an operator to be shrugged off as a crank, yet his simple mechanism of intestinal kinking explained too much by half, and his reports of surgical cures sounded too good to be true. Was there really nothing "more remarkable in the whole range of surgery than the result of removal of the large bowel in a case of rheumatoid arthritis, [t]he transition is so abrupt as to be startling"? Was "the rejuvenation of the body and of all its constituent parts after such operative measures as render the drainage scheme efficient" truly "the most satisfactory result of surgery known to us at the present time"?[39] Many physicians doubted so risky a procedure could yield such extraordinary results.

Thus it was that in the spring of 1913, the Royal Society of Medicine (of London) convened "A Discussion on Alimentary Toxaemia" that was to occupy its members through six lengthy sessions spread over the better part of 2 months. "Alimentary toxaemia," rather than autointoxication or chronic intestinal stasis, was the designated subject because at the time there was also considerable support for the idea that infections of the mouth released poisons into the body, i.e., toxemia could occur at either end of the alimentary tract. The upper end received relatively little attention, however, the great majority of the 60 speakers (experts from surgery, medicine, anatomy, bacteriology, and other related fields) concentrating their attention on the intestines—and on Lane. The issue that precipitated the debate, for it was more a debate than a "discussion," was not toxemia or autointoxication; though some speakers questioned the existence of autointoxication, most accepted it to some degree. Rather, it was the increasing resort to so extreme a measure as colectomy to treat and supposedly cure self-poisoning that demanded a thorough airing of the subject, which meant Lane was the focal point of debate. It was, apparently, a position he relished, for he delivered the lengthiest presentation to the assembly, an authoritative oration on kinks and colectomies that must have had his audience wondering if it would ever end. In the published proceedings of the discussions, Lane's opening session address (he was the fifth speaker) occupies 68 out of 380 pages, nearly 20% of the text; he comprised less than 2% of the presenters.[40]

The proceedings were opened by W. Hale White, a brahmin among London physicians, who set the tone of polite challenge to Lane that would prevail throughout. In the few minutes he took to define the area for discussion, White called into question the evolutionary development of intestinal kinks, the soundness of the clinical connections drawn between stasis and its presumed injuries, and the success of the short-circuit cure: "I, like some others," he said, "have seen some women who are not in the least better for having had it done." Even those who had apparently improved, he proposed, were merely beneficiaries of the placebo effect: "Many of the subjects of operation are neurotic women, and we all know that the immediate effects of operation on them may be extraordinary."[41] Each of the succeeding three speakers also expressed doubts about items that were conspicuously linked to Lane, and though they were unfailingly civil, the surgeon had effectively been put in the dock by the time he took the podium.

And there he remained, most of the 50–odd speakers who followed maintaining a skeptical attitude toward him, and particularly toward the position that aggressive surgery was the best way to treat autointoxication. Several physician participants regretted the too quick resort to the knife they associated with Lane. Dr. Mantle questioned "if the surgeon is aware of what can be done by medical means" (laxatives, enemas, diet, exercise), and wondered further, "has medicine lost its healing art, that an organ when unhealthy, either must be removed or put on a siding as no longer of any use?" No, was another speaker's response, medicine had not lost its ability to heal, "and we may hope that one result of this discussion will be that we shall keep 'the drainage scheme' of our patients in sufficiently good order as to render surgical interference unnecessary." (Lane must have been stung by such remarks, since he had repeatedly stated in his papers on the surgical treatment of stasis that he turned to the operating room only after all medical measures had failed to help a desperate patient.)[42]

Such comments spoke not just to the risk and uncertainty of surgery, but equally to the implication that the colon was of no value to the human economy, an unnecessary organ that could be removed or short circuited ("put on a siding") with impunity. Indeed, Lane had stated as much explicitly on more than one occasion, that the colon was "a serious defect in our anatomy." Now he had to answer. How could anatomists have been so blind, anatomist Arthur Keith asked? Why had they not been able to see that an organ that "was an intrinsic part of every air-breathing vertebrate, that . . . reached a high degree of development and specialization in every mammal that included a vegetable element in its diet, [that was] a great structure which has served that long chain of ancestors, carrying man's lineage through the secondary and tertiary periods of the earth's formation and assisting man to become the dominant and universal species of the world," was in fact "a useless structure"? All Lane had demonstrated with his surgeries, Keith submitted, was that "no colon is better than a diseased one." What had not been shown, however, was "that a man without a colon is in a better state than the man with a healthy colon. It will be time enough to relegate the great bowel to the list of useless structures," he concluded, "when that much is proved."[43]

Physician James Goodhart pushed the point even further, urging the normality of not just the healthy colon but the *full* colon. Denouncing the "poison-bag theory of the colon," a view of it as "a mere sac in which food lies passively and rots," he contended it was in truth an active organ, one from which nutrients (not toxins) continued to be absorbed into the system. His interpretation of the evolution of the colon was that it had adapted over time into "an organ for *delay* and *storage*," a veritable "Gladstone bag" (a popular form of luggage at the time) for the body to carry about its essentials. Far from being "a mere cloaca full of noxious contents, . . . that . . . can make no effort to expel them," it "*wants*" its contents, "it *needs* them, until very low down in the intestinal canal," and at that point it was quite capable of expelling them without assistance if it had been properly taken care of through life. Surgery, however, was not the way to take care of it. "Greatly as one must admire the skill of Surgery in marshalling its facts," Goodhart proposed, "and the energy and courage with which it has obtained them, we may, I am sure, be allowed to question its inferences, for, if not, we may almost be persuaded to weep for humanity that it ever emerged from the four-footed beasts, for so dire are the effects that are pictured of the upright posture." Were Lane correct, one might as well add colectomy instruments to the home medicine chest.[44]

It was not just at the Royal Society of Medicine that Lane was being challenged. Many outside the Society questioned the wisdom of resorting to surgery to combat autointoxication, and doubted its effectiveness. An American physician,

for example, also credited the remarkable recoveries reported by Lane to the placebo effect and the power of suggestion. The evidence of improvement after having "some changes made in their . . . colons or cecums or sigmoids," he submitted, was "out of court. The osteopaths can show us that. So can the chiropractics
[sic], so can the Christian Scientists." Such was the power of faith, he continued,
that he could take a group of patients all complaining of the usual symptoms of
stasis "and gouge holes in their lumbar muscles and have them whole and hearty,
singing my praises within a year."[45]

Faith, furthermore, was reinforced by nature. Most of Lane's patients were
low in health when they came to see him. "These he puts to bed and purges for
the operation," a New York medical professor pointed out; then "there is the low
diet for several days that must follow all laparotomies [abdominal operations], then
comes the three or more weeks bed rest of the body and building up generally
because of no expenditures in physical or nervous energies." Should anyone be
surprised such patients felt improved? And should anyone expect the feeling to
last? In America, the New York physician noted, where "many enthusiastic surgeons have performed these operations," the "cured cases" were requiring medical attention again, for the very same symptoms, but now "after having passed
through the route of dangerous surgery and contributed to flattering surgical
statistics."[46]

What most worried critics about the dangerous and ultimately useless surgery for autointoxication was that there was so much of it, and there threatened to
be much more. "An epidemic of operative surgery" loomed on the horizon by the
1910s, "the immature surgeons of two continents," inspired by the "brilliant advocacy" of Arbuthnot Lane, set to "inaugurate an era of short-circuiting, performing this or the yet graver colectomy for all sorts and conditions of disease in all
sorts and conditions of men, women, and children, on the smallest possible pre-
text." "If this policy prevails," a British medical editor worried, "an intestine of
the natural length will before long be as rare as an appendix" (the turn of the century had witnessed an epidemic of appendectomies). That might not be so disturbing, were all the intestinal shortenings to be performed by Lane. But "the size of
the abdominal wound, and the lengthy exposure of the abdominal contents make
an ideal operation impossible for the average surgeon," a Scottish practitioner
pointed out. "And it is the average surgeon who will supply the registrar with
[mortality] statistics," he reminded, " not the Lanes." An American commentator
spoke more bluntly still, charging Lane with having "given into the hands of the
many undiscerning a series of surgical procedures, awful at their best, but terrifying in the practices of the many who do not discriminate."[47]

One of the critics of the popularity of Lane's operation, by the way, was
widely supposed to be George Bernard Shaw, whose 1906 play *The Doctor's Dilemma* featured a surgeon named Cutler Walpole, a man who made his fortune

operating on upper-crust ladies to remove their "nuciform sac." An invented bit of anatomy, the sac was supposed to be "full of decaying matter—undigested food and waste products—rank ptomaines." The similarity to Arbuthnot Lane and his belief in chronic intestinal stasis and colectomy seems too close to be anything but intentional, though Shaw stoutly denied that Cutler Walpole had been inspired by Lane (he gave the honor instead to "a laryngeal specialist who extirpated uvu-las"). Be that as it may, when the character Mrs. Foljambe demanded Walpole to take out her nuciform sac after her aristocrat sister-in-law "had the biggest sac I ever saw removed," it was because she possessed "the genuine hygienic instinct. She couldn't stand her sister-in-law being a clean, sound woman, and she simply a whited sepulchre." It certainly appears that Shaw detected a cult of colectomy chic in English society. (For fashion-conscious Mrs. Foljambe, insult was added to surgery when Walpole opened her and found that, "By George, sir, she hadn't any sac at all. Not a trace!")[48]

Physicians observed the same trend. The age now belonged, in a London physician's phrase, to the "abdominal woman," a female conditioned to let "abdominal troubles colour her life and personality," women generally "neurotic" or with "unstable nervous systems, who are much more given to thinking about their insides than about getting into the kingdom of heaven." Her mind in "perpetual revolution round her umbilicus," she traveled a long road to "chronic abdominalism" that was "paved with operations," while her estimate of the skill of her surgeon rose and fell "with the number of kinks which he can discover in them [her intestines]." A self-absorbed hypochondriac, the abdominal woman was "always discovering fresh symptoms," never admitting "any improvement in her condition," carting about "a box full of roentgen-ray plates" to dramatize the congested state of her intestines. She was "a veritable vampire, sucking the vitality of all who come near her: . . . half an hour with her reduces her doctor to the consistence of 'a piece of chewed string.'" Practitioners who were not psychiatrists, an American doctor stated with the abdominal woman in mind, "seem to have the idea that all crazy people are plainly insane, and all locked up in asylums. Nothing is farther from the truth."[49]

For his part, Lane brushed aside all opposition to his operation, whether medical and theatrical, as typical British conservatism: "the profession, especially in this country, . . . saw, or imagined it saw, faults or fallacies in anything new, and took no trouble to find out if there was anything true in it." American surgeons, he believed, were more open-minded and progressive, and "would deal with [intestinal stasis] scientifically and effectually." Actually, the American profession was for the most part dubious of colectomy, though in his unpublished autobiography, composed near the end of his life, Lane still relished the ovation he received from surgeons at a 1911 meeting in New York—"the whole body rose and cheered me over and over again"—and the assurance of the conference organizer that "no other man in America but Roosevelt would get the reception you have had here."[50]

But that was 1911. By 1920, professional opinion would shift from cautious approval to ridicule and condemnation, surgery to alleviate chronic intestinal stasis would decline markedly, and the abdominal woman (and man) would fall back into medicine's shadows. A Guy's Hospital physician speaking on the topic of "the sins and sorrows of the colon" in 1922 was happy to announce that the colon, for so long "more sinned against than sinning," was enjoying a respite from its sorrows. The epidemic of surgery for autointoxication had peaked; from 40 colectomies performed at Guy's in 1914, the number of operations had fallen to only one in 1920, and none the following year. Furthermore, on a recent trip to the United States, he had been informed that colectomy was no longer done there for constipation. Even Lane yielded to professional pressure and abandoned the colectomy cure by the early 1920s (that is not to say he lost his conviction that stasis kills; rather, he turned to less risky ways of fighting, as will be seen in a later chapter).[51]

But it was not just Lane's surgery that was called into doubt at The Royal Society of Medicine debate. There was the matter of those infernal kinks, too. More than one speaker dismissed the evolutionary hypothesis ("I cannot follow Mr. Lane's ingenious explanation of the formation of these adhesions, nor do I think it is correct") with the observation that intestinal adhesions and kinks are to be found in fetuses; surely those weren't the result of upright posture. In summary remarks at the close of the final session, White actually teetered on the edge of ridicule, calling on anatomists to dissect apes and penguins and other upright animals to see if their intestines have kinks; giraffes might prove especially enlightening, he suggested, as their "bodies approach the vertical." Furthermore, if penguins and giraffes are found to be kinked, "it would be of great interest to know whether such animals have intestinal stasis." And finally, what of bats, he ventured, animals "that spend so much of their time with head downwards. . . . Are there what might be called reverse bands in bats" (and, one wonders, would reverse bands cause diarrhea)?[52]

Even if kinks did cause stasis, one also had to wonder whether stasis caused toxemia. Several speakers stressed that no one had yet demonstrated that any of the toxins produced in the gut could be found in the bloodstream, hence "we may be reasonably sceptical about 'copraemia,' 'faecal fever,' and other alleged results" of stasis. In an echo of the eighteenth-century physician previously quoted on the vagueness of "vapours," a bacteriologist suggested that much of the appeal of autointoxication was that as a diagnosis it could "drop so easily from our lips and soothe our minds with the feeling that at least we have a name for these things even if we know nothing about them"; such labels for sickness "are in truth but confessions of ignorance."[53]

The Royal Society of Medicine debate exposed autointoxication theory to its first serious questioning, a process that would continue through the ensuing decade and result in the dismissal of notions of poisoning from intestinal stasis. One line of attack was the criticism advanced by participants in the Royal Society discussion that the proponents of autointoxication had never managed to demonstrate the presence of any one of their virulent toxins in the human bloodstream; their proof of the condition was exclusively clinical, a history of intestinal stasis in patients presenting with any combination of a broad array of symptoms. "There is no real evidence to support the theory of intestinal toxemia," an American gastroenterologist wrote in 1919, and "the pathologic findings can be explained more easily in other ways."[54]

There was, however, considerable evidence to cast doubt on the absorption of toxins from clogged intestines. How could an autointoxication theorist account, for example, for the man described in a 1902 issue of the *Journal of the American Medical Association*, a man constipated from childhood, who often went months between bowel movements. At one stretch, his period of defecatory abstinence lasted a bit over a year. Yet while his abdomen became distended and he experienced some pain and eventually weight loss and weakness, he was able to work at his job throughout, and quickly returned to full health when a movement, induced by enema, did occur (it was measured as eight gallons, and was cause for "much rejoicing in the family"). If there were any truth to autointoxication, it was argued, this man's deterioration should have been much worse. Considered alone, of course, he might be thought of as the exception that proved the rule. But there were many more such cases to be found in medical literature, many people who came out none the worse for extended bouts of the most obstinate constipation (the case just described did ultimately come out worse, the man dying suddenly 6 months after his giant movement "while sitting on the stool"). More telling, though, was the immediate recovery of such people once their bowels were finally voided. If their minimal physical problems had been due to toxins absorbed from the putrid mass in their bowels, the problems should have continued a good while longer, since the poison would keep circulating for some time after the emptying of the intestines.[55]

That was the reasoning that informed several experimental tests of the theory of autointoxication. In 1922 American physician Arthur Donaldson, to pick an influential example, persuaded five men accustomed to a daily bowel movement to voluntarily refrain from defecation for 90 hours. By the end of that time, all were experiencing the symptoms usually ascribed to autointoxication: foul breath, depressed appetite, headache, mental sluggishness, irritability, etc. Enemas were then administered to four of the subjects (the fifth had a spontaneous evacuation), and "all were promptly relieved of their distress." Only a mechanical explanation, not a chemical one, could account for such sudden disappearance of symptoms. To test the hypothesis that the discomfort of constipation was caused by physical distension of the lower bowel, Donaldson packed each subject's rectum with cotton and produced the same battery of headache, sluggishness, and other symptoms; all cleared up at once when the cotton was removed (American Walter Alvarez performed similar experiments on human subjects 2 years later, with the same findings and conclusions). Donaldson even forced cotton into a dog's rectum, then determined the animal's blood pressure. The pressure went up significantly soon after the cotton was inserted and stayed at the elevated level until the cotton plug was removed, when it immediately fell to normal. Such findings made it possible to argue, of course, that Lane's patients improved after surgery because he had in effect unplugged their rectums. Indeed, X-ray examinations revealed that more than one patient whose symptoms had been completely relieved by a short-circuit operation still had a colon filled with feces, but was no longer suffering from autointoxication. "Delay in the colon," Donaldson concluded, "does not necessarily produce such a desperately toxic mess as some people would have us believe." Another physician expressing the new opinion described autointoxication as a mix of "mad, maudlin, jumbled, mystic, undigested" ideas, a "sophomoric" conception, a "theory of disease we would suppose a young medical student would originate."[56]

All this meant, as Alvarez put it, that "we should be slow to accept the enthusiastic claims of rough and ready surgeons who have short-circuited a few colons." By the early 1920s, Arbuthnot Lane had become a butt of ridicule in his profession, a profession that had once revered him as its most gifted surgeon. Lane, a Canadian physician joked, had long argued that tuberculosis could not establish a foothold in a person unless he was weakened by intestinal stasis. Yet cattle were as heavily afflicted with tuberculosis as people, and how could a cow, "with its dozen and more evacuations per diem," be said to suffer from intestinal stasis? Would Lane argue that bovines "suffer from displacement of the abdominal viscera due to the assumption of the 'all fours' position?" Was not Lane guilty of forming an "obsession" with "a half-truth" and riding that "horse to death"? An American critic was even less forgiving, laughing that "a marked incapacity to perform any mental exertion" was commonly cited as a feature of autointoxication. "[So] writes Sir Arbuthnot. . . . Has he had his own colon removed, may we ask?"[57]

But if Sir Arbuthnot's peers were finding him a source of merriment, much of the British and American public were taking him and other stasis theorists dead seriously. At the level of popular belief and behavior, constipation phobia was entering its golden age.

4

THE SORROWS OF THE COLON: PHARMACEUTICAL TREATMENT

NO DOUBT THE SIGHT of a diurnal evacuation of cylindrical proportions is an objective evidence of health, . . . and it carries comfort and even happiness to many a wistful heart. But there are other thousands who, looking to procure their daily bread of confidence, are disappointed with the result, and what then? They go away discontented, suppose themselves constipated, and slide into the curse of pill-taking.

James Goodhart, 1910

NO ORGAN OF THE BODY is so misunderstood, so slandered and maltreated as the colon. . . . The colon is slandered every day in the advertising columns of the popular press, which accuse it of sins it never commits, and the mass suggestion which results from constantly reading about the disastrous effects of intestinal intoxication results in most of the lay public and many of the medical profession joining in these slanders. By promoting the sale of purgatives and encouraging the use of various other methods of irritating the colon, these slanders result in maltreatment. No wonder that the colon is unhappy.

Arthur Hurst, 1935

In the year 1917, Walter Alvarez, a San Francisco physician respected as America's leading gastroenterologist, was visited by a businessman desperate for help. The gentleman had always enjoyed adequate health, it seems, until the day 6 years earlier when his morning look in the mirror revealed a receding hairline. Rushing to a dermatologist, he was informed that baldness was being brought on by autointoxication, and, never mind that the patient had never thought himself constipated, that it was necessary to effect more thorough emptying of his bowels if he hoped to retain his hair.[1]

With so much at stake, the man began to dose himself daily with laxatives. Hair continued to fall, though, and now true constipation developed as well. What

81

to do? "Before long he was going from physician to physician in search of stronger purgatives," yet his intestines only grew more inactive. One of the physicians he solicited was a surgeon who proposed removing the appendix to stop the intoxication, and by now convinced that his mental powers would be destroyed once his hair was gone, the patient assented. The appendectomy proved useless, of course, but in the process of performing it, the surgeon discovered the man's intestines to be a mess, tangled with "so many Lane's kinks that only a colectomy would now offer any hope."[2]

It was at that point the patient visited Alvarez, hoping the renowned expert might offer a more heartening second opinion. And so he did: "I found him a nearly perfect specimen of humanity with as normal a digestive tract as one could wish to see." To the extent the man was constipated, Alvarez determined, it was due to his daily use of laxatives and the hurried pace of his life. On Sunday morning, the one day he didn't have to dash for the train to the city, "he generally had an unaided bowel movement, which was the main event in his week." The doctor suggested the patient "leave his colon to its own devices" and stop worrying. Initially, the man balked at so drastic a course, "several hours of argument" being needed to persuade him to give it a try. But as Alvarez had expected, "after three days of anxious waiting," his bowels moved, "and they have been moving satisfactorily ever since." Case cured.[3]

The case of the balding businessman stands as a parable about the cure sometimes being worse than the disease, and can be taken to illustrate how readily the bowel-deadening "cure" of purgatives was resorted to in the early decades of the twentieth century: even a little hair loss could drive a person to cathartic addiction once Lane's kinks and intestinal stasis began to agitate popular imagination. Though it cannot be solidly documented that per-capita consumption of laxative drugs did increase significantly beyond nineteenth-century levels, it was the opinion of authorities such as Alvarez that purgative use had gone up noticeably with the onset of autointoxication anxiety. Certainly proprietary medicine manufacturers sharply intensified their promotion of cathartic products after the turn of this century, and the worried/manipulated public responded; purgation was the people's method of choice for escaping autointoxication.

To be sure, physicians all too often abetted the patent medicine industry in instilling widespread fear of constipation, as more than a few rank-and-file practitioners were still making the diagnosis of autointoxication until the end of the 1920s. "As a means to cloak our ignorance in a garment of pretended knowledge," autointoxication was a handy label, one that provided doctors a quick solution to puzzling cases. "Time and again," Alvarez related, "I have been put to the embarrassment of having to point out to some brother physician that his beautiful case of 'autointoxication' was really an aortic regurgitation, a chronic nephritis, a myxedema, a high blood pressure, tuberculosis or some other well known disease."

The term autointoxication is "pernicious," a second commentator railed, it should not be employed "by any self-respecting member of our profession," but should "be wholly expunged from the medical vocabulary."[4]

Yet if better informed and more critical physicians did delete the word from their vocabulary, many others did not. *Intestinal Management for Longer, Happier Life*; *The Lazy Colon*; *The Conquest of Constipation*; *Constipation. How to Cure Yourself*; "Stasis the Destroyer"; *Le Colon Homicide*—these are representative titles from among many books, articles, and pamphlets written by physicians during the decade of the 1920s to warn the public of the dangers of intestinal stasis. The chilling words of the physician who authored the most popular athletic training manual of the 1920s were commonplace. The contents of the colon, he wrote, are "a burden, fermenting, decomposing, putrefying, filling the body with poisonous substances," producing "sewer-like blood." And, a British surgeon added, the "stagnant morass fermenting in his belly" produced still other discomforts for the intestinally static: "His digestion is a mockery, gurgling and groaning in hopeless disability, his breath reminiscent of a Limburger cheese, and his general outlook upon life a pessimistic wail." Yet another practitioner calculated that "constipation is the cause of ninety per cent of disease," and that was the kind of estimate people heard again and again from apparently authoritative sources: "constipation shortens life." For a not insignificant number of doctors, autointoxication was to be seen everywhere: "For the awakened [the aware physician] to walk the streets of London or Paris, or indeed any other large town," and to observe "the greasy skins, the sloppy gaits, and the septic open mouths of the passers-by, is to realise the pathetic universality of chronic constipation." Lay health educators kept the presses rolling too, issuing popularized interpretations of physicians' misgivings under such titles as *Chronic Constipation. The Most Insidious and the Most Deadly of Diseases.*[5]

Alvarez himself lamented the profession's fostering of public anxiety over bowel intoxication in a lengthy review written in 1924. "The layman has taken to this idea very kindly," he said, because "no sooner does he begin going to school than there appears the school nurse . . . to hold up to him the bogey of autointoxication. Later his doctor will ascribe many of his complaints, large and small, to intestinal poisoning." (That the laity did indeed take to the idea of intestinal self-poisoning is corroborated by the example offered by an American public health official of the 1930s, to illustrate the problem of people becoming obsessive about health behavior: "A little boy whose parents had impressed him with the utter goodness of George Washington, with his perfect compliance with all that is right and proper, startled his mother one day by asking, after a period of silent meditation, 'Mums, did George Washington have good bowel movement?'") But Alvarez also appreciated that the medical profession's contribution to sustaining the fear of universal constipation was outdone by the efforts of the patent medicine industry, which exploited that fear to the fullest. "Every newspaper and magazine which he picks up," Alvarez stated, "will tell him of the terrible results that will follow if he fails to buy so and so's laxative pills, patented syringes, paraffin oil, sour milk, agar or bran."[6]

If only the pressure to buy had been confined to newspapers and magazines. During the 1920s, a new agent became established that supplemented, if didn't surpass, the historically prevalent advertising medium of print: radio. It was bad enough that "it is impossible to look anywhere without seeing an advertisement for a laxative," a writer in *Scientific American* complained in the mid-1930s, but "it is also impossible to listen to the radio more than a few minutes without being implored to attend to your bowels." "Just as we had learned to skip the . . . advertisement so artfully sandwiched in between the news of World affairs," a physician elaborated, "the radio has made bowel information a prelude, postlude and intermezzo to even the music of the masters." More than one laxative manufacturer actually sponsored an entire show. Eno Effervescent Salt, for example, attracted "millions of radio listeners . . . every night" to its Radio Crime Club dramatizations of mystery novels. Another radio hit was Feen-a-mint's "Danger Fighters," a series of Saturday evening recreations of great medical discoveries. Was such advertising effective? Eno's show was "a smash hit," and "already sales are soaring." The files of the American Medical Association reveal laxative products were pushed upon the public in a variety of other ways, too: mass mailings of free samples, distribution of packages at fairgrounds and similar high-attendance venues, discount sales of remedies at sidewalk "health lectures." In their magazine ads, manufacturers often invited readers to send for a more detailed booklet that itemized and explained the ravages of intestinal stasis; one even shipped his booklet, "The Inside Story of Constipation," in a tightly closed envelope with the warning not to break the seal until recipients had steeled themselves for the "very frank statements on constipation" to be found inside. Even the psychology of the healing evangelist was brought into play: Elmer Fowler's Constipation Cure was offered gratis to the poor, and to others on the basis of donation. Recipients filled in and signed a pledge card, sending no money until they had been cured of "serious colon poisoning," but then, Fowler hoped, were generous in their gratitude. "An empty purse [Fowler's] and the cries of the sick are urging that your gifts shall not be delayed a moment longer than necessary," he appealed, yet even then he gave pastors the option to pay only half their pledge if they supplied him with a list of congregation members he could contact. Fowler's, it comes as no surprise, was not one of the more successful laxative ventures.[7]

The content of advertising matter circulated in these ways was essentially open to any claims, no matter how far-fetched, the manufacturer chose to make. To be sure, by the 1920s legislation had been enacted in both Britain and the United States to curb some of the excesses of the patent medicine industry. America's 1906 Food and Drugs Act, for example, prohibited false labeling of patent medicine products. But a 1911 Supreme Court decision declared the rule did not apply to therapeutic statements, and although an amendment to the act was quickly passed to close the loophole, outlawing curative claims that were "false and fraudulent," the Sherley Amendment had little effect. It was not simply that it was very difficult to prove that an advertising claim deemed false was also fraudulent (i.e., known by the manufacturer to be untrue); the greater problem was that neither the Sherley Amendment nor any other provision in the 1906 act applied to advertising material beyond the label. It was the ad placed in the newspaper or slapped onto the billboard, after all, not the fine wording on the bottle's wrapper, that led people to buy and take a medicinal product. The Federal Trade Commission, established in 1914, attempted to fill this breach and suppress exaggerated and misleading advertising (of all products, not just patent medicines), but it had no more power, or success, than the enforcers of the Food and Drugs Act. "Advertising agencies," a physician complained in 1934, "have now for many years flagrantly exploited a trusting and poorly informed public" in carrying out their "Crime Wave in Cathartics"; this "ruthless poisoning of an entire population is, or ought to be considered criminal," he concluded. In a contemporary's eyes, the advertising of patent purgatives was "a disgrace to our modern civilization."[8]

The Food, Drugs and Cosmetics Act that Congress passed in 1938 granted the Food and Drug Administration increased power to regulate proprietary labeling, but political considerations kept the regulation of advertising in the hands of the Federal Trade Commission. The Wheeler-Lea Act of 1938 did ostensibly enhance the Federal Trade Commission's powers over advertising, but in practice manufacturers quickly learned to lead the Commission in circles. The cumbersome mechanism of filing a complaint against advertisements "misleading in a material respect," waiting for a response from the advertiser, conducting a hearing, and at last issuing a cease-and-desist order that became binding only after 60 days, allowed the manufacturer to continue the objectionable ads for months, even years. By the time a desist order finally took effect, a critic had recognized as early as 1940, "the advertiser has used the challenged advertising to the limit; he discards it and embarks on a new and equally deceptive campaign." Thus when the author of a 1927 attack on the abuses of advertising took up the subject again in 1954, 16 years after the Wheeler-Lea Act, he could only moan that "the advertising of . . . patent medicines was perfectly terrible in 1927, and it is terrible today." The story was substantially no different in Great Britain.[9]

It was also the case in both countries that print advertising advanced to a new level of sophistication during the early twentieth century, copy becoming more clever and subtly manipulative, illustrations more eye-catching and persuasive as drawings gave way to photographs. Underlying both copy and illustrations, furthermore, was an appreciation of the awe with which the public bowed before science in this age of the telephone, motor car, and aseptic surgery. Whereas nineteenth-century patent medicine promoters had commonly presented their remedies as cures blessed by some long healing tradition (a wise grandmother's secret recipe, an herb used for centuries by American Indians, Turks, or the Chinese), twentieth-century copywriters extolled drugs that were as new as the radio, the result of the very latest breakthrough in medical science. What cathartic manufacturers in particular aimed for in their ads was to convince readers and listeners that constipation threatened their survival, and to persuade them that purgatives (their particular brand of purgative, to be precise) were the critical weapon for fighting off the assaults of autointoxication. Hence despite medical opinion makers' repudiation of intestinal self-poisoning, the lay person of the 1920s and '30s was being bamboozled more craftily than ever before to dread it as the great scourge of civilization.[10]

"Ask yourself this question," the makers of California Fruit-Bits urged consumers in 1934: "Am I Being Poisoned by Constipation? . . . Most people in this age of refined foods and sedimentary living [presumably the copywriter meant sedentary living] are constipated in some degree," the ad then asserted. And if constipated, they were being poisoned, for "uneliminated filth forms a sticky coating on the walls and in the folds of the intestines," a fecal deposit (so perhaps he did mean sedimentary) which, it was explained, slowly decomposes, releasing poisons of putrefaction into the blood stream. "What could be more repulsive," another laxative ad asked, "than to have one's intestines filled with rotting, foul-smelling, undigested food matter? Is not this very thought revolting?"[11]

Other laxative products of the day were touted under similarly alarming headlines: "Constipation. The Monarch of all Diseases"; "Constipation . . . the most formidable enemy of public health"; Constipation—"the worst disorder which afflicts humanity"; "Constipation . . . the shortest road to old age, wrinkles and decay"; "Constipation . . . the Great American Disease." Everywhere the man and woman in the street turned, they encountered that basic message, one presented with particular force by the manufacturers of Floradex: "A Clean Colon is More Important than a Clean Face," a 1936 ad averred, then illustrated the point through a diagram of the intestinal tract on which an arrow was pointed at the colon, accompanied by an upper-case announcement that *there* was "WHERE MISERY IS MANUFACTURED."[12]

Patent medicine ads did often acknowledge (in accordance with medical teachings) that people manufactured all that misery themselves, by eating too much refined and processed food, taking too little exercise, worrying too much, being too busy to promptly answer nature's calls—in short, by living in modern, civilized society. Americans saw themselves as particularly civilized: that was what made constipation the Great American Disease, and why even medical scientists could pronounce the United States "probably the most constipated nation on the face of the earth!" British commentators, of course, disputed such statements: could the colonials truly be more costive than they? Which nation was indeed the more constipated (a distinction impossible to determine at this remove, in any event) is not the issue, however. What matters is that there should ever have been competition for such an honor. If "most constipated" was deemed an achievement (because it connoted "most civilized"—"civilization is synonymous with constipation," an English author stressed), then the commitment to maintaining and enjoying civilization's ways of life must have run quite deep on both sides of the Atlantic.[13] However menacing constipation might be, it was a risk one had to run to preserve the pleasures of modernity.

That did not mean the risk could be ignored. But there was a civilized way to deal with it, patent medicine ads proposed; one needn't revert to a physically demanding preindustrial lifestyle. Instead, it had to be accepted that civilization would breed its curse, then the curse could be neutralized with civilized remedies, remedies that required no sacrifice of modern comforts. A 1927 Sal Hepatica magazine ad pulsing with the sophisticated excitement of a cocktail party offered readers a choice between the old and new styles of living. Remember the days of ragtime and the horseless carriage, they were asked: "What a life the world led then—and what a different life it lives today. The euchre party that brightened up a month has become an almost nightly bridge gathering. Radios and motors, restaurants and clubs have changed the complexion of life. Now as never before life is lived to the utmost. Few of the precious moments of life are wasted." Nevertheless, there was a serious drawback to such intense living: "Nature doesn't like it a bit! Too much food—too little sleep—too much nervous excitement derange the long-suffering mechanism of the inner man." Enter autointoxication, "which is to blame for many of our modern ills." So, the ad man asked conspiratorially, how would you rather stay free of autointoxication? By a chasteness that wastes life's precious moments, or by living to the utmost, then gaining absolution with a convenient, painless daily medicine?[14]

Medicine was far from the only answer. As subsequent chapters will detail, every conceivable remedy from mineral waters to rectum expanders was zealously marketed over the first third of the century. But with constipation, as with all other ills, medicine was the most satisfying answer. Pills and draughts could be taken with minimal effort and inconvenience (there were even laxative tea bags available—Steep-A-Lax), and they agreed with the universal human conviction that cure is better than prevention. "Do you suppose," a realistic Kentucky practitioner asked in defense of laxatives in 1911, that "when you tell a woman that in the morning at precisely five minutes to nine, not nine, but five minutes to nine, she is to go to stool, that she is to live on prunes, etc., and drink a great deal of water, take a certain amount of exercise, do you suppose that she will heed that advice?" That "does not relieve in my practice," he answered, and it seems unlikely that advice to follow a regulated life was heeded in others' practice, either. Pills were the preferred form of relief, on both sides of the Atlantic (although this chapter will concentrate on the American purgative industry, all the same themes were played out in Britain).[15]

Manufacturers made laxatives seem so appealing by making constipation seem so inescapable and terrifying. It was commonplace for ads to baldly assert that three-fourths or four-fifths or 90% of Americans or Britons or Europeans suffered from constipation, and for reasons that were near impossible to avoid if people wanted to live in a civilized society. "Life Is Like a Game Played By Rules," Eno ("the world-famed effervescent salt") dictated; "You Cannot Ignore the Rules and Yet Win the Game." But the rules were not that easy to follow, a balanced diet and regular exercise being a bit too demanding for many players. Fortunately, there was another rule: "the daily clearance from the system of intestinal waste," without which "the others are of little avail." Indeed, by presenting daily laxation ("Eno first thing in the morning") as the "key rule to health," the manufacturer encouraged buyers to think they could do just fine in "The Game of Life" playing by that rule alone. Sal Hepatica ("the [Sal Hepatica] saline cocktail improves the morning outlook") employed the same strategy, a 1927 ad urging readers to make resolutions for the new year "to exercise regularly, . . . eat sensibly," and not "cut the corners on sleep and rest." But first, the "Memo to Myself" prompted, "to start the good work of keeping myself physically fit, I'm going to get a bottle of Sal Hepatica—today." As it had with the guests at the cocktail party, Sal Hepatica forgave people for not disciplining themselves to adhere to a life of moderation, then offered them laxation as the modern substitute for temperance; in effect, moderation was made obsolete by assurances that the effects of immoderation could be easily and inexpensively cured. "Hundreds of thousands of men and women," the ad reported, take Sal Hepatica "regularly . . . to keep themselves physically fit—to help them meet the exacting demands of this quickstep life."[16]

Those who ignored this new hygienic responsibility and fell out of step would pay dearly for their negligence, at least if advertising copywriters had anything to say about it. The ad writer's assignment was to come up with the most appalling, stomach-churning descriptions of autointoxication possible, so every conceivable combination of "foul" and "corrupt" and "decaying" and "vile" and "poisonous" found its way into a laxative advertisement sooner or later, and consumers were forever being warned that "more people die of diseases caused . . . by constipation than in war and by fire, flood and famine." The winner of the competition to terrify people into becoming customers was the creator of the hideous, vomiting ogre "Bowel Bloat," which confronted readers of ads for Cascarets, the "Candy Cathartic Best for the Bowels." (Fig. 4-1) "A horrible, slimy monster that makes man's life a misery," Bowel Bloat was born in the "putrid, rotting matter" of the constipate's overburdened gut, and was the embodiment of "nasty" and "disgust-

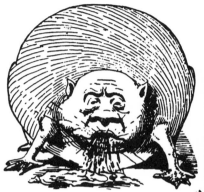

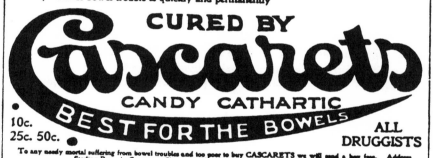

BOWEL BLOAT

A horrible, slimy monster that makes man's life a misery.

After eating: a bloated belly, belching of gas from the stomach, a foul, ill-smelling scurf on the tongue, dizziness, headache, a sour rising and spitting up of half-digested food, — it's Bowel Bloat.

When the bowels stop working they become filled with putrid, rotting matter, forming poisonous gases that go through the whole body. If you don't have a regular, natural movement of the bowels at least once a day your fate is bowel bloat, with all the nasty, disgusting symptoms that go with it.

There's only one way to set it right. Clean yourself out gently but thoroughly and tone up your bowels with CASCARETS. Every form of bowel trouble is quickly and permanently

CURED BY
Cascarets
CANDY CATHARTIC
BEST FOR THE BOWELS

10c.
25c. 50c.

ALL DRUGGISTS

To any needy mortal suffering from bowel troubles and too poor to buy CASCARETS we will send a box free. Address Sterling Remedy Company, Chicago or New York, mentioning advertisement and paper.

Figure 4-1. A 1920s advertisement for the laxative Cascarets, exemplifying the scare tactics employed by purgative manufacturers [Friends of the Bishops' House, *Headlines Idaho Remembers*, 46, Special Collections Division, University of Washington Libraries, Negative Number UW 17931].

ing." (To be fair, the constipation commentaries of well-meaning medical authors and health reformers could be rather unsettling, too, though even the description "fouling of the whole body from a putrid, filthy, poisonous sewer in our abdomen" was not quite up to the mark of Bowel Bloat.) As late as 1942, Alvarez was still complaining that there was "so much fear and anxiety" affecting the public, "that the physician must begin his treatment with . . . particular efforts to lay the ghost of intestinal autointoxication."[17]

The image of inward filthiness and nastiness naturally tied into the early century's preoccupation with external cleanliness. The discovery that germs cause disease and the realization that they breed in dirt had given a tremendous boost to the popularity of bathing. Through the 1920s society actually attached greater health value to washing the skin than the practice deserved, encouraged in their reverence for dirt removal by the advertisements and even the names (Lifebuoy, for instance) of the soaps and other products created for the booming cleanliness market. Laxative manufacturers were quick to carve themselves a niche in that market too, for inner purity could be presented as a realm of cleanliness unto itself, with even more profound implications for health. Nineteenth-century proprietary remedies had frequently touted themselves as blood purifiers, a type of inner cleanser, and blood purification continued as a common claim of laxative products into this century. One of the grandest of the Victorian blood purifiers, Brandreth's Pills, was still around in both America and Britain (and two dozen other countries), having "gained multitudes of new users with every passing [was the pun intended?] generation." Still "purely vegetable," but newly improved, like a fine claret, by being aged in wood for 2 years, Brandreth's removed poisons from the bloodstream as effectively as ever, but now it would also "cleanse the system" overall. Indeed, for some time Brandreth had been boasting, "I can cleanse the inside of the human body as perfectly as water does the outside."[18]

Washing and scrubbing the digestive tract, or giving it a bath, was the new version of inner purification recommended by the purgative industry in the 1920s and '30s. It was *the* marketing strategy of Nujol, a mineral oil laxative. "*Internal cleanliness*" was the company's motto: "You Will Enjoy Work or Play—if you have Internal Cleanliness"; "Age is not measured in Years if you form the habit of Internal Cleanliness"; and "All you long for Health, Happiness, Success are the Reward of Internal Cleanliness." One particularly effective series of ads was set in the bathroom, a suitable enough location for laxative promotion, but with the tub and sink highlighted rather than toilet. A man in his bathrobe carrying a towel is reminded that inner cleaning is "far more important than your bath," a woman in her robe drawing her bath is told that "cleanliness demands more than bathing," and a beaming lad leaning over the sink with washcloth to face is told that without that inner bath, "health, even life itself, is threatened." But Nujol hardly had the internal cleanliness field to itself. "If You Would Have Health, . . . Be Clean Within," a rival advised; "You are as Healthy as Your Insides are Clean," another decreed; and a third laxative said it all with its name: I-Clean-U Health Tea (Fig. 4-2).[19]

A further attraction of the internal cleanliness theme, from manufacturers' perspective, was that since external cleanliness was now accepted as a daily (not

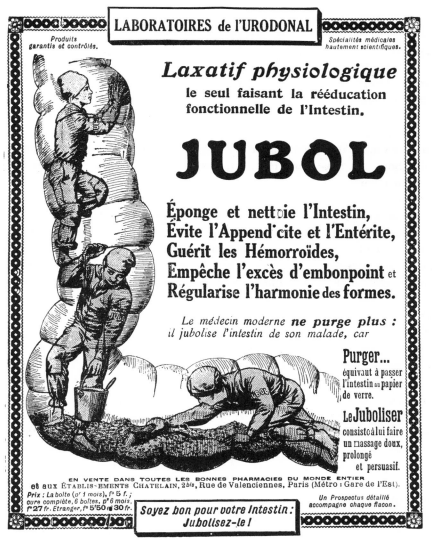

Figure 4-2. Advertisement for the French product Jubol, which claimed to sponge and wipe the intestine, giving it a "sweet, prolonged and persuasive massage." "Be good to your intestine," the ad urges. "Jubolize it." [The William H. Helfand Collection, New York].

just Saturday night) obligation, it was reasonable to suggest that a laxative be taken daily too. "Use Vi-Lax every day," consumers were enjoined; "Take Nujol as regularly as you brush your teeth or wash your face"; Laxative Repeaters for Large Eaters "can be REPEATED every day for a lifetime without producing the least harm"; another company supplied signs for pharmacy windows that asked, "Have you had your Kruschen Salts this morning?" Eno Effervescent Salt described itself as "a routine laxative" and a "Health Drink," and its drugstore window displays featured the emblem of a crowing rooster above the caption "First Thing Every Morning." For some, even daily was not enough: "a large unformed evacuation after every meal," an English physician commented, "is the chief object in life of many men and women at the present day." Consequently, as another British doctor phrased it, "a large proportion" of patients were convinced that "they could not possibly get on without the habitual use of purgatives."[20]

Purgative manufacturers wielded a single stick—autointoxication—but they offered no end of carrots. First was the assurance that purgation had moved into a new, more civilized age, beyond the benighted days of yore when it was accepted that cathartic-induced movements were necessarily prodigious in both bulk and number (remember Mr. Smith worrying, "will all my body runne out here?"; see Fig. 4-3). Up-to-date constipates could anticipate stools that came gently (if they took Moveze), singly, and on schedule (Time Fuse Tablets). It now became better business than ever for manufacturers to denounce rivals' products as harsh and irritating ("Don't TEAR your 'insides' out with rough cathartics") and insist that their own remedies were not ("not a gripe in a carload" of Rinoline). Boston Brown Beans for Bilious Bipeds wooed buyers with promises: "While you are sleeping I am at work. . . . Not an ache or a pain nor a sound out of me. I am modest and gentle and deal kindly with people in order to do them good." Offering a laxative that worked while the user slept was another way of exploiting the theme of civilized purgation, and many manufacturers did, among them the makers of Nature's Remedy: "NR To-Night, Tomorrow Alright"; and TAPS, to be taken after Taps had been played for the day: "Take a tip—take a TAP." Yet while neither an ache nor a pain should accompany the evacuation, the expulsion still had to be thorough; the same ad that guaranteed no griping included the testimonial of a satisfied customer: "It put me on the pot and almost knocked the bottom out."[21]

That rousing an experience could be seen as habit forming, however, so laxative makers also had to promise consumers their products were not strong chemicals that enslaved the colon to artificial stimulation. Rather, they were like Nujol, which "promotes natural, healthy movement"; or Lacricin, "Nature's True Assistant"; or Fruisen, the self-proclaimed "laxative of Millionaires" that gave "a bowel movement as close to natural as humanly possible." For some, the name alone ensured a purely physiological action: what could be safer than Peristalso, Naturalax, and Natures Lawlax? A natural movement also implied regularity, a

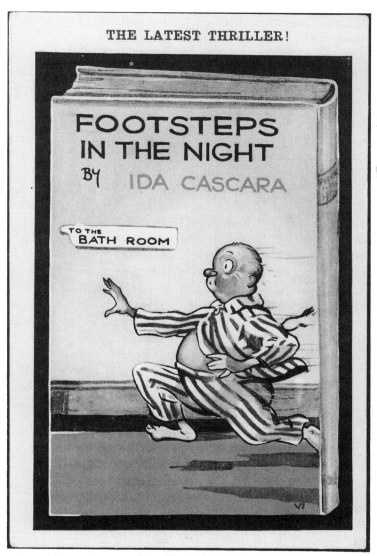

Figure 4-3. Caricature of the effects of cascara and other laxatives [The William H. Helfand Collection, New York].

predictable time of evacuation. Civilized laxatives should not catch users by surprise, or put them *hors de combat* with repeated actions. "It's Never Mentioned,"
an ad for Jiffy-Lax whispers to the grimacing woman with hands clasped to head.
"You never mention that you have been late at the office because you had taken a
laxative the preceding night and could not leave the house until your system was
in order. You feel foolish making the excuse that you were late on account of a
headache caused by your bowels not moving." With Jiffy-Lax, one need never
again be embarrassed or make excuses. Insert the gelatin tube's nozzle into the anus,
give "a generous squeeze with thumb and finger," and wait—briefly. According
to the ad, "It acts in a minute," or even less. At least one user was so impressed
that he submitted an endorsement to the American Medical Association, happily
announcing that Jiffy-Lax "results in an instantaneous bowel movement." "It is
like an enema *without the messy equipment.*"[22]

Yet the upper end of the digestive tract seemed an even easier entry to consumers' pocketbooks. One of the major innovations of early twentieth-century
laxative entrepreneurs was to tie purgation to the pleasure principle, by marketing products that were more palatable than the old standards and backing them
with advertising assurances that in the modern world medicine no longer had to
be nauseating in order to work (Fig. 4-4). "Ain't you glad"? a grade school boy
asks his sister in a 1923 ad for a fig-and-date laxative. "Ain't you glad we don't
have to take any more castor oil? Since Mother found out about Jam-O-Lax she
doesn't give us nasty old castor oil any more." Instead, it's explained, the kids are
given Jam-O-Lax to spread on crackers, or even to eat straight from the jar. "It's
so good," the boy beams, plus, "it keeps us well." His sister joins him in hoping
that "the Mothers of all little boys and girls will get it for them."[23]

Jam-o-Lax, in fact, was only one of countless marriages of active drugs with
attractive foodstuffs. There were also Fruisen, a blending of the old reliable senna
with fruit, and Lax-Krax, a honey and senna-filled cracker. Another of the old
reliables, Epsom salts, could be enjoyed with lemon flavoring and water in the form
of Epsonade, though lemon fanciers could also opt for Citro-Nesia or Citrolax,
"The Lemonade Laxative." Laxa Raisins combined two laxatives with chewy dried
grapes, and even nasty old castor oil was chemically scrubbed clean of bad taste,
then doctored up to make positively flavored concoctions such as Dr. Fitch's Kasta
Kookies and Lacricin, a "Milk of Castor Oil" purporting to taste like whipped
cream.[24]

The most delicious disguise of all, however, was chocolate, the attractive
ingredient in Kastor Jems, Cascarets, Co-rex, Laxybar, Laxaphen, Chu-Lax, Tru-
Lax, Tryalax, Auto-Laks, Carbolax, Coco-lax, and many more, including, of
course, Chocolax. Even one of the oldest of patent medicines, Brandreth's Pills,
began to offer consumers a choice between the "Plain" original flavor and "Chocolate Coated." The active component in most of those chocolate cathartics, as well

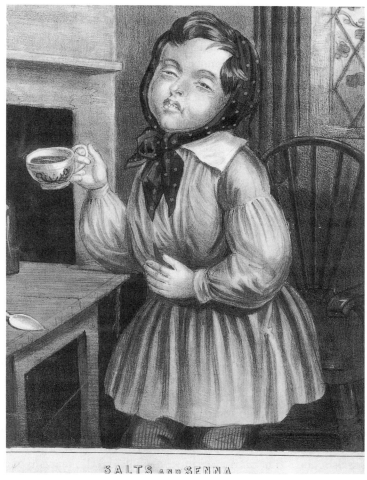

Figure 4-4. Caricature of the unpleasant taste of "salts and senna" and purgatives generally [The William H. Helfand Collection, New York].

as other laxative confections, was the new reliable: phenolphthalein. The most popular aperient substance of the twentieth century (it belongs to the category of stimulant laxatives), phenolphthalein was first marketed in Germany in 1900 under the trade name Purgen. There quickly followed Purgo and Purgil, Purgatin and Purgatol, Purglets, Purgylum, Purgettae, Purginetto, Purgolade, Purgophenpastillen, and Purgierkonfekt; Laxativ, Laxine, and Laxinkonfekt brought up the rear, and these were only the German products. The drug firms of other European countries were soon turning out their versions: Laxatol in Austria, Purgamenta in Hungary, and Laxoin in England. The New World did not lag far behind. "It was not long," an American physician could complain by 1910, "before the enterprising manufacturers in this country saw in it a potential gold mine and now nearly every proprietary drug manufacturer in this country has coined a proprietary name for it and is exploiting it, either alone or in combination with one or more other laxatives, and with more or less unwarranted claims." (Combinations with other laxatives included aloes, cascara, calomel, even prunes, as in the product Prunoids; a rival preparation, Prunol, pulled out all the stops, blending together phenolphthalein, prune juice, and mineral oil). Phenolphthalein was, as Purgen promoted itself, "The Laxative of the Future." By the 1920s, phenolphthalein manufacturers had conceived of virtually every possible catchy name from A to Z for their products: Analax, Biolax, Boal's Rolls (also known as "The Luscious Laxative"), Cathartones, Gall-ogogue, Homolax, Magic-Lax, Regulax, Rhythmin, Sweetlax, Triolax, and last, though hardly sounding like least, Zam Zam.[25]

The onomatopoeic directness of Zam Zam was the exception; the rule was the enticing gentleness of Rhythmin and Sweetlax. In fact, the most aptly named of the phenolphthalein products were two of the earliest ones, Purgierkonfekt and Laxinkonfekt: confect was the critical concept from the start. Phenolphthalein's lack of flavor made it a perfect base for sweet coatings. Thus Purgolax was sold as a fruit pastille, Purgen as vanilla-flavored tablets, and many other brands were camouflaged as chocolate or mint. Not surprisingly, the phenolphthalein industry quickly came to experience an identity crisis: were the new laxatives medicine, or were they dessert? Laxybar's label assured purchasers it was "Not a Confection, [rather] a Medicine," but it simultaneously urged the buyer to "Eat it Like Candy." Similarly, Kastor Jems, whose packaging glowed with the faces of dozens of happy children, affirmed that its recipe of "Pure Castor Oil in Delicious Chocolate Bon Bons. . . . Looks and Tastes Like Candy." Ex-Lax may have been the best-selling brand of all precisely because it so convincingly presented itself as the most delicious. "The world eats more chocolate sodas than any kind," one radio blurb began; "more chocolate cakes, and when Nature needs the assistance of a laxative, chocolate wins again. The world uses Ex-Lax. It's such a joy to take, like eating a piece of smooth, velvety, delicious chocolate." In fact, another ad maintained, "It tastes like the most delicious chocolate you ever ate. . . . You will wonder . . . how anything tasting so good, can do so much good."[26]

But Ex-Lax wasn't just delicious. It was also "as delicious as it is scientific." Phenolphthalein manufacturers had to be careful not to let their products be misperceived as only candy. Ultimately, they had to be recognized as medicine, preferably as new, improved medicine, which required them to be the result of modern scientific research. Samples of Feen-a-mint (a mint-flavored phenolphthalein chewing gum) distributed to more than ten million families in the spring of 1933 bore the image of a scientist in his laboratory over the legend "science produced this little gift for you." Chewing, research had shown, "spreads the laxative evenly and naturally through the clogged system . . . right down to where it does its work." Actually, as the 1933 sample booklet elaborated, science had discovered that it was Nature's own pleasure principle that did the work: the saliva produced by chewing "is Nature's distributor. It carries pleasant-tasting food where Nature intended it to go. . . . Hence, medicines in pleasant-tasting chewing gum act better!" At the same time, the pleasurable act of chewing released nervous tension and further freed the body to function naturally (one example was the use of Feen-a-mint as "an agreeable antecedent" to surgery, "when a clean colon is so essential . . . because gum chewing distracts the patient's mind and Feen-a-mint does the desired work"). All these considerations taken together confirmed that although "it took science a long time to find it out, . . . today we know the best medicine . . . is the one that tastes best."[27]

Ex-Lax, in the meantime, was pushing a similar argument. The printed material supplied with Ex-Lax samples distributed in 1929 gave as the first of six answers to the question "Why Ex-Lax?" the reply, "Because it is a scientific laxative." It was, in truth, a "scientifically timed laxative," one that (unlike "harsh cathartics [which] are too quick and violent") "takes just the proper time to act thoroughly, yet safely." Application of its chocolate coating "*by the exclusive Ex-Lax process* makes the laxative ingredient more effective." As Feen-a-mint had done with gum, Ex-Lax used chocolate to make the pleasure principle serve the work ethic; by declaring that the chocolate somehow potentiated the phenolphthalein, Ex-Lax assuaged any guilt customers felt about taking the pleasant way out.[28]

Sales of phenolphthalein products rose steadily, until by the early 1930s, Americans were consuming nearly half a million pounds of phenolphthalein annually (laxatives were by far the most common source of the substance, though proprietary manufacturers bent on impressing buyers with the physiological activity of their product also employed phenolphthalein in remedies for colds, flu, rhinitis, and menstrual irregularity, as well as putting it into mouthwashes, toothpastes, and even a "laxative health bread" called Viti-Veg). The best-selling brand of laxative by the 1920s was Ex-Lax (Feen-a-mint came second), a fact the company frequently pointed out to retail pharmacists. "Ex-Lax customers come back again and again," ads in pharmacy trade journals reminded, "and buy lots of other things in your store." In short, by moving Ex-Lax, the druggist moved all his wares, not just his customers, while inadvertently adding a second meaning to the company's slogan "You can't get stuck if you stick to Ex-Lax." Ex-Lax, in fact, seems to have been the most widely recognized proprietary product of any type. The files of the American Medical Association's Bureau of Investigation contain hundreds of letters from consumers from the 1930s on, requesting information on the efficacy and safety of the full range of patent medicines (not just laxatives) flooding the market. These letters typically inquire about several brands—as many as 30 in one letter—yet at least half the time, Ex-Lax is the very first item listed.[29]

Ex-Lax sales were so high (and ever climbing, from 23 million boxes in 1929, for example, to 46 million in 1935) primarily because its manufacturer so shamelessly exploited the juvenile market.[30] Ex-Lax hardly stood alone in that regard. The most reprehensible element of the phenolphthalein boom of the early century was the industry's encouragement of parents to believe their children needed laxatives on a daily basis, and its offering of candy cathartics to make the normally taxing job of dosing a child easy. Phenolphthalein manufacturers reformulated adult consumers into a mix of one part patient and one part parent in the hope they could thereby double their take.

This is not to suggest that children of the pre-phenolphthalein centuries were not subjected to regular purgation. They were dosed the same as adults if it appeared that depraved remains of concoction were seeping into their system, and were sure to receive a thorough inner cleansing in the spring and fall, after seasons of extreme temperature had stressed the delicate humoral balance in their still developing young bodies. In the early twentieth century, however, young ones fell under an even heavier assault of cathartic therapy. Advertising warnings of the dangers of autointoxication suggested both that children were more easily injured by slow bowels, because they were younger and less sturdy, and that they were more likely to be constipated, due to inattentiveness to hygiene. "A very frequent spectacle to mothers," a British laxative ad reminded, was the "painful" sight of "a little child sitting on its stool, straining its bowels for a passage, until the veins of the forehead stand out like cords; while the face and neck of the little one is flushed and suffused, the eyes bloodshot, and the eyeballs fixed and glaring" (Fig. 4-5). Painful straining in the short run, steady deterioration from intestinal stasis in the long—that, by the laxative industry's account, was the melancholy fate of children whose bowels were left untended by parents.[31]

And so, a popular health writer could complain as late as the 1930s, "the modern technic of rearing unrepressed, inferiority-complex-free children" was not entirely modern after all. The rod was now spared in their upbringing, "but, alas, the cathartic bottle occupies just as important a place in a child's growing up as it ever did." During the first two decades of the century, odds were that the bottle contained castor oil, particularly if the child were still an infant. Indeed, "the castor oil bottle is always to be found in the nursery of the new-born baby," at least one physician believed, and the comments of numerous other contributors to medical literature indicate that *always* was not that far off. Certainly dosing babies with castor oil was a "routine practice," in the words of a second doctor, and one "much to be deprecated." But if "sins of commission in the infant are great, and of the sins the act of giving purgatives is the greatest," a third doctor's opinion, one would never have guessed it from the advertisements for castor oil (or other laxative products). All too common was the sort of message presented by Lacricin (*Lac* from the Latin for milk, and *ricin* for *Ricinus communis*, the castor

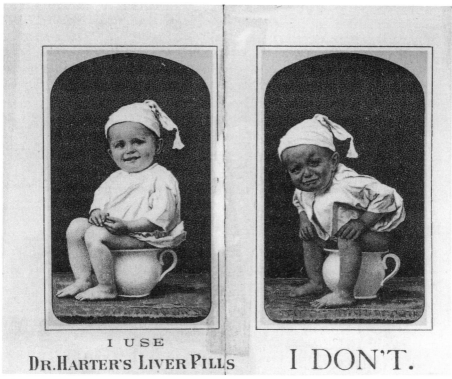

I USE
DR. HARTER'S LIVER PILLS   I DON'T.

Figure 4-5. Advertisement for Dr. Harter's Liver Pills [The William H. Helfand Collection, New York].

plant): a cherubic, diapered toddler stands beside his toy train and looks up trustingly at the hands of his loving mother measuring out a dose of the Lacricin that will make him well.[32]

He trusts mother because "the castor oil taste is gone." Lacricin's boast was that it had submerged the bitter taste of the oil beneath the flavor of cream, and indeed, there were any number of both "tasteless" castor oils and flavored ones, not to mention all the other purgatives cum confections. It was a remarkably dense laxative manufacturer who failed to see that important as pleasant taste was for adult consumers, it was far more attractive when extended to youngsters. After all, the administration of unpleasant medication to children was certain to degenerate into one of those "scenes of single combat" described by Oliver Wendell Holmes in the 1860s, "in which infants were wont to yield at length to the pressure of the spoon and the imminence of asphyxia" (Fig. 4-6). To be sure, pre-twentieth-century parents sometimes tried to get around child-dosing conflicts by

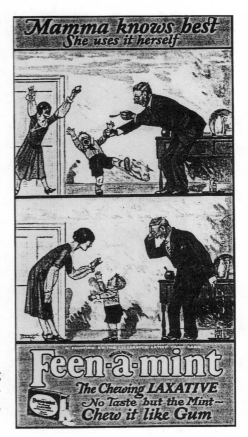

Figure 4-6. Advertisement promoting
Feen-a-mint for the treatment of hard-to-
dose children [from *American Druggist*,
June 1933, p. 134].

purchasing one of the few brands of sugar-coated purgative pills on the market,
but for the most part, it appears they expected their children to take their medicine like men. During the opening years of the twentieth century however laxative producers determined that autointoxication might be fought more profitably
if they stooped to flattering the tastebuds of younger patients, and none flattered
more than vendors of phenolphthalein. More than any of the cathartics previously
available, it could be made appealing to young palates, and thus be marketed as a
double-duty drug: it saved parents headaches even as it saved their children from
autointoxication.[33]

The two themes ran intertwined through all phenolphthalein advertising.
First, laxatives were essential for children's health. Leaflets accompanying Ex-Lax
samples mailed to homes during the 1920s, for instance, maintained that "most
children's ills are directly due to constipation." Ex-Lax, though, "has solved the
problem. . . . It cleans and regulates their little systems by its gentle action, . . .

and keeps them well and happy." The phrase "keeps them well" was calculated, of course, to suggest a preventive, not just curative, role for the laxative. Two sentences later, the point was made explicit, when parents were urged to use the tablets as "an inexpensive way to guard against sickness" (and just three sentences after that, "expectant and nursing mothers" were told their "developing child" or their newborn would be poisoned by the mother's blood or milk if the women didn't keep themselves free of autointoxication through Ex-Laxation). When it came to maintaining children's health, Ex-Lax was the American way: "*pour bonne sante,*" declared a multilingual brochure aimed at acculturating new arrivals from Europe; "*para conservar la salud,*" and "*zur Erhaltung der Gesundheit.*"[34]

Without too much prompting, one could have read "for the preservation of health" to mean that Ex-Lax was no mere laxative but a health food, even a daily nutritional requirement. In that case, perhaps the most serious threat to child health was laxative deficiency. That was the subliminal message put out by more than one brand of phenolphthalein. Co-Rex, a chocolate and phenolphthalein bowel corrective stated, "any family can keep in healthier condition by sprinkling the delicious shreds of Co-rex on foods." The youngster whose food did not receive its diurnal sprinkling might, in this light, be seen as sick even when exhibiting what, for a child, is normal behavior. Little "Betty is pouting again!" in a 1928 Feen-a-mint ad; she is pushing her plate away, leaving her food untouched, teetering on the edge of tears. "Deep in her heart every mother fears these curious, finicky moods that children have. And every mother knows what is the matter, too" (the matter was that "the poisons of fatigue . . . get bottled up in children's bodies," where "they mean bad, irritable tempers, dreary little heads, woebegone faces"). Bad temper was not to be removed by "harsh . . . laxatives," though, for those would "shock delicate little bodies." The shamelessly sappy references to children's "little bodies," their "delicate little systems," and like mawkishness aroused mothers' protective instincts and milked their solicitude to the last drop. If cleaning "their little systems . . . helps them to be well and happy," what sort of mother, or father, would deny their child that protection? How could a parent shrug off the reminder that the requirements of health "are *doubly important* to a child"?[35]

And how thoughtful of manufacturers to meet that doubly important need with medicines the child would actually accept. "Mama says it's medicine," the radiantly smiling girl in a 1934 Feen-a-mint advertisement says, "but it's just like the nicest chewing gum I ever tasted." As usual, Ex-Lax was not to be outdone: "youngsters just *love* Ex-Lax," parents were told; "instead of struggling against taking it, they regularly ask for it." "Youngsters actually beg for Ex-Lax," other ads stated, they "actually *enjoy* taking Ex-Lax. And it's just as good for them as it is for the grown-ups."[36]

When medicine was that good, why wait for mother to administer it? Surprisingly, the first known case of a child confusing phenolphthalein with candy did not occur until 1908, but after that American and British medical journals regularly published accounts of youngsters suffering severe purging after accidentally overdosing on candy laxatives. Popular health literature warned parents to keep these medicines out of the reach of children, but even the most thorough precautions could be undone by the nostrum-makers' marketing strategy of sending out samples to entire neighborhoods. Once the news of free candy got out, children raided mailboxes as if Halloween had come early: a typical experience was that of the Schenectady, New York 10-year-old who "was markedly prostrated, very weak, pale and had considerable abdominal cramps [after going] about from house to house gathering samples" of Vim Lax, a phenolphthalein-activated chewing gum. In 1932, a 10-year-old California boy died after consuming a box of Ex-Lax chocolates, and his physician attributed the death to phenolphthalein poisoning. In fact, phenolphthalein is not acutely toxic, and it's likely the laxative drug simply aggravated a more serious underlying condition. Even so, one has to agree with the physician in the case: "let drugs be drugs," he wrote AMA officials, "and candy be candy."[37]

I have interviewed a number of people who passed through childhood in the 1920s and '30s, and it's clear that letting drugs be candy was a highly effective tactic for laxative manufacturers. One man recalled only too clearly "my mother's horror that her sons might be irregular," which at first meant "that castor oil was ever at the ready. With the advent of Ex-Lax," though, "cleaning out the system became less forbidding." Such memories are corroborated by the commentary of the 2362 children who submitted letters of praise for Ex-Lax in a 1930 juvenile opinion survey published in *Junior Life* magazine. A Minnesota girl announced that her "motto for health and success in school work" was "Take Ex-Lax, then relax." The principle worked in Ohio, too, a Zanesville girl reporting that her math grades had improved "since Mother started giving me Ex-Lax every few nights. Some-way Ex-Lax makes me think faster." If some of these "Ex-Lax Kiddies" became mathematicians, others turned into poets. Certainly there was no more eloquent testimony to the profitability of combining pleasure with purgation than that of Danny Nesby, of Dell Rapids, South Dakota:

> A good little boy is named Max,
> Who loves medicine when it's Ex-Lax,
> It's amazingly handy,
> And tastes 'most like candy,
> And should really be sold in big sacks.[38]

Laxative marketing was not all child's play, however. So ingenious were manufacturers that they could promote the image of big sacks of chocolates in one breath, and the use of purgatives as weight loss products in the next. The Roaring Twenties were also the Dieting Twenties, the decade in which this century's ob-

session with slimness emerged full-scale, as it were. "Reducing has become a national pasttime," a magazine writer marveled in 1925, "a craze, a national fanati-
cism. . . . People now converse in pounds, ounces, and calories." Then as now,
dieting was not to most heavy people's taste; to many, it was more appealing to
practice a kind of inverted bulimia, in which presumably excess food was rejected
by the body through the colon instead of the esophagus. Obesity cure quacks ca-
tered to this weakness, one of the best known, Lucille Kimball, promising to "make
your fat vanish by the gallon." Instead of demanding bothersome dieting and exercise, she sold pills of a secret composition that "simply converts your fat into an
emulsion and passes it through your liver, into your colon and out with your
waste." And plenty of waste there must have been, for her pills were a combination of aloes and Epsom salts (rival Marjorie Hamilton relied on purgative mineral waters and enemas).[39]

Among laxative manufacturers at least one actually placed obesity above
autointoxication and made weight control the primary function of the product.
Kruschen Salts (an English brand) was partly presented in conventional laxative terms: "removes all the waste matter that has been clogging the system,
purifies and refreshes the blood, . . . reminds your liver and kidneys of their
duty." But that was the fine print in Kruschen's advertisements. The large print
was "The SAFE, Healthy Way to Lose FAT," "The Modern Safe Way—Right
Way to Lose Fat," and "Why not strip off that unbecoming fat—get rid of
double chins, chubby hips and ugly rolls of fat"? Many ads said nothing at all
about laxative effects, describing the salts (dissolved in hot water "first thing
every morning") only as "a splendid daily health drink—prescribed by physicians." Customers bought Kruschen to combat fat, not autointoxication. "Any
time we see a woman come in that looks five pounds overweight," pharmacists
at the Owl Drug Store in Quincy, Illinois reported, "we just reach for a Kruschen,
because that's what she will ask for." And why shouldn't she ask for it, when
Kruschen, which advertised in such fashion-setting periodicals as *Vogue*, *Van-
ity Fair*, and *Cosmopolitan*, packed its copy with testimonials of women (and occasionally men) who had lost 20, 50, even 100 pounds: "I took 2 bottles every
month for a year and 3 weeks. It amounted to $25 for reducing 102 pounds but
it was worth it" (Fig. 4-7). Just in case any women doubted it was worth such
an expenditure, Kruschen ads included not only the obligatory "before" and
"after" pictures of ordinary customers but also artfully posed nude photos of
"gloriously attractive, slender Kruschen figures." To hear physicians tell it,
however, Kruschen figures were the sick ones. The use of any brand of laxative
for the purpose of weight control was repeatedly condemned in both medical
and popular health literature, and various forms of injury to the intestinal tract
attributed to the practice. At least one physician linked a case of colon cancer to
the weight-obsessed woman's daily use of "loads" of purgatives.[40]

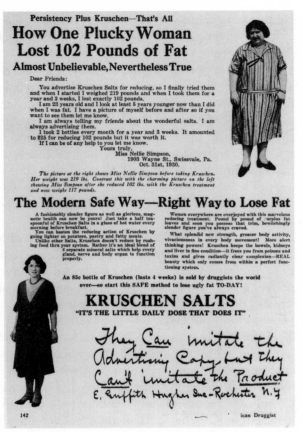

Figure 4-7. Advertisement recommending laxation for weight loss [from *American Druggist*, March 1931, p. 142].

If other companies were less outspoken about their laxative's value for weight loss, they were every bit as bold as Kruschen in promoting the remedy as a beautifier. Nineteenth-century purgatives had sometimes done the same; Beecham's Pills, for instance, placed a lovely young maiden over the caption "a beautiful complexion comes from within." Arbuthnot Lane had related beauty to inner cleanliness much more insistently, and the relation had become part of popular autointoxication lore by the 1920s. Laxative producers were determined not to let the public forget that beauty began in the intestines. Unwittingly imitating the Beecham's ad, Nujol put a pretty young woman's face above the lines "a clear, radiant, youthful complexion, what else but internal cleanliness can produce it?" "A clean system is the originator of charm," it continued, because "science now knows that poisons from intestinal sluggishness are the cause of personal unattractiveness. . . .

No wonder that through faulty elimination the skin becomes sallow, muddy, roughened, blotched or disfigured with pimples or other blemishes." Such statements were multiplied many times over in ads for other cathartics (Fig. 4-8). Sal Hepatica, for example, imagined a woman "blessed with the lineaments of a goddess . . . gowned by Lanvin, and hatted by Agnes" who nevertheless fell short of beauty because of autointoxication: "attractiveness, that elusive quality, depends most of all on *internal cleanliness.*" And unlikely as it seems, laxative products apparently did make good on such claims occasionally. "Thanks to TUTT'S PILLS," a Nebraska man wrote the manufacturer. The pills were "used by my wife for a very torpid liver," he explained, and what an extraordinary change followed: "If you had seen her before using them and see her now, you would not think her the same person, she is so much improved, and I am beginning to think she is a good-looking woman."[41]

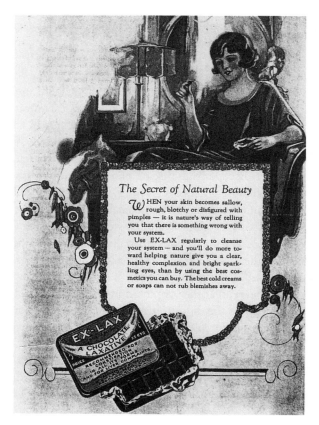

Figure 4-8. Advertisement promoting laxation for beauty [Warshaw Collection, Archives Center, National Museum of American History, box 9, file 25].

If women wanted to become good-looking, men wanted to succeed, adver-
tisers supposed, and it was just as easy to construct a plausible linkage of inner
cleanliness with business success as with beauty. Getting ahead in the world required motivation, intelligence, energy, and stamina. But intestinal stasis caused
depression, dulled the mental processes, and drained the body of physical vitality. "Tired . . . before the day's tasks begin!" described the worn-looking man
throwing on his overcoat as he rushed away from the breakfast table in a 1927 Sal
Hepatica ad. "Driving his brain, hurrying his meals, slighting his exercise, the
business man invites Auto-Intoxication . . . and Auto-Intoxication . . . keeps thousands of men from doing their best work." In an inset, one of these thousands is
shown at the office later in the day, wearily supporting his head with his hand while
the papers on his desk go unattended. But "Successful Breadwinners," Nujol
pointed out, "Know the Value of Internal Cleanliness."[42]

Purgatives even staved off marital discord. It wasn't just that the plain-Jane
wives and poor provider husbands created by constipation were apt to find fault
with one another, but more fundamentally, that the "constant, chronic bad temper" caused by autointoxication, that feeling of "savage irritability with life" ate
away at the affection and understanding between partners. In "Murder at the Breakfast Table," a 1928 Feen-a-mint ad, an enraged husband stands menacingly over
his cringing wife. "Suddenly, it happens! A quick retort, a slamming door. . . . "
As it turns out, actual homicide wasn't committed, just a steady withering of affection: "Love isn't killed at once that way, but murdered slowly, day by day."[43]

Success and sex appeal, even marital harmony, were only icing on the cake
of health and longevity. Escape from disease and premature death was what the
laxative industry pushed most aggressively. Judging from testimonials, both those
sent to manufacturers and those mailed to medical agencies such as the American
Medical Association, it was freedom from disease that the public thought it was
buying. A letter from Mrs. Martha Rasmussen to the AMA typifies the too-common
popular acceptance of the proprietary industry's teachings. "When the digestion
is in good working order," she told the doctors, "than it dond throw no extra work
on the kidney and the heart and other organs, and keeps the blood in good working order but just as soon as the digestion get wrong than it poisons your whole
system and causes cancer insanity nerves nous infantile peralisic and causes all kind
of ackes and pains." She herself took two laxative pills every day, along with an
egg and turpentine enema; that these preserved her in health was demonstrated
beyond doubt by the fact that when she had tried to go off the pills the previous
summer, "my knee got loose jointed and I got to feeling so tired I finely gave up
my Job."[44]

The bulk of laxative promotion was aimed directly at the public, but advertising budgets also provided liberally for promoting the product to medical professionals, pharmacists in particular. The retail druggist's recommendation, manu-

facturers appreciated, could be an unusually effective marketing tool. Not everyone could be expected to fall for such transparently self-serving ads as were placed in newspapers and aired over the radio. All but the most cynical, however, might surrender to the influence of a presumably disinterested health professional, every neighborhood's scientist, the trusted corner pharmacist. In truth, druggists were hard pressed to remain dispassionate about the sales of patent medicines. In these years before chain drug stores, the pharmacist who owned and operated his own business had to scramble to turn a profit. Proprietary remedies, much in demand from customers enticed by advertising, supplied the druggist's largest single source of income, so whatever qualms he might feel about a product on a scientific basis, it was virtually impossible to resist proprietary manufacturers' requests to stock and sell, even recommend, their products: "For 31 years," Sal Hepatica reminded pharmacists in 1926, their remedy "has been the intimate friend of every cash register."[45]

The trick for laxative manufacturers was to make enlistment in a particular product's cause attractive—i.e., profitable—to the retail druggist. It was, in fact, a trick quite easily turned, the only challenge being to come up periodically with ingenious variations that separated one's own product from the huge pack howling for the pharmacist's favor. Reduced wholesale prices, and even free merchandise, were common devices to secure large-volume purchases from druggists. So were multicolored window displays supplied by manufacturers, with the assurance that they would lure customers in from the street. (Who could resist, for example, the "Believe it or Not!" exhibit revealing that "if all the Feen-a-mint sold in one day were stacked . . . the boxes would tower 1260 feet and be taller than the EMPIRE STATE BUILDING"?). Once hooked this way, customers could be landed with the promise of modest gifts distributed with each purchase, or with the chance to win luxury items in a contest. Nature's Remedy, a laxative popularly known as NR, gave early 1930s buyers free calendars, flower seeds, checker boards, and thermometers. At the other extreme, Feen-a-mint offered "a brand-new Plymouth Sedan" to some lucky winner, with 100 baseballs autographed by Babe Ruth going to second-place finishers (and to each and every contestant, "a lifelike Babe Ruth mask"). In an ad directed at druggists, the "Babe" himself begged to be put "to work in your store," explaining "here's a set-up that's not only going to sell a lot of Feen-a-mint, but is also going to bring thousands of people into drug stores all over the country. What about *your* store? Where are the people in *your* neighborhood going to get their information?" (Fig. 4-9).[46]

One place they could get it was from their physicians. Patent purgatives also were promoted to doctors, through ads in medical journals, materials mailed to individual practitioners, and at parties and receptions hosted for the profession. At least one company, the manufacturer of Feen-a-mint, offered "a selected list of physicians" the opportunity to purchase preferred stock in the company, and

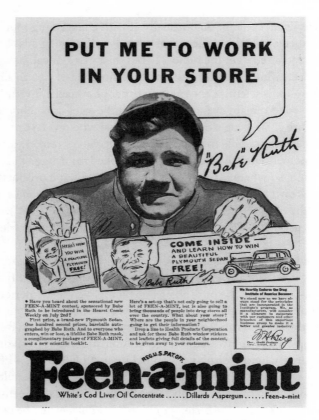

Figure 4-9. Advertisement using Babe Ruth to recruit
pharmacists to the promotion of laxatives [AMA, box
342, folder 12].

receive a bonus of additional stock free. But even without the inducements of the
proprietary industry, doctors would have prescribed cathartics for their patients.
Those who believed in autointoxication, at any rate, would see the time-honored
reliance on purgation as more desirable than ever. As a result, a London practitioner remarked at the beginning of this century, "when we [physicians] are called
upon to treat" constipation, "we run the patent pill man very closely."[47] Such complaints of therapeutic backwardness tainting the profession reappeared frequently
in medical literature through the 1930s.

   The exchanges made at the 1911 Louisville meeting of a national medical
association suggest the magnitude of the challenge faced by progressive physicians
attempting to wean colleagues from their commitment to purgation. A speaker

from Indiana presented a "Protest Against the Routine Use of Purgatives" in which he deplored "the bad precept and example of the medical profession." A visit to the physician, it was charged, "practically always" culminated in a prescription for a purgative. That sad fact was not just "an opprobium [sic] to the profession," he argued, but also a certain way to ensure that patients would lend credence to patent medicine ads and take still more laxatives on their own. Some in his audience disagreed. "Perhaps the people in Indiana are not so constipated as they are here in Kentucky," one doctor responded. In his opinion, "six-tenths of the people are constipated," constituting "a great army of suffering humanity," and "what are you going to do for them if you do not unload the bowels"? Immediately the speaker was confronted by another physician, a brother Indianan no less, who offered his opinion that constipation "is one of the most pernicious and intractable troubles that besets the human family," that "the vast majority of humans are chronic rectal constipates," and that "I would not denounce as roundly the usefulness of purgatives." No sooner did the objector sit than a doctor from Cincinnati stood to suggest that "a widespread custom that exists for years is usually founded on some truth," and to profess his own faith in "a free calomel purge, followed by a saline cathartic." (He and at least one other member of the audience also resorted to "the Lane operation" in obstinate cases.) The conflict would continue for decades, a London physician complaining as late as 1937 about "Ritual Purgation in Modern Medicine." Many a physician, he maintained, "purges any unfortunate patient who is robust enough to stand the strain," his therapeutic method being "often a magic ritual . . . rooted in archaic and primitive beliefs rather than physiology and pathology." Physicians who administered purgatives in the name of autointoxication, he submitted, were "exchanging the laboratory jacket of the twentieth century for the panoply of the witch doctor and the exorciser."[48]

Ritual purgation, whether physician-prescribed or self-selected, was as risky as it was irrational. The great sorrow of the colon alluded to at the beginning of the chapter was not the kinks Lane ascribed to it but the battering it took from the purgative drugs consumed by people determined to overcome their kinks. Laxative addiction and "cathartic colon" were common enough among nineteenth-century patients, despite their physicians' repeated pleas not to bat their bowels about like a shuttlecock. Medical invective against the misuse of cathartics grew even more frequent during the early twentieth century, however, as fear of autointoxication intensified public demand for laxatives, and laxative advertising intensified public fear of autointoxication. The true illness, many physicians agreed, was not autointoxication or constipation, but "bowel consciousness," an obsessive fear that one had or might any day develop autointoxication; "colon neurosis" was another way physicians described the groundless anxiety. "Because of constant bowel consciousness," an American doctor charged, "patients' lives have been made miserable" through "the constant use of laxatives." In his estimate, based on a survey of several hundred patients in New York and Newark, "70% of our public" was "addicted to laxation." Not all placed the percentage quite that high, but physicians in Britain and America frequently bemoaned the enormous number of laxative pills swallowed by the public. As a London MD put it, "the indiscriminate and habitual use of purgatives is one of the most serious menaces to the health of the community at the present day." As with the question of whose citizens were more constipated, American doctors were certain their countrymen led the way in self-abuse. "It is a well-known fact that cathartics and purgatives are used by the American people more than by any other people on the globe," one practitioner stated, while another commentary identified Americans as "the most liberally purged people on the globe."[49]

Whoever the most liberally purged people were, they were probably the most constipated people as well, for the cathartic colon produced by chronic purgative use was essentially a constipated colon, a large intestine so deadened by repeated drug stimulation as to be no longer able to function naturally ("Many people who were habitually constipated," London's James Goodhart observed, "were completely healthy when unharassed by aperients"). For "a large part of the population," one critic scoffed, bowel movements occurred only "under the severe lashing of cathartic drugs," while the author of a 1920 textbook on the proper use of cathartics argued that laxative overuse was "responsible for having made a large number of persons 'colonic cripples'—lifelong slaves to pills." The rhetoric was hardly exaggerated. The leader of British gastroenterology, Sir Arthur Hurst (coiner of "the sorrows of the colon"), spoke for many in calling cathartic colon "one of the commonest disorders of the present day," and reported patients who took "gigantic doses" of senna pods or other purgatives "every night. One woman had for years taken nightly a 'handful' of Carter's little liver pills, 30 being an average handful." "The life of the average cathartic habitue," an American physician added, "is often made miserable and is as lacking in happiness as that of many sufferers from chronic organic disease."[50]

Perhaps the champion colonic cripple was the Illinois woman who appealed to the American Medical Association in 1931. "I have tried acidophilus milk, yeast, mineral oils, enemas, cacara [cascara] liquid, the usual run of tablets, phenolax, senna leaf tea, saline laxatives . . . etc.," Mrs. Patterson wrote. "I have been thru two clinics the last five years, and took the diet list for constipation and stuck to it, but that *laid me out*—I got bilious and took Flu and Bronchitis each year that I left off the laxatives. I am now back on pills, but find they often contain something to quicken the heart and to cause gripping [griping] in bowels and bladder—would greatly appreciate your help." The physician who responded advised her to see her family doctor, which she did, but only to have more mineral oil prescribed: "So I am resigned," she wrote a week later. It was the Mrs. Pattersons of the world that an American gastroenterologist had in mind when he joked that "if it were not for the practice among the laity of relieving constipation by purgatives, over half his practice would be lost." (Some of the practice of the gastroenterologist, it should be noted, came from another form of laxative abuse, people's reflex taking of cathartics to relieve sudden abdominal pains. Often the pains were due to appendicitis. An inflamed appendix is easily ruptured when subjected to the increased intestinal motility stimulated by purgatives, and death will often result. A 1932 survey of recent appendicitis deaths found that over 90% of victims had taken a laxative as treatment.)[51]

Try as medical writers did to persuade people to give up laxatives, they encountered overwhelming resistance. It was not just the erroneous notions instilled by advertising, but equally the lay person's trusted common sense that defeated physicians' educational efforts. When someone took an active cathartic, her entire bowel, not just the region near the rectum, was emptied. That meant that next day there would be no waste near the rectum to be eliminated naturally, she would not have a movement, would thus suppose herself constipated again, and take another laxative. Physicians despaired of convincing patients that they merely needed to wait a few days for the colon to fill naturally: "it required considerable persuasion to have her stop cathartics," was the recurring medical lament, "as she said that her bowels would never move without help" (just as the balding businessman who consulted Alvarez required "several hours of argument" to be talked into stopping his laxatives). Alvarez, incidentally, came up with the best analogy for explaining the normal process of elimination to the laity. Think of the colon as "a short railroad-siding holding three cars," he suggested. "Normally, each day a new car comes down and bumps one off at the other end, so that three always remain." But when a purgative is taken, "a car will come down with such force that it will bump all the cars off and then go off itself to leave the siding empty." Thus, even if cars come down normally again, it will take four days before a car "will be bumped off at the end because the siding is filling up." The laxative user "does not dare [wait] because he thinks it would be dangerous."[52]

The danger of autointoxication continued to worry both the profession and the public through the 1930s. As late as 1942, Alvarez complained that patients were being "badly frightened" by their doctors "by being shown in his x-ray films the shadow of a colon that appeared to have several bad kinks in it," and that therefore required treatment with cathartics or other measures. The sorrows of the colon were thus little lighter at mid-century than at the beginning, and the words of an American bowel specialist still rang only too true: "the food canal," he sighed, "is a soft tube with a hard life."[53]

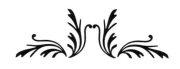

5

WASHING OUT
THE INNER PERSON:
THE WATER CURE

THERE IS SOMETHING very curious and very funny about the mineral-water mania. If a man, digging about in a dirty swamp, finds a filthy hole in the ground which sends up a disgusting smell, he gets down upon his knees at once, sticks his nose into the hole, and, suddenly drawing away almost suffocated with the stench, he shouts out to his companions, "Come here! Come here! Oh, boys, smell of that! That's a big thing! Ain't that strong? almost knocks a fellow down! . . . There ain't a spring in Saratoga that takes hold like that. Talk about this farm being worth nothing—I wouldn't sell this spring alone for a hundred thousand dollars. I tell you that will knock your dyspepsia and consumption and things higher than a kite."

Isn't it the strangest hallucination? Nine people in ten have a notion that if water only smells bad enough it must be "awfully healthy." If the stuff only makes them "crawl all over" as it goes down, they seem to think it is surcharged with salvation.

Dioclesian Lewis, 1872

IS IT ANY WONDER that people die of premature old age, of apoplexy, paralysis, dropsy, consumption, and the thousand and one maladies that scourge humanity . . . when occupying nearly one-half of the abdominal cavity is an engorged intestine reeking with filth almost as foul as carrion, and which is being steadily absorbed into the circulation? . . . And yet there is a simple and effective method of dealing with this trouble . . . of thoroughly cleansing and purifying that important organ, the colon, without the least demand upon the vital forces, and that is by Washing It Out.

Charles Tyrrell, 1920

New York City resident Andrew Vena was in sound health. Even so, "it would not be a bad idea," he decided in December of 1930, "to take a little percuation [precaution] to keep healthy." From what he had read, as well as heard from "public health lectures" delivered by laxative salesmen along Sixth Avenue, there was now "stamped in [his] mind" the belief that virtually all disease originated from constipation. It followed that preservation of health required "keeping the bowl clean . . . cleaning the collen and keeping it clean," practicing "internal bathing." To that end, he purchased a J. B. L. Cascade, a popular brand of enema equipment pervasively advertised as the most effective provider of the "Internal Bath," and began to use it weekly as a "safety measure." Ten months later, still vigorous and free of illness, he was convinced the Cascade had been money well spent.[1]

But then Mr. Vena came across a publication from the American Medical Association, "Mechanical Nostrums and Quackery," and "was shocked and supprised indeed" to learn what medical experts had to say about the Cascade. The device was an expensive folly, he read; it exploited an erroneous popular belief (autointoxication), it was potentially dangerous, and it was altogether an unconscionable bilking of a nervous public. Vena wrote the AMA at once, asking to be told "that it 'ain't true'," but knowing in his heart that it was. "It seems to me that this world has become so crooket," he said, that one no longer knows "where to turn for truth, what to believe, who to trust, how to keep out of traps and falling victim to schemes of deviltry. Much of everything seems to be a matter of racketeering, frauds, fakes, catchdollar tricks, falsehood and all the like. Yeeeeee Gods!"[2]

Still, Vena asked, even if the Dr. Tyrrell who marketed the Cascade was a quack, was it not true that "by preventing constipation I will prevent much other trouble caused by self-poisoning?" And if so, must it not then also be true that regular enemas, whether taken with the Cascade or any other model, would do "much towards preserving my present good state of health?" Looked at that way, "it seems to me that the Cascade is a good device . . . regardless of it[s] origin or of the man who makes it and his past or even his present." So, he ended, would the Association advise him to discontinue using the device "and discart it alltogether? If so, could I get my money back for it—$12.50, or is my name doomed to remain on Tyrrell's list of victims? Tell me squarely," he begged, "and on the level. I'm not afraid of the truth, I want it."[3]

Mr. Vena's ambivalence—respecting authoritative opinion that the Cascade was useless, but unable to deny all he had heard about the dangers of autointoxication or to dispute his own common sense supposition that cleaning his "collen" should protect him from disease—was a common predicament for the American and British public of the 1920s and '30s. Medicine's representatives were outspoken in their condemnation of autointoxication theory, enemas, laxatives, and other colon remedies. The American Medical Association received many more letters regarding the Cascade, and invariably responded with dismissals: "utterly quack-ish," for example, and "[the product of] deceit, misrepresentation and quackery."[4] Yet so much of what people read in newspapers and magazines and heard on the radio insisted that autointoxication was real. Which was the more frightening gamble: throwing away $12.50 and ending up on some quack's list of victims, or throwing away one's life and ending up on autointoxication's much longer list? Like Vena, people wanted to hear the truth, but they were likewise confused about where to turn for truth, what to believe, whom to trust. In the end, too many failed to take account of how "crooket" the world had become; they succumbed to auto-intoxication scaremongers, often putting their trust particularly in colon therapists who appealed to the intuitive notion that internal bathing must be the most direct and natural method of keeping the bowel pure and the body healthy.

The belief that washing out the inner self would ward off disease was an ancient one, expressed over centuries both as willingness to submit to enemas such as the Cascade and as readiness to drink the waters of mineral springs. Both prac-tices prospered during the early years of the twentieth century as options for com-batting autointoxication, and the use of each will be considered in turn. One should begin with mineral waters, as the waters served, in effect, as a bridge from phar-maceutical purgation to enema cleansing. Indeed, mineral water might be thought of as a cross between cathartics and enemas; since the waters generally contained purgative salts, they flushed out fecal waste while simultaneously sanitizing the colon walls.

Consumption of mineral waters is associated historically with spa therapy, the treatment of illness at natural springs. Initially, the preferred spas were those built around hot springs, warm waters in which the sick could relax and let the heat "open the pores, resolve, attenuate, digest, consume, and draw forth super-fluities."[5] That was the common rationale, in this instance given for the spring in England's Bath. A health resort used since pre-Roman times, Bath became *the* destination for socially advantaged hypochondriacs during the eighteenth century. By then, however, cold water springs were becoming as popular as hot ones, at least those found to have a significant mineral content. The sulfurous and other odious tastes of mineral springs had always satisfied the good-medicine-must-taste-bad preconception, while magnesium sulfate, sodium sulfate, and other cathartic salts appealed to the purgation-is-regeneration conviction. During the seventeenth century, a much more sophisticated interpretation of the waters' benefits was made available by the doctrines of iatrochemistry (medical chemistry), an outgrowth of alchemy that proclaimed the superior efficacy of mineral drugs prepared in the chemical laboratory. Mineral springs thus seemed to provide a natural comple-ment to the mineral drugs synthesized in the iatrochemical lab; spa waters seemed to be nature's vehicle for chemical compounds that could correct pathological chemical imbalances in the body. More compelling—the proof of these theoretical musings—was the fact that mineral waters did appear to purify the body. They forced the same evacuations (sweat, urine, vomit, and feces) as the medicines from the iatrochemists' crucibles. The impact of the iatrochemical promotion of mineral waters was to make the *minerals* as important as the *waters*. Drinking the waters, which had been downplayed in favor of bathing in them, now became a critical part of the spa regimen, especially in England, where so few springs were naturally hot.[6]

With nature's minerals as much as laboratory ones, purgation was the acid test of efficacy, and purgative power alone ensured the popularity of more than one spa. Epsom, for example, the Surrey town now known for its Derby, emerged as a popular weekend resort for Londoners in the mid-1600s because of the "bitter purging salt" found in its springs (magnesium sulfate is still sold by the ton as Epsom salt). Just how purging the bitter salt could be was suggested by the 1650s poet who related that "Some drink of it, and in an houre, Their Stomach, Guts, and Kidneys scower." As the writer elaborated on his experience visiting the well, however, it became apparent that a full hour of grace was actually the blessed exception. He and a friend had been persuaded by an elderly resident to take a cup for their health's sake, he reported, but no sooner had it passed their lips,

> Till Gut by rumbling, us beseeches,
> My boyes, beware, you'l wrong your Breeches.
> Ah, doth it worke? the old man cryes,
> Yonder are brakes to hide your thighes.
> Where, though 'twere near we hardly came,
> Ere one of us had been to blame.

Epsom water, he continued, was as powerful as it was fast, and though he claimed to have set the spa's distance record, even the least athletic of imbibers made his mark on the landscape. "Close by the Well," it was explained,

> you may discerne
> Small shrubs of *Eglantin* and *Fern*,
> Which shew the business of the place;
> [For there the greensward's upper face]
> Is yellow, not with heat of summer,
> But safroniz'd with mortall scumber.

Finally, in these days before the mail-order catalog, cleansing oneself of scumber took a classical form:

> Here lies *Rome's Naso* torn and rent,
> Now reeking from the fundament. . . .
> Here did lye *Virgil*, there lay *Horace*,
> Which newly had wiped his, or her Arse.[7]

To be sure, John Mennes's advice "To a friend upon a journey to Epsam Well" was a vulgar piece. Its puerility, however, was the point. When people considered the Epsom experience (or, in following centuries, treatment at Cheltenham, Harrogate, or other spas), they did not meditate raptly on the etherial healing virtue of nature's universal fluid; they thought rather in the crudest terms of rumbling guts and explosive ejections. Taking the waters meant taking a purge.

What Epsom was to the seventeenth century, Cheltenham was to the nineteenth. And though Cheltenham had faded as a spa by the time autointoxication appeared, the Cheltenham experience undergone by so many in the 1800s should be considered at least briefly before returning to the twentieth century. Not only was it a fashionable alternative for colon cleansing in Georgian and Victorian society, it constituted a style of treatment that would continue at other spas into the Edwardian era and the age of autointoxication.

A market town nestled into the northwest corner of the Cotswolds, Cheltenham came to rival Bath after George III sought relief there in 1788. The ailing monarch selected the spa partly because "Farmer George" preferred its rural tranquillity to the bustle of Bath, but more, no doubt, because "a moderate dose" of its water, as a spa survey of the time phrased it, "acts powerfully and speedily as a purgative." In fact, that hardly did the waters justice, not if one is to believe a pair of engravings now displayed in the Cheltenham Art Gallery. The first picture, executed in 1802 by one Giles Grinagain, suggests "The Rapid Effects of the Cheltenham Waters" by installing a smiling patient securely in a water closet, while half a dozen other recent imbibers queue in tight-lipped desperation outside. "Pray Sir make haste," the first-in-line implores. "Oh! dear Me! What a while he is about it," the next-in-line mutters, while the man behind her urges their leader, "Pray speak to him again." At the end of the queue a woman with clenched fists sighs, "Oh! dear. Oh! Oh. Oh—Ah! Ah! It's all over!" The soldier ahead of her has shown more foresight. Walking away from the group, he announces, "I had better go up Stairs and take a Pot—or I shall certainly go off at Half-Cock." Just ahead of him, a German visitor, hands hugging his belly, makes the most pointed observation: "Neber vas so gripe in all my Life—dise Shitten-ham Vaters are very operatif."[8]

The 1823 "Effects of the Cheltenham Waters" expresses again how very operative the waters were. A tottering parade of well-dressed water drinkers is shown hastening away from a pump room. Every face stretched with worry, the bent-over drinkers, top hats askew and skirts pulled close, hurry in tight, short steps toward an attendant dispensing sheets of paper. A young boy with his hand pressed against his bottom howls as he looks about for a parent. The only relaxation to be seen is on the face of a man peering through the leaves of the background shrubbery in which he has taken shelter and unburdened himself. The legend beneath warns that "tis NECESSARY to quicken your MOTIONS after the Second Glass. Get home as fast as you can." There was even a joke that a tomb-stone in the town churchyard bore the epitaph:

Here I lie, and my two daughters,
We died from drinking the Cheltenham Waters.[9]

Representations of the water as dangerously overactive were dismissed by the spa's boosters as satirical exaggeration, of course. In all the promotional lit-erature for Cheltenham, the only violence done by the water was to disease: "We should not be bestowing too high an encomium upon [the waters]," one defender maintained, to say "that they approach the nearest of anything in nature to an universal remedy, or 'panacea'" (the claim can still be tested by the tourist who dares; Cheltenham water is available for sampling at the Pump Room in Pittville Park). For the panacea to work, though, invalids had to live hygienically once they arrived at the spa, and that was not so easily done, there being so many tempta-tions to balance the round of therapy with the social whirl. Like Bath and other stylish spas, Cheltenham had its own Master of Ceremonies, a gentleman who orchestrated a full schedule of diversion for the town's visitors—a weekly cotil-lion, twice-a-week card playing, thrice-weekly theater, periodic animal baitings, and billiards and bowling at all times. The town was a place where "old people can be seen going to the grave with a pack of cards in their hands," one critic joked, where at no age, a second noted, were invalids content merely to "send for their bottle of water from the pump"; they must also have "their bottle of wine from the tavern; and think that Hygeia and Bacchus may be safely associated." Turned into a center for horse racing as well in the 1820s, Cheltenham's ascent to "high celebrity, and pre-eminent station . . . in the rank of Watering Places" was due in large measure to its being "The fount of health and mirth, The merriest sick re-sort on earth."[10]

One could hardly make merry on the non-naturals. Spa doctors advised moderation at the table and with the bottle, but acknowledged that with most pa-tients the only regularity to be accepted into their lives was that of the daily schedule of taking the waters. Hence the most had to be made of those morning hours be-fore the card and other games began. Well operators opened their doors at seven to encourage an early-to-rise philosophy (early-to-bed was out of their hands). Drinkers were given two or three pints of water, then encouraged to stroll the gardens and wooded grounds, to the accompaniment of woodwind and string bands. How many debauch-grogged patients actually reported for therapy in the morning? According to the doctors, they came in droves: "No sooner has the lark ceased his first morning carol, and the general choir of birds succeeded [another hygienic stimulus], than the 'busy hum' commences at the well. . . . The walks begin to be filled" between six and seven, and "from seven till nine they are crowded. . . . The visitors throng with avidity towards the water: and such is the general anxiety to imbibe the virtues of this celebrated spring, that many ladies and gentlemen bring their own glasses, for the sake of being more speedily accomodated." For the truly serious, this morning journey to the shrine would be repeated daily for the 4 to 6 weeks the cure required. Even after leaving Cheltenham, one could continue to enjoy its waters, for a Mr. Thompson ran a laboratory in which he evaporated water from more than 70 wells to isolate six different salts that he bottled for sale throughout Britain and for export "to the eastern, western, and other parts of the globe." Other nineteenth-century spa towns operated much the same (including American ones, such as Saratoga Springs, New York).[11]

Cheltenham's glory days drew to a close during the second half of the century (the chic Rotunda, where the spa's clients had amused themselves at so many balls and concerts, at last became The Rotunda Pub), and the town evolved into a magnet for retirees and horse-racing afficionados. For a time, French, German, and other continental spas became the favorites of mineral water devotees. With the onset of Arbuthnot Lane's campaign against intestinal toxemia, however another English health resort assumed leadership in the battle to escape autointoxication: Harrogate, a London gastroenterologist announced in 1922, was now "the Mecca for the sins of the colon."[12]

The Yorkshire town of Harrogate had flourished as a spa since the 1500s, known particularly as the "Stincking Spaw" because of the high sulfur content of its springs; the rotten-egg odor of hydrogen sulfide gas hovered over more or less all of Harrogate's wells. Consequently, the recollections of the spa's patients over the centuries are an amusing juxtaposition of encomiums to the water's healing powers (the springs were also rich in purgative salts) and shudderings over its smell and taste. In the seventeenth century, for example, Celia Fiennes, something of a *cognoscenta* of cathartic springs, found the aroma of Harrogate water to be "so very strong and offensive," so "like carrion or a jakes [toilet] . . . that I could not force my horse near the Well." She did force herself near it, drinking a quart on each of two consecutive mornings and discovering it "to be a good sort of Purge if you can hold your breath so as to drinke." So notorious was the stinking spa that its water was disparaged even from the pages of fiction. Smollet's Matthew Bramble, who journeyed to Harrogate in search of health when Bath failed him, only to be disappointed again, had this to say: "I have drank it once, and the first draught has cured me of all desire to repeat the medicine." Its taste, he grimaced, "is exactly that of bilge-water," so vile "I was obliged to hold my nose with one hand while I advanced the glass to my mouth with the other." Even "after I had made shift to swallow it," Bramble complained, "my stomach could hardly retain what it had received. . . . I can hardly mention it without puking."[13]

Yet if Harrogate sounds less than invigorating (the women employed to draw water from the springs, who spent their lives bathed by malodorous fumes, were described by a seventeenth-century visitor as having skin "like bacon rind" and looks that could "vie with an old Bath guide's ass"), the sulfur water's foulness actually enhanced its appeal as therapy. Because medicine was supposed to taste bad, Low Harrogate, where the most offensive wells were concentrated, grew much more rapidly than High Harrogate. Development of both ends of town accelerated during the Georgian and Regency eras, when the spa was transformed into a place of great architectural charm. Despite the steady decline of spas through the Victorian age, Harrogate remained an attractive destination for higher society in the north of England. Its zenith was reached, however, during the first two decades of this century.[14]

"Never had the town been so rich and elegant," it was written of the 1911 season, "never had so much money flowed into the municipal coffers, never had the future looked so bright," because never had there been such demand for intestinal cleansing without cathartic drugs, nor a spa offering so many ways of satisfying that demand. It was not just that Harrogate enclosed a full 88 natural springs, each reputedly distinct from all others with respect to sulfur and magnesium content, thus making it "by far the most remarkable and generally useful Spa yet discovered in this or any other country." There were also "upwards of one hundred different curative methods" obtainable, methods that went well beyond the standard practice of drinking as much of the sulfureous water as one could force down. First were the many baths. The Harrogate springs were not naturally thermal, so had previously not invited bathing the way Bath did. By 1900, however, the mineral waters were being heated artificially, so that Harrogate could compete with Bath and the hot springs on the Continent. Depending on the spring from which the water was taken, one could order a sulfur bath, a saline sulfur bath, or an alkaline sulfur bath. In addition, there were peat baths (using water impregnated with peat from nearby moors), foam baths (the foam was created with a stream of either oxygen or carbon dioxide, and allowed the patient to withstand higher temperatures), and effervescent saline baths (effervescence was produced by mixing sodium bicarbonate and hydrochloric acid with the bath water). There were various hydrotherapeutic douches, or showers: the Aix Douche, the Vichy Douche, Tivoli Douche, Trough Douche, Needle Douche, and the Scotch Douche. There were several steam and hot air baths, different forms of massage, and treatments involving electrical stimulation. There was the "paraffin wax bath," and one of the most highly touted procedures, the "Harrogate Mud Pack," that used a local radioactive mud the therapists called "fango" (a comparable selection of water therapies was available at some American spas). Given so great a variety of treatments to direct against human debility, there may well have been some measure of truth in a Harrogate booster's claim that while visitors "may arrive in bath chairs or on crutches, they very quickly scamper about like young lambs."[15]

Harrogate's physicians believed the lion's share of credit for the rejuvenation of invalids belonged to a final treatment, the one known as the Plombières douche. Plombières was a popular hydrotherapeutic resort in the northeast of

France where, in 1898, staff physicians had introduced a "douche horizontale" that utilized a rubber catheter inserted about 9 inches into the intestinal tract, through which a liter or more of warm water (107°F) was introduced at high pressure. The tube was then withdrawn, the bowels evacuated, and the tube reintroduced for a second and, if necessary, third or more treatment. Even the minimum of two administrations seems to have been something of an ordeal: "The whole proceeding," according to a British physician who received care at Plombières, "was most uncomfortable and, at times, extremely painful." Other patients agreed, "many remark[ing] how they dreaded" repetition of the horizontal douche once they had experienced it.[16] Thus in the early 1900s, the Plombières method was revised along more humane lines (less water, lower pressure), and it quickly caught on in spa circles throughout Europe. The "Plombières douche" became the modish person's choice of internal bath.

This was true in Britain especially. Indeed, "the Plombières system of rectal irrigation has recently become alarmingly popular in this country," a London physician wrote in 1910. The reason it had become so popular, of course, was Arbuthnot Lane, whose vivid images of death and deterioration wrought by intestinal stasis were more than enough to goad many patients beyond their dread of "extremely painful" colon irrigations. The method was associated with several spas in particular, notably Bath, Buxton, Llandrindod Wells, but most of all, Harrogate, a place "where many thousand Plombières douches are administered every year," a doctor estimated in the early 1920s. The spa's medical staff preferred to identify the procedure as "The Harrogate System of Intestinal Lavage," believing that their use of the resort's distinctive sulfur water lifted it above the French method. By either name, that was the treatment for which "large numbers of cases of functional disorders of the alimentary canal find their way to Harrogate from all parts of the world."[17]

The Harrogate lavage was introduced to the spa in 1905, just at the time Arbuthnot Lane was bringing intestinal stasis to the nervous attention of the profession and the public. Thus while it was "originally given almost entirely for colitis," its use was soon extended to "the numerous ailments thought to be due to, or associated with, intestinal toxaemia." After just a few years, 15,000 patients annually were receiving the irrigations. What the Harrogate interpretation of Plombières involved was having the patient lie on her right side to receive an injection of warm (102°F) sulfur water through a soft rubber tube (every patient purchased her own tube on arrival at the spa, "for obvious hygienic reasons"). After a while she would be turned onto her back, then onto her left side: "evacuation then takes place," clearing out the bowel so that subsequent injections "may have a better chance of thoroughly cleansing and acting upon the intestinal mucous membranes." Lavage attendants immediately inspected every stool and made a written report of "the quantity, colour and character of the feces and mucous, and the presence or otherwise of casts, blood, undigested food, parasites, etc.," then repeated the process until "the rectum and colon are thus effectually washed out." The Harrogate system failed to improve on the Plombières method in at least one way, however, as indicated by the fact that the lavage was followed by the patient being moved to a 98°F sulfur bath in which a "submarine douche" of 110°F water was "sprayed on the abdomen and lumbar region." The purpose of this after-treatment was "relieving pain in the large bowel, and in the pelvic organs in women." Yet whatever abdominal discomfort patients experienced was more than balanced, it was believed, by the bactericidal properties of the sulfur, which presumably destroyed the toxin-producing germs in the colon.[18]

With the irrigations being given only on alternate days, the typical duration of the lavage cure was 3 weeks. The time must have passed pleasantly enough, however, for the treatments were administered at the Royal Baths, a building opened in 1897 and "replete with every possible bathing luxury, . . . equal, if not superior, to anything of the kind in existence." The Royal Baths included a large room for drinking the waters while strolling about and listening to the orchestra that performed on the bandstand; there was also a covered garden for taking more strenuous exercise. Life outside the Royal Baths was most agreeable as well, with music, balls, and *thés dansants* at the many hotels, golf, tennis, and badminton facilities, even "excellent hunting with several different packs." When the cure was complete and the patient returned home, waters for preventive maintenance could be purchased through the mail; that from spring number 88 was particularly recommended, in part because "it mixes excellently with spirits."[19]

The rejuvenation of clients at Harrogate, and other spas, was due much more to the pleasures and relaxation of spa life, the respite it gave them from the business and social pressures of their normal life, than to intestinal lavage or sulfur water. Furthermore, water cure therapy was "a mental attitude of discipline," a "stimulating psychic atmosphere" that converted the patient to "the great cause of his own salvation." With his treatment "a new and palpitating joy to him," the spa patient learns to "prattle about specific gravities, indicans and aromatic sulphates. . . . He talks glibly of *petrissage*, alternating currents, and the *douche ascendante*. He becomes an expert on diet, and will harangue you by the hour on calories[and] on purins." In short, the patient gets better by becoming "the most persistent and intolerable of social bores." Nor does his recovery last. How frequent it is, an American doctor commented, that "the remarkable cure effected at the spring becomes a dismal failure shortly after the return of the patient to his usual pursuits and environments."[20]

Up to the mid-1910s, however, medical skepticism about the efficacy of the Plombières douche was outweighed by the enthusiasm of physicians who believed it, in conjunction with the rest of the spa regimen, to be the surest way of countering autointoxication. There were the spa physicians themselves, of course (one could find "no more confirmed advocates of this particular health regime," the Harrogate Medical Society stated around 1920, "than medical men who have experienced its benefits"), but there were many more in general practice who prescribed the Harrogate cure for any patient who could afford it; one of the rare Harrogate physicians who believed the Plombières method was overused attributed the excess to "doctors throughout the country demanding it," and his opinion was often confirmed by others.[21]

"In the New Utopia," a disciple of Arbuthnot Lane predicted in 1918, "where stasis will be regarded as a sin more sinister than sedition, and surfeit more unseemly than schism, fasts will cease to be the farcical fantasies of a few faddists and will become facts; the function of the police will be the purveying of paraffin; pilgrimages will be made, not to Palestine, but to Plombières." His true intent, of course, was that pilgrimages would be made to Harrogate. But already autointoxication was falling out of professional favor, and drug therapy entering an era of revolutionary expansion that would relegate spa therapy and like traditional methods to quaint obsolescence in most physicians' minds. Medical opinion quickly shifted toward the view that Plombières therapy "caused more colitis than it ever cured." That did not stop patients from diagnosing intestinal toxemia for themselves, however, and prescribing a stint at the spa, so Harrogate regained some of the business it had lost from World War I. It was but a temporary revival. The renown of the Plombières douche spurred enterprising healers to open local (hence cheaper) facilities for intestinal lavage, making a trip to Harrogate seem an unnecessary expense and inconvenience. Other forms of spa therapy were fading in public estimation as well, as Victorian institutions came to seem increasingly old-fashioned and out of harmony with modern tastes. All watering places encountered hard times with the economic crash of 1929, and Harrogate suffered more than most, thanks to the managerial ineptitude of its director of the Royal Baths at the time (the man was summed up by one of the town's physicians as having "the aspect and deportment of a horrible bounder"). By the 1940s, the meetings of the Harrogate Medical Society and the Wells and Baths Committee were dominated by exasperating discussions of how to keep the spa prosperous.[22]

The solution, it turned out, was to no longer keep it a spa. George Bernard Shaw, ever the cynic, had foreseen such a devolution, observing that spas generally "are under a steady economic pressure which eventually and inevitably changes them into more or less expensive hotels"; their "inception in therapeutics," he jibed, must sooner or later lead to a "culmination in golfing." In 1940, an American doctor confirmed that the process was indeed well along. Sharply falling business at spas was due "mainly to lack of medical support in recommending patients for cure," resulting in financial deficits that spa managers attempted to

offset "by emphasizing the entertainment values of the spa," turning facilities toward "recreation instead of re-creation." That drift toward frivolity further alien-
ated physicians, making them even less likely to refer patients, thus sinking the
spa ever deeper in red ink. Harrogate went under, as a spa, in the 1940s. From mid-
century on, the hotels that had formerly housed thousands of pilgrims to the shrine
to sulfur water were turned toward the conference and convention trade, and to
tourism generated by the town's development of itself into "Britain's Floral Resort." The Royal Baths where so many had submitted to the purifying ritual of
the Plombières douche were redeveloped into a civic center, and the Royal Pump
Room that had once rung with the revelry of well-heeled health seekers became a
store, next a restaurant, and at last, a museum that would attract nearly as many
tourists as it once had patients. By the last quarter of the century, this "Queen of
Watering Places," the "town endowed by nature with the richest variety of natural mineral springs in the world," had been reduced to a convention center that
"crams the shelves of its shops and supermarkets with inferior foreign waters and
allows its own to slumber in utter neglect."[23]

But one did not have to travel to Harrogate, or to any other spa, for that
matter, to find shop shelves crammed with mineral waters. One of the most common ways spas struggled to keep their head above water financially was to bottle
their mineral waters and package the salts from those waters for distribution and
sale to the general public. The sale of water from Harrogate's spring number 88
has been mentioned. Water from another well was also bottled, and sold under
the name Aquaperia. Drawn from a clever bit of word play that merged "aqua"
and "aperient," Aquaperia claimed to be "The Harrogate Aperient Mineral Water."
This use of a catchy trademark name and the aggressive promotion of the product to druggists and the public were, unfortunately, all too common tactics, and
are indicative of the degeneration of mineral water therapy into just another branch
of proprietary medicine charlatanism in the early twentieth century. "The men-
dacity of many of the advertisements for mineral springs," an American physician wrote as late as 1938, "rivals that of the claims for 'patent medicines' in their
palmiest days."[24]

Spas had sold waters and salts to consumers at large since the 1600s, to be sure,
but such commercialism increased manyfold in the era of autointoxication. Aquaperia
ads hint at the newly glutted mineral water market by asserting that the Harrogate
brand is superior to "Foreign Mineral Waters." What Aquaperia's proprietors had
in mind were the bottled waters from many of the Continental spas—Carlsbad,
Vichy, Hunyadi Janos—that were advertised with relentless pressure throughout
Britain and the United States. "Going to Carlsbad this summer in search of health?"
an ad directed at Americans asked, knowing all the while that almost no one who
saw the ad would go. "Thousands go" (proof of the water's virtue), "Many cannot
go" (a show of solicitude for everyman), so "Carlsbad is coming to them."[25]

Everything else was coming to them too, for not only did the managers of long-established fashionable spas such as Carlsbad and Harrogate and Saratoga pounce upon the economic opportunity created by popular worry over autointoxication but newcomers grabbed hold of the coattails of continental resorts and marketed a swarm of Marienbad Tablets, Poudres de Vichy, Pastilles de Châtel-Guyon, and other supposed salts from famous waters; in reality, the products were ordinary purgative compounds such as senna and aloes. Some well-established purgative products likewise added spa appeal to their promotional efforts. Sal Hepatica, for example, had long been billed as a saline, i.e., mineral, laxative. Spa waters acted through their minerals, so it followed that "Sal Hepatica is the American equivalent of . . . European spas." That meant that since "fashionable Europeans, skilled in the art of beauty," had for centuries trusted in spa water to protect their complexion from "the blemishes that come from within," American ladies could now be made to rival the "lovely Viennese women, the cool, lithe-limbed English and the slim dark women of French aristocracy" who "thronged" to Old World watering places. And they could accomplish that without thronging anywhere; the Sal Hepatica "saline method" of beautification could be practiced in the privacy and comfort of home.[26]

Only slightly more respectable were the opportunists who happened to own a piece of land graced with a natural mineral spring or well. Though the waters may have gone disregarded for ages, proprietors now experienced a therapeutic epiphany and saw that their springs were actually cure-alls. From Waukesha, Wisconsin (Corinnis Waukesha Water promised to "restore natural functioning to the organs of elimination") to Mineral Wells, Texas (both Texas Pal-Pinto Crystals and Dismuke's Pronto-Lax eliminated "toxic poisons from the system"), hitherto humble springs were recruited to the battle against autointoxication. But it was French Lick, Indiana that made the most of its healing waters. Latterly known as the hometown of basketball immortal Larry Bird, French Lick enjoyed an earlier fame as a spa. Indeed, it was a spa reminiscent of Harrogate, for French Lick too had sulfureous water, which, an 1833 visitor to the town complained, "emits a very strong offensive odour, and is exceedingly loathsome." Nevertheless, once the French Lick Springs Hotel was opened in 1840, invalids beat a path to its doors. Business boomed, and soon trains from Chicago, St. Louis, and other midwestern cities were being sent on regular runs to haul the sick to French Lick. But like Harrogate, there was a steady shift in French Lick's orientation, from therapy toward recreation. During the Roaring Twenties, the spa was best known for speakeasies, casinos, and brothels, not wholesome and healing springs (Al Capone found the atmosphere of French Lick so agreeable, he considered holding a wedding reception at the local hotel). The town achieved something of a return to respectability during the thirties, but in the ensuing decade steadily abandoned the spa business to dedicate itself to hosting conventions.[27]

Three of French Lick's springs were on the grounds of the hotel, and one of them, the Pluto Spring, was tapped for bottling by the hotel's owner in the late 1890s. But although the Pluto Spring contained both Epsom and Glauber's salts, hence was naturally purgative, Pluto Concentrated Spring Water contained considerable quantities of those same compounds added at bottling. Its potency, in other words, was not to be questioned, and partly for that reason Pluto Water quickly established a secure foothold in the purgative market; within 25 years it became one of the top six sales items in American drugstores. But as with other successful patent medicines, Pluto sold less because it worked than because it was backed by ingenious and inescapable advertising. Its label and all its ads were graced by a little red devil representative of Pluto, god of the underworld (from whence the water flowed). The water was promoted directly to physicians through booklets ("America's Physic") and letters reminding them that "in these days of nervous stress and strain, sedentary life and the automobile," constipation was a near universal problem; that "every intelligent physician recognizes . . . the role of auto-intoxication in the causation of disease"; and that "there is no purgative that will so thoroughly empty the intestinal tract in a shorter time and with as little discomfort" as Pluto Water. "Each day that you practice," doctors were told, "you need a reliable 'colon cleanser,'" and only Pluto Water could gurarantee "a clean alimentary tract from esophagus to anus." Free samples, of course, accompanied each letter.[28]

Pharmacists drew a large share of attention from Pluto promoters too. The company advertised in all pharmacy trade journals ("PLUTO will move off your shelves as fast and as satisfactorily as it removes disturbing intestinal accumulations"), supplied druggists with attention-getting window displays, and provided them with informational brochures to pass out to customers drawn inside by the little red devil in the window. But the public at large bore the brunt of the Pluto marketing offensive. "Constipation was strongly entrenched when Pluto Water entered the lists to combat its disease-breeding grip on the American people," a 1927 booklet stated. But now the water was "eradicating this wide-spread malady," overpowering "intestinal stagnation—the penalty of civilization." And while it was about it, Pluto was annihilating another of civilization's insults: fat. "How to Slenderize the French Lick Way," a booklet issued in 1932, maintained that while dieting and exercise were important measures for getting rid of excess weight, "remember, first of all, that CONSTIPATION is our enemy. You cannot expect the desired results from your reducing program," readers were told, "if the intestinal tract is clogged with body waste." Presumably that was also why a "Pluto highball" was the best method of all for dealing with a hangover.[29]

Pluto's effects and its high visibility made it a popular item for jokes, such as the story of the drugstore handyman whom the pharmacist left in charge of the shop while he ran a short errand. When the pharmacist returned and asked if there had been any sales, the substitute replied he had sold a bottle of Pluto Water to a customer looking for a good cough syrup. Informed that Pluto Water was not intended for coughs, the handyman answered, "I told him to take a half a glass every half hour. After three doses," he guessed, "he'll be afraid to cough!" The Pluto Corporation discontinued bottling the water in the late 1940s and now manufactures cleaning products.[30]

Meanwhile, numerous other mineral waters fought with Pluto for a share of the market. Ads for these are to be found in the American Medical Association's archives, many clearly deserving of the classification "Fake File" with which they're stamped. Sleepy Salts, for example, assured users that their daily "intestinal bath" would allow them to "Drink All the Beer [You] Want—Yet Lose Fat or Keep Slim." Sleepy Salts was also one of the host of mineral waters claiming to be radioactive, but even that mystical property paled beside the cosmic powers of Heal Rays Mineral Water, which was drawn from a well that had been revealed to its proprietor by an angel.[31]

The Harrogate model of autointoxication therapy had emphasized intestinal lavage equally with oral ingestion of mineral water, and that approach was also widely imitated. Introducing water into the rectum in order to empty it had been a standard medical practice since at least the days of the pharoahs ("enema" is derived from the Greek for "to throw or send in"; the same meaning in Latin gave birth to "injection," an unambiguous synonym for enema up to the mid-1800s, when the introduction of the hypodermic syringe gave injection its modern signification). The enema, or clyster as it was also commonly known, remained a popular form of self-treatment for constipation through the nineteenth century. Even Queen Victoria, the very model of propriety, made such demands of her injection equipment that her druggist could hardly keep the royal instrument operational; his account books contain "monotonously frequent" entries for "An Enema apparatus repaired," "Enema apparatus rep^d," etc.[32]

By the end of the 1800s, however, a New York physician could comment that "many persons" had become "constant slaves to the *enema*, the only substitute which they know for the pill." If people did in truth become enslaved to the enema at that time, it was because the fear of autointoxication drove them to look for any measure that might clear their bowels of putrefying waste, and because a small army of mountebanks seized the opportunity to entice them into trying clysters instead of cathartics. Indeed, it was precisely as a substitute for the pill that enema devices came to be promoted so successfully as cure-alls during the early years of this century: by the early 1920s, a medical critic complained that enemas were being "used in season, out of season, internally, eternally and from everlasting to everlasting."[33] The enema could be presented not only as a natural and nonirritating way of clearing putridity from the intestinal tract but also as a painless means of freeing the bowel from dependency on stimulating drugs and allowing it to return to normal function.

"The employment of drugs to relieve an overcharged colon is both unsatis-factory and unscientific," Dr. Charles Tyrrell wrote in *The Secret of Health With-out Drugs*. "Stimulants to defecation are like the applications of the whip to the jaded horse . . . the reaction is diastrous in the extreme." The proper way to dis-charge the colon—nature's way—was "Washing It Out," he stated; to put it "in plain English, the preservation and restoration of health depends entirely upon cleanliness, especially *internal cleanliness*." Elsewhere, he harangued readers to acknowledge that "You're Not Healthy Unless You're Clean Inside," and for that kind of cleanliness, there was only one answer, the enema *non pareil*, "the greatest discovery of the age": the J. B. L. Cascade.[34]

Charles Tyrrell should have known something about health, having had to regain it so many times. Born in the south of England in 1843, he set off at an early age to see the world, traveling to India and China in the 1860s, Australia and New Zealand in the 1870s, returning to the Asian continent (China and Japan) in the 1880s, and along the way spending 2 years in South Africa. He claimed to have "circumnavigated the earth three times," and everywhere he went, illness and injury followed. He was "once dangerously wounded in cutting out a nest of Chinese pirates on coast of Formosa, 1864," suffered "bullet wounds" from an-other, unspecified, adventure in China 3 years later, was ill with jungle fever for 4 months in India, with typhoid for 6 months in Australia (was also "once ship-wrecked on coast of Australia"), and had bouts with "paralysis" in both China and New York. That last attack was the turning point of his life. Arriving in Manhat-tan in 1889, Tyrrell immediately suffered a financial reverse, which led to "men-tal worry" that "induced another attack of my old enemy." Finding himself com-pletely disabled on his left side, he called doctors in, but they "proved powerless to help me." Now looking for help from any quarter, he came across a hygiene handbook by A. Wilford Hall, a lay healer who amassed a small fortune over the last decades of the century dispensing enema therapy. "Being an earnest physi-ological and hygienic student" (hence aware of the budding autointoxication theory), Tyrrell had a go at what he would soon be calling the internal bath. "The result was magical." Within 2 months, he was "on the road to health," what he would soon be calling *The Royal Road to Health*. All that was needed was some "patient and tireless experimenting" with the conventional enema bag, to transform it into the perfected Cascade, then patent it and manufacture it for sale in 1894. From that point on, he was (like his inspiration Hall) on the royal road to wealth.[35]

Thousands were to follow him down that road. But were they in the train of a well-meaning (if overzealous) physician, or were they, as the AMA maintained, blindly following a quack? Tyrrell did have medical training, graduating ("with honor," he boasted) from the Eclectic Medical College of New York in 1900 (though he had been identifying himself as Charles A. Tyrrell, MD, for some years by then). He usually went by "Professor" Tyrrell as well, and it is partly this air of self-importance, the narcissistic creation of a public persona calculated to sway the masses through image rather than content, that gives the professor away as ultimately a charlatan. However genuine his belief in internal bathing may have been, Tyrrell possessed all the other qualifications of the classic quack. He took a pathological theory that enjoyed some degree of scientific standing and public circulation and inflated it into a comprehensive explanation for all the ailments of mortal flesh, supporting his claims with selective quotations from medical authorities while simultaneously translating abstruse medical pronouncements into the language of lay common sense. Doctors have recently discovered that germs cause disease, Tyrrell pointed out, and that intestinal germs cause autointoxication. Doesn't that just corroborate what everyone already knows intuitively, that it could not be healthful that the human gut ("this scent bag of filth") "should always be so full of putrid matter that we cannot abide one moment with it"? The mere thought of it, and "the mind shrinks in dismay, and shudders at the possibility of the 'human form divine' becoming such a peripatetic charnel house."[36]

Creating aesthetic revulsion, making people queasy at the thought of hauling about their scent bags of filth, would no doubt sell a fair number of enema bags. But serious income lay in the generation of genuine terror. Like other quacks, Tyrrell put his warnings of threatened health into the hysterical language of impending doom. The deadly microbe's sphere of action "is absolutely without limit"; he (Tyrrell's selection of gender) is "one of the mightiest of conquerors. . . . He is a foe to be dreaded, . . . forever lying in ambush for fresh victims." And where he likes to lie most of all, filthy parasite that he is, is in the fecal matter in the colon, "a prolific hot bed" in which germs "multiply with the most marvelous rapidity, permeating every portion of the tissue—causing, in fact, DECOMPOSITION WHILE STILL ALIVE."[37]

The only point of driving people to the edge of despair for their lives, of course, is to miraculously rescue them with the one remedy in all of creation that can counteract the universal cause of disease, and that is available only from the salesman whose horrifying utterances have reduced listeners to a state of desperate credulousness. Typically for the trade, Tyrrell's remedy was "a simple device," yet a unique one, cleverly designed to cleanse the intestinal tract in a way no other therapy could rival: "the J. B. L. Cascade is entirely different from any other appliance, for 'flushing the colon,' that has ever been offered to the public." It was not just another enema, the traditional form of injection that required users to lie down while receiving water from a suspended bag, then get up again and make their way to the toilet without losing the contents of the rectum en route. The Cascade, rather, allowed the patient to sit, "in ease and comfort," while taking treatment. A 5 quart rubber bag shaped like an ordinary hot water bottle, the Cascade had a 2 inch–long rectal "injection point" protruding from its center, with a small handle projecting from the point's base by which the user could regulate the flow of water. A treatment involved nothing more than filling the bag with warm water, placing it on a chamber pot or toilet seat lid, and carefully situating oneself on the injection point. When the injection nozzle was opened, water was pushed into the user's body by his own weight, "without the slightest physical effort." Fluid supposedly entered "as a gentle, diffused stream, creating a slowly rising body of water that reaches every portion of the colon." Since the injection points were "so constructed, that the natural constriction of the sphincter muscle holds them firmly in position in the rectum . . . while affording the water free passage into the colon," one did not have to worry about leakage, not even "a single drop." In a matter of minutes (no more than 3 or 4, Tyrrell assured), the transfer of water from bag to bowel would be complete and the user could pull the deflated Cascade from under the body, rise and lift the toilet lid, then sit and discharge the fluid. Immediate discharge was not necessary, however (nor premature discharge a risk), since "the warm cushion" of the Cascade "soothes the system and allays any desire to expel the water." The internal bath could be prolonged well beyond the time limits of the conventional enema, in other words, giving the bowel a much more thorough washing. That was the reason for naming the device the Cascade, to indicate its quantitative superiority to the old fashioned enema, which had long been known familiarly as the fountain syringe. Why lie under a fountain when you can sit on a cascade?[38]

Formally, the instrument was the J. B. L. Cascade, because it was the dispenser of "Joy, Beauty, Life," of all earthly satisfactions whatever. The cure, after all, had to be made equal to the disease, to be lauded with the same exaggerated buncombe that had been used to delineate the terrors of germs and autointoxication. "Its regular practice . . . will give firmness to the tissues, elasticity to the step, color to the cheek, and sparkle to the eye": these were the Joy and the Beauty of internal baths. And the Life? The Cascade "will positively CURE ANY DISEASE"—any disease, that is, "that is not absolutely beyond hope." Tyrrell was not above hedging his bets by admitting not every patient would recover, though still implying that in such cases it was the patient's fault, not the Cascade's. Simultaneously, he made the most of the quackish stratagem of encouraging customers to see disease in every sensation they experienced. Irritability, depression, pain in the lower back, tenderness in the joints, shortness of breath after exertion, headaches, coldness of the extremities, and any number of other everyday discomforts, including the bowels not moving "AT LEAST once a day," were identified as sure signs of autointoxication and of the immediate necessity for an internal bath. Even pregnancy was treated as pathology ("for then intestinal action is always obstructed"), and "well-nourished offspring, . . . easy delivery and rapid recovery" were promised as benefits of the Cascade. The internal bath might actually help one get pregnant, for the maiden who took one regularly could be confident of "a purity of complexion, and a symmetry of form" that would make her "fair and pleasing in the eyes of men." Needless to say, perhaps, the Cascade was indispensable as well for young girls on the brink of puberty and older women facing menopause: in both cases, if internal baths were enjoyed frequently, "the change will scarcely be noticed." Tyrrell was hardly being immodest, it would seem, in promising "lady readers, that they cannot possibly have a better friend than THE J. B. L. CASCADE."[39]

One did not have to take Professor Tyrrell's word for it, though, for, like the multitude of patent medicine hucksters, he counted on satisfied customers to recruit new ones through the submission of testimonials. These were, of course, unanimous in their praise of the Cascade as " a wonder beyond comprehension," "ALL you claim for it," and "something [one] could not be hired to dispense with." "It works like a charm," one correspondent bubbled; "whether one weighs 90 lbs. or 250, it gets there and does the work." Certainly it did the work for Mrs. M. Cutaiar ("I passed a mass of slime and corruption"), for the Rev. J. H. Baird (it rid him of "dark faeces that looked as though it might have been in me for years"), and for an unnamed gentleman who "got rid of an immense amount of putrid foul decaying matter that was clogged hard and fast to the walls of the colon." Nor was the work always so offensive. A man who had been "so bad with rheumatism that I was not able to dress myself for sixteen weeks" purchased a Cascade, took a few internal baths, then got a job teaching school, and soon after "went to Mason City, Iowa, and got married."[40]

Still another indication of charlatanism was Tyrrell's creation of an array of products and services to supplement the Cascade, his patent determination to squeeze every penny possible out of the internal bath. First, however suitable ordinary water might be for external bathing, it would never do for the inner variety. Even the best tap water contained germs, buyers were advised, so unless one wanted to add still more microbes to the swarming masses already infesting his colon, one needed to purify the Cascade water with Tyrrell's Celebrated J. B. L. Antiseptic Tonic ("the most perfect antiseptic and germ-destroyer in existence"). So perfect was the Tonic that it killed germs in the colon as well, striking at the very root of autointoxication. Finally, it applied a healing effect to the walls of the intestine: it "soothes away irritation caused by germ attacks, and tones the muscles to new health" (toned intestinal muscles, of course, were more resistant to constipation). Because of the crucial importance of the Tonic, "I have arranged to make it as inexpensive as possible," the philanthropic Tyrrell offered, selling it "in one pound air-proof cans" for a mere one dollar ("by mail twenty cents extra"). Its composition was conspicuously shrouded in secrecy, of course, an even surer indication it must possess wondrous potency. Not surprisingly (from Tyrrell's viewpoint), the envy of organized medicine over so extraordinary a remedy could not be contained, and eventually a sample of the tonic was whisked off to the laboratories of the American Medical Association for analysis. Only then was it learned that the ravages of autointoxication could be forestalled by combining roughly 12 ounces of table salt with 4 ounces of borax. With a drop of food coloring thrown in, the ingredients of a can of tonic cost nearly a nickel.[41]

Then there was Tyrrell's Rectal Soap, an olive oil–based product ("especially made in Italy") sold "in the form of sticks tapering toward one end," apparently meant to lubricate the anus before exposing it to the injection point. Tyrrell sold a regular Health Soap too, both for cleaning the skin and for use in shaving (one hopes it was differently shaped, so not easily mistaken for the Rectal Soap). He sold a J. B. L. Catarrh Remedy, for sufferers of inflamed nasal cavities and respiratory passages, and even an Ideal Sight Restorer, an instrument that looked like a pair of binoculars designed by a plumber and operated by establishing a partial vacuum over the eyeballs. Though attacked by the American Medical Association as extremely dangerous, the Sight Restorer was advertised as just the thing for every visual problem from nearsightedness and astigmatism to cataracts, glaucoma, and crossed eyes. Even after Tyrrell died in 1918, his company, Tyrrell's Hygienic Institute, continued in business, selling the Cascade on through the 1940s and introducing still more health aids. J. B. L. Lubricant was an improved version of the Rectal Soap, J. B. L. Pile-Ease was a hemorrhoid ointment, the J. B. L. Inhaler cleared stuffy noses, and J. B. L. Nasal Balm healed them. Finally, there was Jabel, "a scientifically correct douche powder for feminine hygiene" that one could also "sprinkle . . . on sanitary napkins to dispel embarrassing odors. Think of the relief it is to know that you are not offending!"[42]

Purchase of a Cascade automatically enrolled the buyer in the Tyrrell Hygienic Club ("Motto—Health and Happiness"), with the perquisite of free consultation for any health problem with one of the expert medical staff at Tyrrell's Hygienic Institute in New York. Furthermore, for every friend a member persuaded to buy the Cascade, the member was awarded the choice of a pound can of Antiseptic Tonic, two boxes of Rectal Soap, or four cakes of Health Soap—gratis. The Cascade itself cost $10 originally, going up to $12 in the 1920s, and the company paraded it before the public with all the ingenuity and persistence of the proprietary laxative manufacturers. Pharmacists, for instance, were provided with booklets, "Why We Should Bathe Internally," to distribute to customers ("They read it, all right, and come back to buy"), and were relentlessly badgered with appeals to give central window space to the 3 by 4 foot sign asking passersby, "Did You Ever Take an INTERNAL BATH?" "These striking displays," druggists were informed by Tyrrell ads, "have drawn crowds, modern sophisticated crowds, who, hardened by experience to every type of advertising appeal, yet have stopped and looked, read—and bought a $12 item in surprising numbers" (Fig. 5-1). The pharmacist was practically guaranteed he would sell at least one Cascade a day,

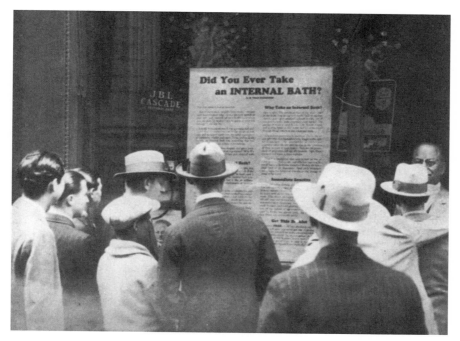

Figure 5-1. New York pedestrians attracted to a window display for the J. B. L. Cascade [from *American Druggist*, July 1928, p. 61].

"including Sundays," with "a man sized profit" in each sale; and if that weren't enough, he could also request a free Cascade for his own use.[43]

Avoiding drug stores was no solution to escaping the Tyrrell advertising barrage. The company mailed "Why We Should Bathe Internally" to private homes, along with a two-page letter that offered recipients the hope of "a new and fuller life" for just $12.30 (the 30 cents was for postage). Consumers who resisted could count on receiving a lengthy follow-up letter in a fortnight, explaining "that you have a constipated condition of which you may or may not be aware, and that you are suffering from one or more of the various disorders that often have their origin in a sluggish bowel," and quoting a United States Senator in support of the Cascade. If that didn't get the hoped-for response within a month, a third letter would be sent presenting "a special offer," an installment plan that allowed one to get the Cascade right away for only $7.30; the remaining $5.00 need not be remitted until the following month.[44]

"The administration of rectal enemas by means of the J. B. L. Cascade is not only unscientific, but may in many cases be dangerous." That was the oft-stated opinion of Arthur Cramp, head of the American Medical Association's Bureau of Investigation, which received numerous inquiries from physicians and lay people alike regarding the value and safety of the Cascade (Cramp retired in 1935; inquiries about the Tyrrell product remained frequent through the 1940s, and one was received as late as 1984). It was expert medical opinion generally that repeated enemas were irritating to the bowel and caused chronic intestinal health problems. Tyrrell's encouragement of people to take enemas routinely, therefore, was advice that "is mischievous to the point of viciousness. The 'enema habit'," Cramp tried to convince the public, "is just as harmful as the 'cathartic habit'," so much so that, to cite another physician's view, "there is no one who is more to be pitied than is the person who is a slave to the enema habit." But even those who were aware of medical warnings, Andrew Vena, for example, were hard to persuade. "For 30 years I have never gone to bed without a perfectly clean colon," an aggrieved attorney wrote Cramp, thanks to "the internal bath"; and, he added with a jab, "I am 64 years old, enjoy perfect health."[45]

To the extent an enema relieved constipation, it no doubt did make the user feel better, even if it did nothing to combat the imagined horrors of autointoxication. Further, people must have wondered, if the Cascade was so bad, why were there so many other products of virtually identical design on the market, all of them selling well, too? There was the Davol Self-Administering Internal Bath ("Best of its Kind. . . . makes the Internal Bath easy, safe and cleanly"), Hunt's Internal Bath ("Auto-Intoxication Doomed at Last"), The Eager Intestine Cleanser ("Compel it [the colon] to perform its duty"), and Williams' Alimentary Douche (subtitled "Natures' [sic] Assistant," it cleared the intestine of "encrusted feces, blood and pus, worms and worm eggs, and, in some cases, maggots"; it had the further advantage of being less "cruel" than competitors, as "it will not break off in the rectum, as other tubes have done"). Cramp's opinion was the same for all makes of internal bath: they were only "a slight modification of a similar humbug exploited by Tyrrell of New York," and "just as potentially harmful" as that humbug.[46]

Not to be overlooked was the Internal Fountain Bath: "My Dear Dr. Jamison," a grateful patient wrote, your Fountain Bath "is simply the best of the best." With respect to convenience, perhaps, the enema device constructed by Alcinous Jamison, MD, New York City, was the best, even though it was never promoted as successfully as Tyrrell's product (not that Jamison didn't try his utmost to frighten the public into purchases: autointoxication turns "the body of nearly every human being" into "a pest-house of absorbed poison . . . from the day of the diaper to that of death"). The advantage of the Jamison Fountain was that the 5 quart rubber bag was horseshoe shaped. With its middle open, the Fountain could be placed directly on the toilet seat instead of the lid, allowing the user to irrigate, then immediately defecate by lifting his body off the injection point (attached to a rigid handle inserted between the legs), pulling the point to the front of the toilet, and sitting again. It was a cycle a person could go through "as many times as one desires without rising from the sitting posture." For people such as A. L. Leubuscher, veteran of more than a quarter-century of twice-daily enemas of the old type, the Internal Fountain was a godsend. "Without rising from the toilet seat, I take from six to twelve injections," he reported, using them as "provokers, relieving the bowels instantly each time."[47]

The Internal Fountain was as versatile as it was efficient, being recommended also as a hot water bottle, a foot warmer, a pillow, and an invalid seat, as well as a vaginal douche (a vaginal "point" was standard equipment, and easily substituted for the rectal nozzle). The equipment was sturdy too: "Whoever your rubber manufacturer is," a customer complimented Jamison, "he certainly is a good judge of rubber." The man had used the device "roughly and persistently," and at "225 pounds, I have given it a very severe test," yet it remained "in first-class working condition." Far more important, of course, was that it put its users into first-class condition (as long as they closely observed Jamison's advice to "gargle" their bowels after each meal). Gratitude for health recaptured resounds through the testimonials submitted to Jamison, and at times breaks out into visions of an entire species rejuvenated. "You have struck the keynote of . . . the healthfulness of the human race," he was told. "A child born of parents who have used the rectum and colon as a fecal storage-house for years cannot be healthy. Its blood and tissues are stamped with the fecal taint as well as with the features of the parents." But just imagine, the writer proposed, "a child born of parents free from any . . . poison and filth from the intestinal canal! Think of a race of men and women free from ancestral fecal taint"—and keeping themselves free of acquired taint by regular use of the Fountain. "Crime and evil-doing will diminish," and the internally cleaned race adopt "a higher and more refined conception of . . . social and spiritual duties."[48]

That anyone could imagine moral salvation to be simply a matter of bowel sanitation suggests how firmly internal bathing captured the autointoxication phobe's fancy. But the internal bath was only one sphere of modernized enema therapy. Just as large was the realm of colonic irrigation, a practice that was essentially the same in purpose—to fill the colon with water—but that employed much more elaborate equipment, and consequently was not amenable to self-treatment. Colonic irrigation required practitioners administering a procedure, rather than manufacturers peddling rubber bags and nozzles. Despite the convenience and privacy afforded by Cascades and Fountains, there was such demand for "colonics" that physicians of the day could describe it as a "rage" and a "fetish": "it seems to have come to such a pass that . . . the citizenship may readily be divided into two distinct groups—those who wash their colons regularly, and those who do not."[49] Not surprisingly, irrigationists flocked to the field from all corners; from the conscientious MD who still believed in autointoxication but wished to purify the bowel without harsh drugs, to the amoral quack who saw a bull market and grabbed it by the horns, an irrigationist of some stripe was never far from hand during the 1920s and '30s.

To many doctors, irrigation, which came into use at the close of the 1800s, seemed to be only a "glorified enema"; but proponents stressed that it served a completely different purpose. Whereas the enema involved merely the introduction of fluid into the lowest reaches of the bowel so as to stimulate the defecation reflex and empty the rectum, irrigation consisted of repeated rinsings of the entire colon with large volumes of liquid, "not to induce defecation, but to wash out material situated above the defecation area and to lavage the wall of the bowel as high as the water can be made to reach." Irrigation, or colonic lavage as it also came to be known, could be performed only after the rectum had been evacuated through the administration of drugs or an enema.[50]

That description makes colonic irrigation sound considerably simpler than in truth it was. As with the skinning of cats, there was more than one way to scour the guts (indeed, "the technic varies with nearly every individual" practitioner, one physician opined), and prospective irrigatees had quite an array of choices set before them. First, one had to select the particular model of irrigation apparatus, and there were many, each designed by an experienced practitioner along the lines he had found most efficient (Fig. 5-2). The basic principle of operation was simple enough: fluid from one or more reservoirs suspended above the table on which the patient rested was fed by gravity through tubing into the recipient's intestines, and eventually expelled into a waste container (the best appliances were connected directly to a drain to the sewer). But the Dierker apparatus used a single reservoir, while the Vattenborg apparatus employed three, and still more variations were to be found in the Schellberg, the Borosini, the Honsaker, the Springfield, the Studa, and other designs, including the most strenuous sounding of all, the Gymnacolon. So elaborate were some lavage machines, with such awe did they strike patients, that "they doubtless carry with them a psychotherapy [effect]," doctors recognized, and jested that whether it cured autointoxication or not, irrigation purged anxious patients of neuroses. (Psychoses were favorably affected as well, at least according to a Massachusetts physician who administered "upwards of fifteen thousand colon irrigations" to mental patients during the early 1930s for the "sedation" they accomplished. Typical was the manic-depressive woman who received 835 irrigation treatments between 1930 and 1935; by the end of the regimen, "her manic episodes are less violent, she is tidier in her habits and more moderate in her language.")[51]

The position assumed by the patient during the irrigation was a second matter of differing opinions. Some advised lying on the left side, some on the right, and many recommended the knee-elbow posture as best for "allowing possible kinks to open up and permitting the inflow of the injection fluid." Just what that

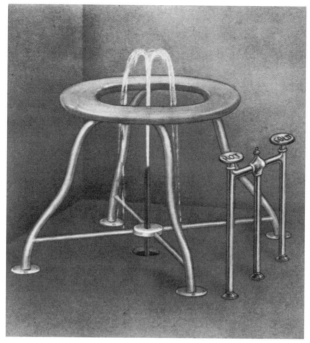

Figure 5-2. A version of the ascending douche for intestinal lavage [from Samuel Gant, *Constipation and Intestinal Obstruction*, p. 258].

fluid should be was still another item for discussion: plain water was the most popular choice, but some irrigators, in certain situations, recommended a weak solution of either table salt or baking soda, and/or various antiseptic compounds, including hydrogen peroxide, potassium permanganate, and silver nitrate. The volume of fluid varied from one practitioner to the next. One or two quarts per irrigation was the standard range, but some patients "boast of their ability to inject as much as two gallons into their bowels. They are to be pitied." Another concern was the temperature of the fluid, for though most practitioners agreed that it should be at or a bit above body temperature (as high as 104°F), the fact that they so frequently had to remind other irrigators not to use too hot or too cold a mixture, as well as to deliver it at low pressure, suggests that on occasion patients received more of a jolt than expected from their colonic. Even an uneventful treatment typically took from half an hour to an hour.[52]

Finally, an issue of much interest to patients, and of much contention among practitioners, was that of the so-called "high irrigation" method versus the "low irrigation." Some operators claimed to achieve lavage farther up the bowel by means of maneuvering a long delivery tube all the way to the beginning of the large intestine. The standard length of tube was 52 inches, though skeptical physicians charged some operators with using tubes "of length sufficient to irrigate all the way from Dan to Beersheba." That required a technician with "an educated touch that guarantees . . . extreme gentleness," but in such an operator's hands, the tube could be passed "to the cecum in less than five minutes as a rule, . . . with absolutely no discomfort to the patient." Most physicians laughed at such statements, maintaining that the tube could not be pushed past the acute angles of the intestine, and would simply curl up in the lower bowel. Other physicians acknowledged that with some models, the tube could be manipulated through the colon by a skilled operator, but denied that anything would be gained by the procedure. A tube inserted only 3 to 4 inches into the rectum would deliver fluid all the way to the cecum if the patient were placed in the proper position (lying on his side with knees drawn up). There was, in short, no difference between the supposedly "high" irrigation and the common variety: "such misleading terms" as high colonic, one of the most respected authorities on irrigation demanded, "should be abolished." Indeed, others suggested, the long tube itself, not just the terminology, should be abolished, as a threat to patients. Having more than 4 feet of tubing forced into one's intestines could not be a pleasant experience: "One's sympathy goes out . . . to the patients on whom the beginner attempts to gain the necessary practice and skill."[53]

One hopes there was enough sympathy to go around for clients of the short tube too, for they also ran risks. From nausea, cramps, and anal irritation at the mild end of the side effects spectrum, to bleeding hemorrhoids, abrasions of the intestinal wall, and tears of the rectal valve at the other, a number of untoward reactions could result from even this less-intrusive form of irrigation. Furthermore, there was considerable skepticism within the medical profession that any good ever resulted from the procedure. By the 1930s, most physicians no longer believed in autointoxication, and doubted that real gastrointestinal problems would benefit from lavage either. The majority demonstrated a "prevalent tendency to ridicule" that frustrated irrigation's proponents, they "frowned upon" colon cleaning, and "generally regarded [it] with a feeling of irritation." It was mere "colonic calisthenics," one doubter joked.[54]

Snide dismissals of that sort—and they were common—betray an emotional overlay on the objective medical evaluation of lavage. Even the most sober and fair-minded physicians found it difficult to be dispassionate about colonic irrigation and evaluate it purely on its merits, because of their anger at the rampant exploitation of public gullibility by bowel purity hucksters. There was a "monstrous fad," in one outraged MD's words, a "racket," in another's, of "commercialized irrigation specialists" and "conscienceless fakers" operating "colon filling stations" and "colonic laundries." "It is not unusual," one physician observed, "to find under the plate glass of the dresser in a hotel room a card on which these colon experts announce their willingness to lavage the colon before the guest retires." Colon specialists ran a wide gamut in terms of credentials, from opportunistic members of the profession ("self-styled 'gastro-enterologists'") who presided over "elaborate suites of offices with one or more 'colonic lavagatories'," to the well-meaning but misguided lay person ("sometimes a nurse, sometimes a widow, or sometimes simply a member of the great army of the unemployed"), to "the out-and-out charlatan" who lured dupes in from the street with colon-cleaning contraptions of such imposing design (tubes, stop-cocks, drains, lots of glass and chrome) as might win the admiration of Rube Goldberg. In all categories, there was "thriving business."[55]

One of the most thriving businesses was the American Colonic Institute in Chicago. The windy city had more than its share of colon laundries, the Chicago Institute for Colonic Therapy, the Intestinal Bath Company, and the McNemee Method of Colonic Irrigation and "intestinal normalizing" being just three that gave the Colonic Institute a run for the public's money; there was also a National Institute for Colonic Therapy, owned and operated by the same people who ran the American Colonic Institute (the latter was located at 5 North Wabash, the former a block away at 5 South Wabash). Chicago physicians were, of course, quite upset by this proliferation of irrigation establishments (as were the MDs of New York, Philadelphia, and just about every other American city): "This 'new' colon therapy rests on no basis of fact," one complained, "is employed by none of the country's leading gastro-enterologists, and is permitted in no institution of recognized standing. But, Chicago must fall in line as a 'progressive' and have its 'Institute.' Barnum was right!" Doctors' derision hardly bothered the American Colonic Institute. From its headquarters on North Wabash Avenue, the Institute sent out regular personally addressed mailings to area physicians urging them to refer their "patients suffering from chronic intestinal stasis" for the "prompt relief [of] colonic therapy": "We are equipped with modern apparatus and facilities to give colonic irrigations in a scientific manner." That was what they all said, of course, but the Colonic Institute said it best when it came to articulating the era's turn of mind with respect to sickness. In its booklet "Colon Therapy," a freely distributed advertisement masquerading as science, the firm's "Medical Director" quoted the ominous words of Victor Hugo on the ultimate dependence of human happiness on the erratic humor of the bowels. "The serpent is in man," the novelist wrote. "It is the intestine. The belly is a heavy burden; it disturbs the equilibrium between the soul and the body. . . . It is the mother of vices. The colon is king."[56] Colectomies, purgatives, and internal baths were not the only methods of appeasing the king, however; they were, sadly, only the beginning.

The Culture of the Abdomen: Physical Therapies

THERE ARE PEOPLE, and they are many, . . . who hoard their feces as a miser hoards his gold. A certain amount is daily and laboriously given to the world, but, in comparison to what remains behind, the amount is mean, physiologically insufficient and therapeutically ineffectual. When young, these people carry their avarice upon their earthy, oily and pimply faces, in middle age they become anemic, scant of breath, exiguous of skin and abdominally opulent. Old age they never reach.

People who were intended by Nature to surpass the Psalmist's three score years and ten, fall victims to their own colons at fifty or even under. . . . It is only the very fittest who can support into middle life a system by which the image of the Deity is converted into a hot-bed of human manure.

Leonard Williams, 1917, 1918

PEOPLE . . . need to be told that their skin marked with liver blotches, their pudgy abdomens, rheumatic joints and disorganized liver secretions and many other ills . . . have their source in a great majority of cases in ignorance of abdominal hygiene.

Charles Campbell and Albert Detweiler, 1925

San Franciscan S. F. Loughborough was yet another of the early twentieth-century's martyrs to constipation. In the space of just 20 months in 1903–4, he paid out $95 to doctors for their advice and evacuant drugs, and spent another $110 for patent medicine cathartics—to no avail. He was "robbed," he complained, "by ignorant pill prescribers" whose medications left him "worse off than when I began using them." Not only was he now more constipated than ever, all the straining at stool he had done in the interim had given him a severe case of hemorrhoids. But as is so often the case at the nadir of a person's existence, serendipity waited just around the corner. On his next foray to the Owl Drug Store, he came upon a set of Dr. Young's Rectal Dilators, a product advertised specifically for constipation and hemorrhoids. With nothing to lose but a few more dollars, Loughborough bought the set and commenced a course of dilation that very evening.[1]

An easy course it was not. The dilators, phallic-shaped and made of hard rubber, came four sizes to a set, graduated from 2 and ½ to 3 and ½ inches in length, and from ¾ to 1 and ¼ inches in diameter at what Dr. Young called the "bulb" (Fig. 6-1). They were not fundamentally different from the bougie, an instrument long used by physicians and surgeons to open constricted passages and known to stimulate the defecation reflex when introduced into the rectum. But the bougie was prescribed and administered by professionals for a very limited range of conditions; Young's and other rectal dilators were presented directly to the public with encouragement to self-prescribe the device for virtually every ailment, and then self-administer it. Dilator self-treatment began with the application of vaseline, or better, Dr. Young's Pile Ointment ("the very best thing to use as a lubricant") to the smallest of the instruments, then the assumption of the colonic irrigation position (lying on the side, knees drawn up) and the careful insertion "well into the rectum as far as the flange [at its base] will admit it." One had to hold it in place a few seconds, "until the inner sphincter grasps it," but after that it should be effortlessly retained for the 30 to 60 minutes recommended as morning and evening sessions. Contrary to intuition, Dr. Young maintained there was no cause for a person to worry about moving around after the dilator had been put in place, and since the dilator was "a good promoter of natural, refreshing sleep," no harm would come if the user dozed off before his evening half hour had expired (though presumably that would eliminate the need for a morning treatment). To be sure, one should anticipate some mild pain at first: the Rev. Hezekiah Cook "could hardly stand it to insert the small one" when he began treatment, "and could not endure it more than five minutes. I thought I must give it up, for it made me so sore." But over the course of a week or two, the rectum would adjust to the foreign object, and the user could then move up to the next size, though "it will greatly aid and be less difficult to introduce [the larger dilator] if the next smaller size, well lubricated, is always first taken and inserted and withdrawn several times" to loosen the sphincter. Rev. Cook, it is a relief to learn, was soon able to retain the dilator for an hour, and steadily worked his way up to the largest in intervals of 2 to 3 weeks.[2]

Despite these assurances of safety and comfort, Dr. Young acknowledged that some customers' first reaction to the sight of the dilators was panic, fear they would never be able to accomodate the largest. Nevertheless, he reiterated, "every normal adult of average size should be able in time to insert the largest size without discomfort," and some might even want to take on the "Extra Length" dilator, 5 inches long and more than an inch and a half thick at the bulb (there was

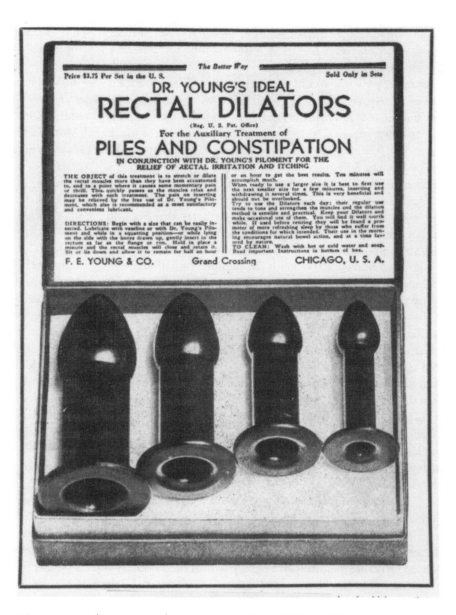

Figure 6-1. Advertisement for Dr. Young's Rectal Dilators [from *Nature's Path*, December 1938].

also an "Infants Size" dilator for sale, as well as a set of four "tubular" dilators; though of regular size, these had a hollow tube running through the core "as a vent for passage of gas"). Yet even after the most formidable of the inserts had been tamed, patience would still be required. "Do not expect the dilators to always overcome in a few week's [sic] time what has been caused by years of neglect and abuse of drugs [cathartics]," Young advised; "Be faithful and Persistent," he urged, and expect 6 to 10 weeks to pass before intestinal health would be restored. The Rev. Cook had faith, and though he had been taking cathartics every day for the past 5 years, to ease constipation so terrible he had "sometimes suffered like a brute" even while using the drugs, his bowels began moving regularly just the second day after his adoption of the dilator. No wonder the dilators came with a money back guarantee, a guarantee that not only would they cure, but they were "practically indestructible" as well.[3]

Mr. Loughborough had no cause to ask for his money back. Like Rev. Cook, he improved immediately. With the regimen of half an hour of dilation at bedtime, and another half hour in the morning (while he shaved), he regained his health in only 6 days: "I find that my piles have been cured, so far as pain is concerned, . . . and my bowels are as regular as government pay." His vigor overall, in fact, was "like that of a frontier buck," so one can understand why he swore that "ten thousand dollars would not tempt me to sell my set if I could not get them duplicated" (Hezekiah Cook specified only $100 in gold as the amount that would not tempt him to sell). Why, Loughborough wondered, "will poor, suffering, sallow humanity suffer the ills and agony produced from this constipation, when such a simple remedy that will not burn up and ruin the intestines" was readily available? Suffering humanity clearly needed enlightenment, so with his newfound vigor, Loughborough became an evangelist, spreading the good news of the dilators about the streets of San Francisco, ultimately interesting "no less than 110 different people in buying them."[4]

That a person would start and end each day with a half hour of rectal dilation is a telling measure of the early century's autointoxication anxiety level. It's an indication as well of the variety of remedies human ingenuity devised to meet the emergency: surely the rectal dilator would have been resorted to only after all other conceivable measures had been tried. In fact, exercise, massage, electrical stimulation, and yet other remedial categories were tested by the public in the early 1900s, there being such a hodge-podge of physical agents and procedures that the following recounting of them is almost certain to cause confusion at times. In truth, if the account is not somewhat confusing, I will have failed to convey just how bewildering were all the options available for satisfying Dr. Young's fundamental dictum of health: "We live," he pontificated, "by peristaltic action."[5]

Rectal dilators (Dr. Young's was hardly the only brand) worked, supposedly, by restoring muscular tone to a rectum grown flaccid by inactivity. Other muscles needed to be toned too, though, specifically those of the abdomen. It was not just that they supported the intestinal organs against gravity's deforming traction (Lane's analysis), but more that "a sound abdominal wall" pressed, even squeezed the colon. "The intestines are muscular tubes," and "muscular tissue responds to the stimulus of massage or kneading." It was through the steady grip of the stomach muscles that the gut was "wakened into activity," that "the propulsion of the bowel contents" was assured, and that "stagnation is prevented." It was widely agreed that to a considerable degree, constipation was "attributable to lack of abdominal muscular activity."[6]

"Whoever heard of a constipated Indian?," one expert on costiveness asked in 1934. He was thinking, of course, of Native Americans of earlier centuries, for pre-civilized races generally were presumed to be physically noble savages, free of constipation and autointoxication, and in large part because of the active life they led. Running, riding, hunting, even gathering tensed the abdominal muscles repeatedly, whereas "atrophy of the abdominal muscles produced by want of exercise" was the status of urban man. Urban woman was even more inactive and soft, despite the early-century increase of participation of girls and young women in athletics. "I cannot allow my daughter to grow up a tomboy" was the far too common attitude of mothers, doctors complained; and though the non-tomboy girl might seem "angelic" to parents, she "will soon be with the angels is the forecast of the physiologist," and largely because of stasis in unexercised intestines. All health advice books insisted that an essential component of the battle against constipation was daily abdominal exercise, devotion to what was often called "the culture of the abdomen."[7]

That phrase paid deference to a popular health movement known as physical culture, the early twentieth-century's campaign to encourage exercise for all aspects of well-being. Physical exertion had always been regarded as a hygiene requirement; it was one of the non-naturals, after all. But during the 1890s, as the unrelenting expansion of city life seemed to portend the elimination of all physical activity beyond writing reports or balancing account books, a widely based determination formed to promote cultivation of the muscular body as the primary source of health. Physical culture took many shapes, from weightlifting for strength, to calisthenics for energy and endurance, to bodybuilding for beauty. For Bernarr Macfadden, it took all those forms. Strongest claimant to the title of father of physical culture, Macfadden (1868–1955) was the Jack LaLanne of the first half of this century (indeed, one of Macfadden's star pupils, Paul Bragg, would become the physical savior and mentor of LaLanne). A weakling as well as an orphan during his Missouri childhood, Macfadden took up dumbbells and distance walking to gradually build himself into the very model of vitality and muscularity. By the 1890s, he was sharing his hard-won secrets of health with all who would attend him as a self-appointed professor of "kinesitherapy," and at the end of the decade expanded beyond his New York base to gain national attention as the publisher of *Physical Culture* magazine. An innate entrepreneurial talent quickly blossomed, and by the 1920s Macfadden was both the author of numerous books on health (*Vitality Supreme*, *Virile Powers of Superb Manhood*, *The Power and Beauty of Superb Womanhood*, to name but three) and the head of a huge publishing empire that churned out true romance, true crime, and other sensationalist magazines in addition to all the volumes on physical culture.[8]

The first man ever to become a multimillionaire by urging people to strain and sweat ("Inactivity is non-existence. It means death. . . . Why not throb with superior vitality? Why not possess the physical energy of a young lion?"), Macfadden included much more than exertion in his philosophy of health. Non-stimulating diet, fresh air, sunshine, sleep,—all the other non-naturals figured into physical culture (his program was, in fact, a revival of Grahamism, except that he regarded sexual indulgence as a path to fitness rather than frailty; sex, Macfadden maintained, was one of the most beneficial forms of physical activity, and his wives attested that he practiced what he preached).[9] His cornerstone, however, was exercise, so when he addressed the question of evacuation and the self-poisoning of the body by uneliminated waste, it was to exercise that he looked for the cure.

"If you are constipated, BEWARE," Macfadden advised on the dustjacket of his 1924 opus *Constipation*; "constipation is the greatest breeder of disease. If you don't kill it, it will kill you." Like other autointoxication theorists, he attributed virtually every illness known to intestinal poisoning, even managing, thanks to his preoccupation with sex, to find a link with uncontrollable libido. Because the feces-expanded bowel pressed heavily upon the adjacent organs of generation, it produced "an irritation which is readily mistaken for . . . passion," Macfaddened confided, adding that "the amount of rape and murder which in this way may have been clearly the result of constipation, is . . . probably far beyond our wildest speculations." At the minimum, it was curious, he mused, that "crime always increases with civilization, and the artificial conditions, rich diet and physical degeneration that go with civilization."[10]

A bulky diet would help to prevent fecal accumulations, Macfadden counselled, but "the real cause of constipation in virtually every instance is the want of vital vigor of the structures and tissues involved," in brief, "muscles . . . lacking in tone." To restore tone, he recommended not only the obvious daily repetitions of sit-ups, leg lifts, and trunk-bending movements to strengthen the abdomen but also a series of a dozen exercises that supposedly stimulated the "nerve centers" that controlled the organs of the digestive tract (Fig. 6-2) (many of these exercises were concentrated on the lower back, in an attempt to activate the spinal cord to higher activity; *Constipation* included 42 pages of photographs of different exercises to prevent costiveness). "Jumping one to two hundred times, as when jumping a rope," could be counted on to combat constipation also, as could slapping of the abdominal muscles for 5 or 10 minutes, "making the blows strong without

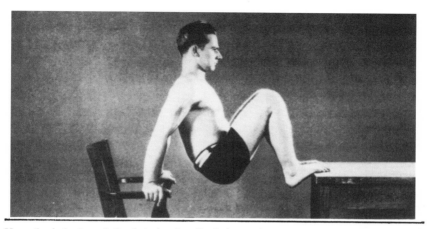

Move the body toward the feet, keeping the body vertical and giving considerable pressure by the thighs into the abdomen. A small pillow may be placed between the abdomen and the thighs to secure greater pressure.

Figure 6-2. One of Bernarr Macfadden's exercises for strengthening the abdominal muscles to guard against constipation [from Bernarr Macfadden, *Constipation*, p. 233].

causing pain." An even more direct workout for the intestines was "the sand cure," which involved the swallowing of 3 to 6 teaspoons of sand (rounded, not sharp-edged, was specified) daily until the constipated gut had been stirred to action. A glass of water was advised for making the sand go down, and "though it is rather unpleasant to have grains lodge between the teeth," Macfadden granted, "all the granules disappear in a short time." Finally, exercise of any kind that induced perspiration was, by Macfadden's way of thinking, a means of purifying the blood, hence undoing the effects of constipation.[11]

Macfadden's books were big sellers, and *Physical Culture* enjoyed one of the highest circulations of any magazine in America. But one did not have to read Macfadden or any of the other physical culturists (and they were legion) to learn that exercise strengthened the body against constipation. Toning of the abdomen was standard advice in the mainstream medical literature on constipation, too. Whether physicians believed that constipation caused deadly autointoxication or simply chronic discomfort, they saw in exercise an effective way to cure and prevent costiveness (Fig. 6-3). "Weak abdominal muscles are practically always associated with intestinal stasis," the authors of *The Lazy Colon* informed the public; "ignorance on this subject is widespread and most disastrous in consequences." They followed that warning with a list of 10 stomach-strengthening calisthenic exercises to be performed daily. Other authorities recommended their own workout programs, everything from similar calisthenics, to goose stepping about the house, to "jumping about the room by a series of short and quick jumps in a squat-

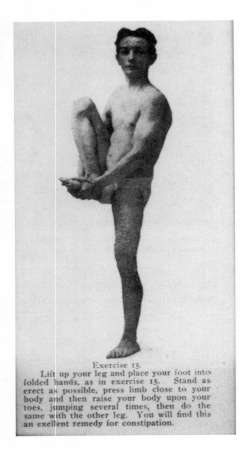

Exercise 15.
Lift up your leg and place your foot into folded hands, as in exercise 15. Stand as erect as possible, press limb close to your body and then raise your body upon your toes, jumping several times, then do the same with the other leg. You will find this an exellent remedy for constipation.

Figure 6-3. Another exercise to prevent constipation [from W. Hubert-Miller, "Physical culture at home," In: *The Naturopath and Herald of Health*, 1904, p. 79].

ting posture"; every abdominal toner from frenzied twistings and turnings while seated in the kitchen chair, to picking up "with much stooping and stretching a big handful of marbles or buttons flung over the floor and under furniture," to driving an automobile over rough roads. Englishman F. A. Hornibrook, author of a book-length *Culture of the Abdomen*, devised a program of exercises specific for constipation that was modelled on the body movements common to the dances of primitive cultures (and was performed to the accompaniment of phonograph music). English constipates could also try Maxalding, a system of "Abdominal-Control Feats" developed by a muscular Londoner named Saldo. The procedure seems to have involved alternate flexing of right and left abdominal muscles (muscles that had been strengthened to Herculean levels by exercise). Saldo and his son even sponsored a "muscle control competition," with a "magnificent silver cup and gold medals" going to the winners. In short, exercise was so frequently recommended as a constipation cure, even some purgative manufacturers recast the image of their products into drugs that gave the intestines a workout instead of a cleanout. Thus Cascarets ("they act like Exercise") claimed not to roughly purge the intestine but to "*strengthen* and stimulate the *Bowel* Muscles instead. . . . A Cascaret acts on *your* Bowel-Muscles as if you had just sawed a cord of wood, or walked ten miles." Physicians, meanwhile, did not limit their recommendations for exercise to books and magazine articles. One of the most outspoken opponents of the routine use of purgatives, for example, gave his constipated patients a page from his prescription pad with not a single drug scribbled on it; instead, there were predrawn stick figures doing sit-ups, push-ups, and prone "bicycling." This physician "considered the sheet put to better use than if I had ordered a large section of our Materia Medica."[12]

The sheet was put to full use, of course, only if patients had the motivation and discipline to follow the exercise prescription. Many did not, or else felt too debilitated by their costive condition to muster the energy. For these cases, passive exercise was the answer, in the form of massage; in the words of one physician, massage was the exercise remedy for "invalids too feeble for self-help." The practice of rubbing and kneading muscles and soft tissue to relax and revitalize is doubtless as old as creation, and was a respected component of ancient medical practice in Asia as well as Europe; Hippocrates and Galen were just two of the classical authorities who recommended massage as a form of gentle exercise. During the nineteenth century, however, massage expanded into an independent system of therapy in association with various "movement cures" (particularly "Swedish movement") derived from gymnastics. This modern massage therapy had established itself on the Continent by the mid-1800s, but not until the 1880s did it gain a secure foothold in Britain and America.[13]

Massage in the late nineteenth and early twentieth centuries employed four basic techniques, commonly identified by their French names: pètrissage (kneading), effleurage (friction), tapôtement (percussion), and vibrisage (vibration). All could be applied to the treatment of constipation, a condition that was easily viewed as a simple physical obstruction that might be pushed out of the way by the application of pressure in the right direction and of the right magnitude. Nineteenth-century massage therapists thus administered various combinations of pètrissage, effleurage, etc., to relieve intestinal sluggishness. And for those who could not or would not afford a professional masseur, there was always the cannonball massage. A frequently recommended procedure, this required, in the words of a Canadian pathology professor, "that they should beg, borrow, or steal a small cannonball and roll it morning and evening for so many minutes over their abdomen." If rolled up the right side of the abdomen, across the top and then down the left side, the ball, it was believed, would stimulate peristalsis; the effect was reinforced by the coldness of the metal, which imparted a tonic jolt to the muscles.[14]

Initially, massage therapy met with determined opposition from the medical profession: "both it and its innovators," an English physician remarked in 1910, "were relegated to the realms of quackery." This was in large part due to the long history of quacks promoting themselves as specialists in the cure of particular ailments (cataracts, for example) or in the use of a single therapy (skeletal manipulation in the form of "bone-setting" had been regarded as a quack practice for centuries). Massage was specialization in that second sense—one treatment for a multitude of problems. Some of its pioneer practitioners, furthermore, were so exuberant in their claims of efficacy as to seem no different than patent medicine touts, while there were also complete amateurs who appointed themselves masseurs and proceeded to give the whole field a bad name through their incompetence. More restrained massage therapists did gradually succeed in getting an objective hearing from the medical establishment, and convincing many physicians that their methods were useful adjuncts to conventional therapies. By the 1910s, massage had, in fact, become "one of the most active mechano-therapeutic agents," and thereafter, at least into the 1930s, discussion of massage methods applicable to constipation was to be found in most medical works on costiveness. In the eyes of proponents, it was "one of the few chances of curing this very distressing complaint."[15]

Different practitioners employed different techniques for massaging constipation away. One example, to provide some idea of how therapy was administered, is the method recommended by an English physician of the 1910s: "The whole abdomen is treated by small circular frictions with moderate pressure, the skin moving with the fingers. Deep stroking of ascending and descending colons is then performed, an occasional break being made for vibration over various parts of the colon. . . . [The treatment] must not now be other than slow, gentle and rythmical, and the vibrations must be well spaced." A variety of other procedures, including some outside the category of slow and gentle ("sacral beating," "gluteal hacking," "concussion of the vertebral spines . . . with a suitable hammer"), could be used to supplement the basic technique of "colon stroking."[16]

Techniques by which a constipated person could massage himself were also regularly provided in manuals for the laity. Thus the physician author of *Intestinal Management* outlined the technique of "internal visceral auto-massage," a "wonder-worker" that was to be used just before defecation to stimulate the intestinal tract into action. Standing with shoulders thrown back and arms to the side at shoulder height, the patient was to "lift the diaphragm as high as possible," then "rotate the hips as rapidly and as forcibly as possible, right and left, six to eight times. . . . This motion swings the bowels considerably from side to side," Dr. Stemmerman explained, "opening kinks and thus facilitates the movement of the contents forward to the exit." A second stage of automassage followed, begun after the patient was seated on the toilet, that required repeated contractions of the abdominal muscles. (Among Macfadden's exercise recommendations, incidentally, were various methods of self-massage of the abdomen.) Even the cannonball was still being suggested into the 1920s, either in its original, uncomplicated version (using a ball as heavy as 25 pounds in some recommendations), or in technology-assisted forms such as the Zander machine ("available at most sanitoriums"), on which the subject "lies face downward, the abdomen resting on a loose leather diaphragm, beneath which a ball set in motion by a motor follows the course of the colon, giving continuous upward pressure." By now, however, the majority medical opinion about cannon balls was that they were too heavy, applying so much pressure that "the colon is frequently sagged out of place." More suitable, it appears, was the Rallie Health Belt, a heavy rubber belt with three thick rubber bands attached to each side; taking the handles at the end of each set of bands, the user stretched the bands out and back, much like a spring chest exerciser, squeezing and massaging the abdomen with each pull.[17]

The colon may also have been sagged out of place by the Kolon-Motor. Attachable to the wall of any room, the Motor featured a round projection that vibrated against the user's abdomen when he turned handles mounted on either side of the equipment. "Every Home Requires This Machine," ads encouraged; "It does away for all time with . . . purgatives, cathartics and other artificial and habit-forming remedies." But the Kolon-Motor was only one model of a host of massage machines. Some were, like it, the inventions of get-rich-quick charlatans, but many more were developed and used by well-intentioned practitioners of massage. Vibration therapy, as it was commonly called, gradually evolved from massage therapy from the 1860s onward, as medical inventors explored ways of rubbing and stimulating body tissues without engaging the expensive services of a masseur. Wooden rollers and slappers (Klemm's Muscle Beater, for example) of various designs were introduced for patients to use on themselves, then more elaborate pieces of manually operated equipment that made a rod or plate (generally of metal or rubber) move back and forth against the body. By the beginning of the twentieth century, electricity had been harnessed for running vibrator machines, and the equipment was in use for stimulating all parts and systems of the body, and treating nearly all diseases (also in use were vibrators run by water pressure and compressed air).[18]

As autointoxication theory took hold, vibra-massage (another name for the discipline, as was, briefly, seismotherapy) was expected to perform its most valuable service as a cure for constipation. The focal point of treatment, naturally, was the abdomen, it seeming obvious that intestinal activity might be stimulated by vibration of the tissue supporting the bowel. Various machines were used, some employing vibrators, or vibratodes as they were known to practitioners, that moved in an up and down direction, others vibratodes that moved to and fro, or rotated, percussed, or oscillated. (The most popular form of the "oscillator" was the ma-

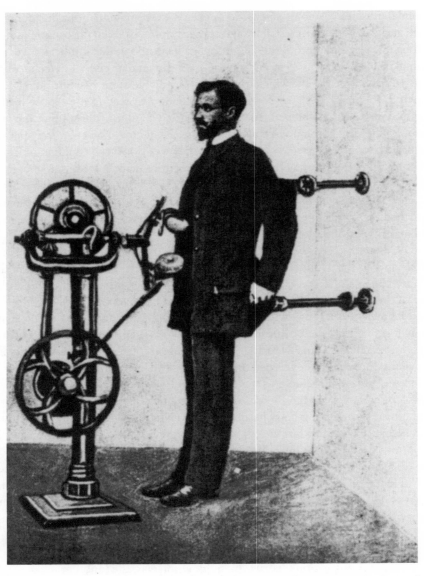

Figure 6-4. Abdominal massage machine [from Samuel Gant, *Constipation and Instestinal Obstruction*, p. 281].

chine with a belt that ran around the user's midsection and gave a "quivering or shaking motion [that] stimulates the colon to renewed activity.") All those applications were made to the lower back as well, to stimulate the nerves that connect to the intestines. Vibratode speed and pressure could be set at different levels, and length of time of application could be varied to adapt the therapy to each patient's needs. In the form of such large machines as the Zander horse (an ancestor of the mechanical bull of recent, urban cowboy vogue) or such versatile instruments as the Chattanooga vibrator, the technology could become more than a bit intimidating. If used according to instructions, though, vibrators must have worked more often than not. The unhappily named Veedee vibrator (modelled after the classic egg beater but with a flat disk at the end of the beaters) was typical in advising purchasers to supplement the Veedee with daily exercise, fruits, vegetables, whole grain bread, and attempts at defecation at a set hour every day.[19]

Lest vibratory treatments seem wholly agreeable, it needs to be noted that they were not limited to external applications to the abdomen and spine. "Lively peristaltic movements" could be stimulated even more surely by application of the internal rectal vibratode. The tool "should be well lubricated," manuals reminded, and "introduced while in motion" (if turned on after insertion, it was apt to create a physical shock or even injury). Three to five minutes of vibration was normally required, both for the standard model (5 or 6 inches in length), and for the 15 inch flexible rubber vibratode required for "very obstinate cases." Another way of dealing with obstinate cases was the vibrating colon tube (up to 2 feet in length) that fed a quart or more of warm water into the bowel as it shook the tissues about; alternatively, warm olive oil might be introduced through the vibrating enema. Among the most obstinate of all cases were those in which the patient's anal sphincter was so tight as to require relaxation and widening before the rectal vibrator could be used. A special pyramidal vibrator head was applied to this purpose, "employed, with fairly rapid speed, and full stroke, for five minutes daily," until the sphincter yielded. On average, most cases of constipation could be cured, proponents believed, "in a few weeks time." In the interim, however unlikely it may sound, rectal vibratory treatment was "absolutely painless, harmless, and productive of the most gratifying results," though only, vibration manuals admitted, "when carefully administered."[20] Perhaps Dr. Young's Rectal Dilators were not so drastic a recourse after all.

Vibrators ran on electricity. Other devices dispensed electricity, delivering current directly to the abdomen in order to promote its physical culture. Electrotherapy had been around in a crude form since antiquity, when torpedo fish and other electrified marine life were sometimes employed to shock the sick. It was not until the mid-1700s, however, that medical electricity began to expand as a field, when the recently discovered phenomenon of static electrical discharge began to be administered to the paralyzed, the epileptic, the blind, and many others who, medical common sense suggested, might benefit from a sudden infusion of electrical energy. There were many failures with the new electric treatments, and many of the claims of cure were dubious. There nevertheless were enough cases of apparent improvement after electrical shock therapy to justify continued experimentation, and before the nineteenth century had reached its midpoint, the discovery of first direct current, then alternating current electricity generated still higher expectations of benefits from electrotherapy. More and more complicated pieces of equipment were developed over the rest of the century, some no larger than a breadbox, others the size of a bed, and all replete with great tangles of wires and electrode attachments of whatever shapes needed to apply to every region of the body's exterior and insert into every one of its orifices. Therapists boasted that their machines could deliver electricity in any number of forms: static, galvanic (direct current), faradic (alternating current), galvanofaradic, sinusoidal, static induction, or high frequency. Textbooks devoted exclusively to electrotherapy were commonplace by 1900, medical electricity departments had been opened in hospitals, and professional associations of medical electricians had been organized. When at their peak of influence in the 1880s and '90s, the practitioners of electrical stimulation were treating just about everything with their equipment, but especially neurasthenia and gynecological problems.[21]

Professional support for electrotherapeutics was beginning to ebb by 1900, however. Since neurasthenia was losing status as a pathological entity, and surgery was suddenly much more effective at dealing with gynecological conditions, medical electricity's area of application was shrinking. The field was also being discredited by the excesses of quacks exploiting public fascination with, and gullibility over, the mysteries of electrical technology of all sorts. The sale of home electrotherapy equipment, and of "electrical" belts, girdles, vests, genital supporters, hats, etc. constituted one of the most profitable categories of the proprietary health device business around the turn of this century. Yet professional electrotherapists' own excesses were probably more damaging. Overzealous predictions of electricity as a near panacea had resounded through the last quarter of the nineteenth century, and as evidence failed to come forth to support expectations of cure, medical electricity's status shrank. It nevertheless maintained a limited position as an adjunct to other therapies, and in that capacity found use as a treatment for autointoxication.

From the very beginning of therapeutic experimentation with static electricity, in the mid-eighteenth century, it had been observed that diarrhea was sometimes produced by electrification. But that was an unpredictable result and a systemic effect, independent of where the discharge or current was administered. By the beginning of this century, stimulation of bowel activity had been refined to a science. Textbooks devoted separate chapters to the alleviation of constipation and the prevention of autointoxication, and rationalized success with theories of activation of nerve pathways, stimulation of mucus secretion in the colon, and even tightening of loose abdominal muscles. There were, of course, numerous variations in technique for achieving these effects, but generally what was involved was the application of two electrodes (positive and negative), one to the abdomen, the other to the lower back. The former would be moved slowly over the colonic tract, from the cecum, up the ascending colon, across the transverse, and so on to the rectum: "the current should be strong enough to cause distinct though not violent contractions of the abdominal wall," electrotherapist Elkin Cumberbatch explained in his 1920s text, and the procedure should be done repeatedly for at least a quarter of an hour.[22]

To that point, electrotherapy for constipation sounds no more frightening than acupuncture does today. But improvement did not always result from the basic method, and if after a month or so of treatment the patient was still costive, more direct stimulation was indicated. "The electrode which is applied to the back," Cumberbatch instructed, "should be replaced by another which is passed into the rectum." Rectal electrodes were standard equipment with all electrotherapeutic machines (they provided electric clysters, in some practitioners' terminology), and were perhaps what another constipation specialist had in mind when he observed that electricity "frequently appeals to the patient [because it] makes him feel that something definite is 'being done'." He must have felt the same comforting assurance when he took a galvanic bath. There was a powerful temptation to combine electro- with hydrotherapy, and there resulted numerous procedures in which the patient sat or reclined in a tub of water while electrical current passed through it: "the current is gradually turned on until a feeling of discomfort is complained of," one text explained, and then it was left on for 15 to 20 minutes.[23]

Unelectrified baths contributed to the culture of the abdomen, also. Cold baths presumably acted as a tonic to the system and encouraged intestinal activity; warm or hot baths sedated the tensed muscular fibers, relaxing them so that feces could advance more easily. Douches in the form of showers or more forceful streams of water directed against the abdomen, lower back, and perinuem were recommended for constipation relief; one practitioner's "ascending douche" came with both hot and cold controls to regulate the temperature of the water the user drove against her perineum. Additionally, hot and cold compresses and packs could be applied to the abdomen to stimulate the system or to soothe an irritable bowel.[24]

"The rapidity with which 'mineral oil,' . . . has conquered the globe," a contributor to the *Journal of the American Medical Association* marveled in 1919, "has been phenomenal. It is now a most extensively used medicinal substance." Arbuthnot Lane deserved much of the credit for the phenomenon, through having championed paraffin oil so energetically. But the patent medicine industry had not stood idly by, and by the end of the 1910s, any number of brands of oil derived from petroleum had been brought to market as constipation cures. They were, of course, promoted with all the same advertising hysteria as purgatives (Nujol's "internal cleanliness" campaign will be recalled from Chapter 4). But mineral oil was not properly thought of as a cathartic. Odorless and tasteless, it was also chemically inert, so did not irritate intestinal tissue or cause cathartic colon. Paraffin oil, or liquid petrolatum, as it was usually referred to in the United States, operated by a simple mechanical process of softening and increasing the bulk of the stools. As Nujol ads put it, oil "promotes natural, healthy movement." Physicians agreed, thinking of its action as falling into the same category as exercise or electricity: oil stimulated and facilitated the normal workings of nature, and so helped restore the natural culture of the abdomen. One brand of oil even named itself Hyginol.[25]

There was no shortage of other brand names (a "half hundred," was one physician's guess), but nearly all identified themselves additionally as belonging to one of three categories: American oil, Californian oil, and Russian oil. American oil was a relatively light, or low-density product, derived from the lower-molecular-weight hydrocarbons, and refined from crude oil produced in states other than California. Californian oil was considerably heavier, while Russian oil was put out in both light and heavy forms (Parke, Davis sold American Oil, Squibb Californian Oil, and Schieffelin Russian, among some of the major producers). Yet whatever the label said, most of the liquid petrolatum sold originated in California.[26]

Preferable as mineral oils were to chemical purgatives, however, they were not without drawbacks. "A disagreeable feature complained of by many," one clinical researcher found, was that there was "sufficient leakage from the anus to keep the neighboring skin continually in a greasy condition, and sometimes to stain the clothes." Indeed, leakage was a continual complaint ("most annoying," one set of oil guidelines called it), so much so that "does not produce leakage" was a required bit of false advertising for brands that wanted to stay competitive. Emulsified mineral oils were produced to obviate the leakage problem, and physicians sometimes recommended vaseline, an even more viscous petroleum product, as a non-leaking substitute for mineral oil. Many people found the texture of vaseline too disagreeable, and for that matter, even mineral oil was unpleasantly bland, and many had to sweeten it with honey or molasses or otherwise disguise it as in mineral oil mayonnaise for the dressing of salads. The stools produced by petrolatum were no more attractive, being "mushy, obviously greasy," and having "a peculiar odor described as sour." Nevertheless, some oil users became habituated, as dependent on their daily dose as if they were taking phenolphthalein or senna (as indeed sometimes they were, it being common practice to blend such laxatives with the oil). Thus an English physician reporting on cases at the end of the 1930s was able to cite a 38-year-old woman who had taken paraffin oil every other day since childhood, and a 7-year-old who had been given oil twice a day since birth.[27]

The list of methods for the culture of the abdomen went on and on. Intestinal antiseptics that supposedly killed the germs that caused autointoxication were an option. Indeed, Bouchard, the 1880s pioneer of autointoxication theory, had tried to disinfect the digestive tract with naphthol, and subsequently other researchers had tested several compounds. None had proven effective, though, and by the 1910s physicians were disparaging the administration of intestinal antiseptics as "frequently attended by disastrous results owing to their tendency to produce further irritation." Medical disapproval did not stop the commercial production of alleged antiseptics, of course, nor did it interfere with the marketing of preparations of bile, of various hormones or enzymes, or all of the above as stimulants to intestinal activity ("Pancrobilin supplies the physiological tools that Nature demands to assist her in functionating properly"; "Constipation, the physician's *bete noir* [sic], can be conquered by Pancrobilin"). There was even psychotherapy, strengthening the patient's mind to overcome his reluctant matter. From building up the constipate's faith that he truly could recover if he persevered, to motivating him to take time to attend to nature each morning, to eat right, and to exercise, to administering sugar pills that were described as strong cathartics—doctors worked on patients' psyches any way they could to effect a more positive frame of mind to counter negative bowel habits.[28]

Virtually all of the above methods of warding off autointoxication were employed by the numerous self-described "drugless healers" who appeared in the early years of the century. Various systems of "irregular medicine" (what lately we have been calling alternative medicine) had been developed in the nineteenth century as rivals to mainstream medicine, and all had put forward their own distinctive therapies for constipation (hydropathy, the treatment of all illness with water, had shown particular concern for costiveness). But the drugless healers of the early 1900s recognized in autointoxication an enemy demanding a much greater effort than predecessors had made. Most of the drugless clan also identified themselves as practitioners of naturopathy, a system of practice that grew out of hydropathy, as well as German water-cure and nature-cure traditions. Organized in the late 1890s under the leadership of German immigrant Benedict Lust, naturopathy sought to cure the full scope of human ills with natural agents (herbs, water, air, sunlight, electricity, massage, and others), agents that supported and stimulated the body's own natural healing mechanisms. Constipation and autointoxication were frequently addressed by naturopaths of the 1920s and '30s, founder Lust himself issuing more than one warning in the pages of *The Naturopath*, the widely circulated magazine he edited. Alarms sounded by other eminent practitioners ("constipation is a monster that slays more humans than all other causes known to science today"; most people "are perambulating cesspools, as vulnerable as a powder magazine"; "the decomposing waste in the 'sewer' of the average civilized man compares to vomit about as vomit compares to a bowl of fresh, fragrant vegetable soup. . . . Can we wonder why life becomes such a horrible nightmare to so many") were buttressed by advertisements in naturopathic publications for regulating foods, colonic irrigation equipment, vibration devices, electrotherapy instruments, and herbal laxatives. There was even a distinctively naturopathic laxative, Kneipp's Laxative Herbs Number Three. Sebastian Kneipp was a renowned late nineteenth-century German water cure specialist who first cured Lust, then "commissioned" him "to go to America and teach his system of Natural Healing." The "exclusive formula" for an all-natural laxative ("Know the Joys of Internal Cleanliness") was entrusted to Lust as well, who made it the stock intestinal remedy at the large naturopathic health retreats he ran in New Jersey and Florida, and sold it by mail order from his Original Health Food Store in New York City.[29]

Constipates determined to find a drugless solution to their troubles could also consider apyrotrophy and Ehretism, two dietary systems that were closely allied with naturopathy. Apyrotrophers ("unfired-fooders") had discovered that the application of heat to food denatured it and made it subject to inner fermentations that led to constipation and autointoxication. Eugene Christian, apyrotrophy's chief spokesman, awed readers of *The Naturopath* with his boast of averaging 1000 cures of constipation a year with raw fruits and vegetables. (Apyrotrophy has survived to the end of the century, today's raw food advocates disseminating their message through websites such as www.rawtimes.com., and still warning that "cooked foods clog the intestines and colon, leading to such ills as cancer and diabetes.") Arnold Ehret, on the other hand, touted the virtues of "mucusless" foods. The very first principle of his "mucusless-diet healing system" was that "*every disease*, no matter what name it is known by Medical Science, is *Constipation*." To be sure, Ehret's "constipation" could occur in any organ or vessel, in any part of the "pipe system of the human body"; it was simply an obstruction with waste matter—what he called "mucus"—derived from improper food. Mucus was by far the most common, however, and most dangerous in the intestines, and had to be combatted with non-mucus-forming fruits and vegetables, as well as purging whole wheat "mucuslean bread." Periodic fasts rounded out the system. Finally, naturopathy figured significantly in the treatments prescribed by Edgar Cayce, the notorious "sleeping prophet," who diagnosed patients through "readings" performed while he was in a trance. Many of the approximately 6000 clients on whom he did readings were found to be suffering with autointoxication and told to relieve their troubles with some combination of purgatives, enemas, massage, and special diet. Eventually Cayce established a referral relationship with naturopath Harold Reilly, sending more than 1000 patients to the Reilly Health Institute at New York's Rockefeller Center between 1930 and his death in 1945. The "Cayce-Reilly treatments," as they became known, purportedly worked wonders using colonics and castor oil. One autointoxicated woman began treatment with "so much gas I could have supported all of Con Edison. . . . By the end of the week I sang a concert and felt fine." Another, a physician's wife no less, was jaundiced from intestinal toxins when she received her first colonic; before long she "had to buy new lipstick because the shade of lipstick I had used to go with my yellow color looked terrible with my new white skin."[30]

Drugless healers' inclination toward dietary promotion of abdominal culture was paralleled by the solution to autointoxication presented by one of the early century's most prominent health reformers. Horace Fletcher maintained it was not what one ate, or whether it was cooked or not, but the physical process by which one ate it that determined if intestinal toxemia would develop. For Fletcher, it was the jaws that had to be exercised, not the abdomen; his approach to dealing with the germs of autointoxication was not to disinfect them or electrocute them but to starve them.

That is not to say the man starved himself, for contrary to the defining character of the species "food reformer," Fletcher was a *bon vivant*. Born in 1849, in Massachusetts, he began an extraordinary life of adventure by shipping out on a whaler at age 15; by the time he turned 50, Fletcher had circled the globe four times and pursued more than 30 distinct occupations. And through it all, whether training sharpshooters for the Japanese army, managing a New Orleans opera company, serving as Paris art correspondent for a New York newspaper, or sailing with a crew of Chinese pirates, Fletcher ate well. So well did he eat, that by the age of 40 his 5 foot 7 inch frame had expanded to an unwieldy 217 pounds, and life insurance companies were refusing his business. His health wasted (he had been an all-round athlete as a young man), he tried out various unorthodox "cures" over the course of the 1890s, but without success. He finally turned to hygiene for relief, but that, too, was at first unavailing, there being so many inconsistencies and contradictions among the authors he consulted. Only when Fletcher determined to find an answer through the use of his own reason did progress come.[31]

Starting from the premise that nature does not make mistakes, he proposed that any condition short of physical perfection must be the result of human transgression of natural hygienic law. Adding the premise that the physical basis of full health is proper nutrition, he next concluded that all bodily weakness must stem from improper treatment of food while it is still in the mouth, since once it's swallowed, food passes out of human control and into the hands of unerring nature. Fortunately, nature's intent as to how food should be treated in the mouth, that "three inches of personal responsibility," is evident in the sense of taste. Taste, Fletcher the dyed-in-the-wool gourmand argued, is put into food for human enjoyment, and nature intends every bite be retained in the mouth until the last atom of flavor has been extracted. The great source of human frailty, therefore, must be incomplete mastication of food, the swallowing of nourishment before it has been reduced to the state desired by nature and thus required by the body.[32]

An eminently practical man, Fletcher at once put his theory to the test, henceforth carefully chewing every single bite until all sensation of taste was withdrawn. On beginning the trial in June of 1898, he had a waistline of 44 inches; by mid-October, his waist had shrunk to 37 inches, his weight had dropped to 163 pounds, and he felt better than he had in years (the more conventional interpretation of this improvement in health is that the time required for complete mastication, and the accompanying jaw fatigue, greatly reduced the quantity of food he consumed). Further, in the process of losing weight, Fletcher had found a rationale: he had discovered that mastication built health because it prevented autointoxication. As food was chewed to pulp, he learned, it naturally flowed to the back of the mouth where, as the last bit of taste was released, it was suddenly and involuntarily swallowed. There was an innate swallowing impulse, Fletcher decided, that was nature's mechanism for taking over responsibility for food once preparation in the mouth was complete (complete mouth preparation could be an arduous process; a stalk of green onion once parried more than 700 chews before yielding to Fletcher's swallowing impulse, though with most foods fewer than 100 accomplished the job). Not every bit of food was swallowed, though, for often a small portion of nonliquefied sediment was left behind and had to be spit out. This was evidence, in Fletcher's terminology, of nature's "Food Filter," the power of the body to discriminate between nutritious and non-nutritious matter and reject waste before it was taken into the stomach.[33]

The most convincing evidence of the efficiency of nature's food filter occurred in the form of what Fletcher called "tell-tale excreta." It might seem on first thought that there should be no excreta to tell tales. If the food filter turned back any innutritious matter before it was swallowed, and if Fletcher was also right in assuming the food that was swallowed was completely digested and absorbed, no waste should reach the colon to be excreted. In matter of fact, some did. There wasn't much: the relatively small amounts of food Fletcher swallowed, and his preference for low-fiber victuals kept his intestinal contents to a minimum. He nevertheless did void excreta, but only on occasion (every 1 to 2 weeks was his schedule) and in small quantities (2 to 4 ounces). To Fletcher's way of thinking, that was not constipation, but the rhythm that nature intended for everyone. His stools, furthermore, were not composed of food waste (none had been swallowed), but detached particles of intestinal lining and condensed solids of digestive juices— "dandruff of the alimentary canal," he called it.[34]

His excreta told their tale, though, not by their frequency, nor by their quantity, but with their odor: "HEALTHY HUMAN EXCRETA," Fletcher exclaimed, "ARE NO MORE OFFENSIVE THAN MOIST CLAY AND HAVE NO MORE ODOR THAN A HOT BISCUIT." (Lest that seem an indefensible claim, he unblushingly presented an objective scientist's eye-witness description of two of his defecations, complete with testimony that they were indeed no more disagreeable than fresh biscuits.) Fletcher was never more eloquent than when rhapsodizing about the refined qualities of his own feces, never more vehement than when voicing his disgust with the "offensive excreta" voided by everyone else. The noxious odor of the products of most bowels told a story of inner putrefaction, of autointoxication, of "sewer gas," he said, permeating the bodies of hasty eaters. The absence of odor in his stools told a tale of no putrefaction, of no autointoxication to undermine the health conferred by nature.[35]

Fletcher bombarded the public with books throughout the first decade of the century, and was a very well-known figure not just in his own country but also in Britain. His recipe for health demanded unusual dedication, and on the surface seemed more than a bit eccentric; "Fletcher," Mr. Dooley said, "thinks so much iv his stomach that he won't use it. . . . Fletcher's idee is that th' human stomach is a sort iv little Lord Fauntleroy. If ye give it too much to do it will pine away." Fletcher nevertheless commanded careful attention because of the results he achieved for himself. Once he lost weight, "the Great Masticator" (his popular nickname) returned to the athletic endeavors of his youth, where, to even his surprise, he found he was able to carry out exceptional feats of muscular endurance with no program of physical training beforehand, and no effects of fatigue or soreness afterwards. Eventually his claims of extraordinary physical efficiency were tested—twice—by the professor of physical education at Yale, a physician whose scientific reputation was beyond reproach. In both tests, performed when Fletcher was 54 and 58 years of age respectively, he was put through the exercises required of university athletes, and performed "with an ease," the professor remarked, "that is unlooked for." Fletcher surpassed the records of Yale undergraduates for number of repetitions of contractions of various muscles against resistance, actually doubling the record in the test of his gastrocnemius (calf). "Mr. Fletcher performs this work with greater ease and with fewer noticeable bad results," Professor William Anderson summarized, "than any man of his age and condition I have ever worked with." It is no easier today to account for Fletcher's muscular endurance. He was quite exceptional, a "physiological puzzle," as a contemporary nutritionist called him (indeed, none of his followers were able to duplicate his athletic accomplishments, and at least one, a man who spent a year and a half Fletcherizing, experienced a decrease in endurance; his typing skills declined as well, but his ability at chess improved). Fletcher was not puzzled at all, though. His endurance was simply a sign of perfect physical efficiency achieved by the elimination of "putrid decomposition" from his alimentary tract. His strength came from the conquest of autointoxication.[36]

Fletcher also attracted attention through the social philosophy he erected upon his system of hygiene. His "Physiologic Optimism" promised not only greatly lengthened and more energetic life for individuals but grand improvements in living conditions for society as a whole as people were restored to a physiological state of nature. Physical health would generate moral health, and an economic system that had always rewarded greed and ruthless individualism would be transformed into a capitalism of courteous competition in which everyone could succeed, thanks to the physical endurance and efficiency bestowed by proper mastication.[37]

Fletcher's idealism, his hatred of economic and governmental corruption along with physical decay, and the emphasis he laid on both social and bodily efficiency won him a following among other progressive thinkers. Upton Sinclair, the socialist novelist, practiced Fletcherism for awhile, as did Henry James, who announced himself a *"fanatic"* for the regime and distributed copies of Fletcher's works to his London friends ("munching parties" were a popular diversion for the London elite for a season, with guests being expected to devote 5 minutes to the chewing of each bite; such fetes were common enough that *Punch* memorialized them in a cartoon showing a solemn group of "hygienic enthusiasts" slumped around a sparsely laid table "Working Out Their Own Salivation"). Yale economist Irving Fisher credited Fletcher as an inspiration for his founding of the Health and Efficiency League of America, an organization whose health education programs included advice to eat more slowly. John D. Rockefeller endorsed Fletcherism. And for every celebrity who took up careful mastication, there were many more who chewed away quietly beyond public notice (including, it was reported, some of the inmates of Sing Sing). Fletcher estimated that 200,000 Americans were attempting to follow his precepts by the 1910s, and even if that figure was inflated, and even though few managed to practice his system in all its rigor for any extended period of time, he did heighten public awareness of the need to eat more slowly and chew more attentively, and so helped wean Americans and Britons from the "gobble, gulp and go" table manners of the nineteenth century. The standard textbook of hygiene for high school and college used during the first half of this century, Fisher and Fisk's *How to Live*, continued to cite Fletcher as the discoverer of the importance of thorough mastication through the 21st (and last) edition of the book, in 1946. As one of his obituaries declared, "Horace Fletcher taught the world to chew."[38]

But if Fletcherism and all else failed, there were always those dilators, intimidating in appearance, perhaps, but fully reassuring in rationale. Dr. Young, the most prominent spokesman for the rectal dilation school of therapy, offered a most persuasive (to the lay person) explanation of why stretching the sphincter brought health. Backed by a diagram of the sympathetic nervous system that showed a great cluster of nerve endings in the pelvic region, his theory rested on the premise that any dysfunction or weakness in the rectum would pass through adjoining nerves to the solar plexus, the concentrated network of nerves behind the stomach, and result in "nerve waste." The solar plexus (alias the "abdominal brain," in Young's terminology) affects the action of the heart, and therefore circulation, so ultimately every organ and tissue could be injured by disturbances in the rectum. There were, Young admitted, other parts of the body that might disrupt the solar plexus, but "fully nine out of ten cases . . . may be traced to the lower bowel and its outlet."[39]

Tragically, there was one nearly universal form of rectal disturbance: loss of sphincter tone. In effect, that translated into constipation, for nature's method of maintaining proper tone in the rectum was "the stretching of these rectal muscles at least once daily by a natural movement of the bowels." Feces were nature's rectal dilators, the diurnal expansion they caused forcing the intestinal walls to develop muscle tone, thus insuring a fully functioning solar plexus. Since the constipated person's rectum did not get its daily workout, costiveness resulted sooner or later in sickness. Young did not deny autointoxication ("self-poisoning from the absorption of decomposing foodstuffs . . . explains many diseases and accounts for many deaths"), but to his way of thinking the fundamental problem with constipation was that it allowed the rectal sphincter to go lax. After all, if sphincter tone were restored through mechanical dilation, constipation would be relieved, normal regularity would return, and autointoxication would cease.[40]

It was absolutely essential, however, to relieve constipation by dilation instead of cathartics. If drugs were used for the purpose, they might rid the bowel of decomposing foodstuffs, but because purgative-induced evacuations were watery rather than firm, they would do nothing to restore rectal tone. Cathartics were "villainous," an "utter folly" that "play[ed] the very devil with the alimentary canal from swallow to sphincter," such that "every dose taken removes you that much further from a cure." Cathartics were not, in short, something to spend money on when dilators would actually cure, and cost far less money in the long run. Young nevertheless marketed his own brand of Laxative Tonic Tablets as "the Intelligent Treatment of Constipation"; mildly laxative rather than harshly purgative, the Tablets also possessed tonic properties, and were for use "in obstinate cases [of constipation], especially of long standing" to help get dilation therapy started. For most people, it should be added, constipation had a sequel. Because of the loss of tone occasioned by bowel inactivity, most sufferers also developed piles (hemorrhoids) at the anal opening due to poor circulation and the irritation of cathartic drugs. Young believed this injury to be so common, that he recommended thinking of the anus as the body's "pile bearing inch," and created both a Pile Ointment (lubricant and medicine in one) and Pile Tablets to soothe the damaged veins while the dilators restored rectal tone and health. If testimonials can be counted as truth, Youngian therapy worked as dramatically against hemorrhoids as against constipation. To cite just one case, a Baltimore man who had "suffered from the bleeding, itching and protruding piles for many years," who for "many days and weeks [had been] unable to attend to my business on account of the pain," who often "couldn't walk or sit," bought the dilators and was made new in a matter of days: "every man, woman and child." he enthused, "should have a set of Young's Rectal Dilators if they want to be relieved and cured of that terrible malady, the piles."[41]

R. H. Bragdon had a different prescription for every man and woman, indeed for anyone "who desires to be strong, well and happy, to grow old backwards and be energetic and successful." It was his own device, the "Safe and Sane System of Cure and Prevention of Constipation," the Sphincter Muscle Expander. "Do not confuse . . . with *Dr. Young's or any other* Rectal Dilators, which are *altogether different!*", Bragdon demanded, but the Sphincter Expander does not, in fact, sound that different from the Rectal Dilator. It came in three sizes instead of four (small, medium, large), and was made of enamel instead of rubber, but it was employed in exactly the same way as Young's product (for confirmation, see Bragdon's free booklet "Sphincter Muscle Expansion"), and cured everything just as quickly and certainly. There were, moreover, numerous other variations on the expansion/dilation theme that likewise differed only in terms of number of expanders and material of construction. There were aluminum dilators, for example, and—hard to believe they would have sold—glass ones. There were even wax dilators; people whose priority was saving money saw no reason why a household candle shouldn't work as well as any manufactured insert. At the other extreme were technologically advanced devices such as Benko's Adjustable Rectal Dilator, seven dilators to be more precise, that differed from one another only in length. "Adjustable" referred to the instrument's width, which could be increased considerably after insertion through a screw mechanism similar to that employed in the carpenter's vise. "Nicky" the Dilator Perfect ("your best friend") was comparably designed, while the Pneumatic Dilator relied on a rubber bladder that was inflated by hand squeeze bulb after insertion (Macfadden recommended treatment of "sphincter spasms" with a model that was similar except for having an attachment that made the bladder vibrate). Finally, Vestvold's Improved Photo-Electric Dilator was plugged into an electrical outlet so that the long metal cylinder could deliver infrared radiation to the colon and destroy the bacteria that caused autointoxication: "the discovery of these rays opens up a new field in the realm of deep therapy."[42]

To be sure, physicians sometimes introduced objects into the rectum in order to trigger the defecation reflex. The finger, the bougie, the proctoscope, even inflation of the rectum with air, oxygen, or carbon dioxide were employed for the purpose (Fig. 6-5). One prominent (and imaginative) gastroenterologist even poured marbles through the sigmoidoscope to get results. But it was one thing, doctors cautioned the public, for trained professionals to tamper with the rectum, and quite another for lay people to do such things to themselves. Proprietary medicine dilators were attacked by the medical profession not just for their nonsensical curative claims but even more for the dangers they posed to the user ("an

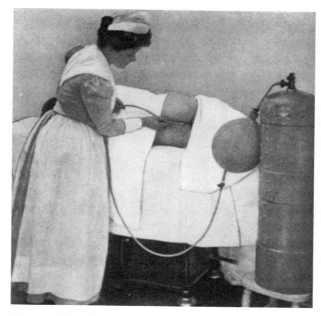

Figure 6-5. Administration of the intestinal oxygen bath [from Samuel Gant, *Constipation and Intestinal Obstruction*, p. 297].

instrument for self-torture," one doctor called it, "bequeathed to our time [by] the inquisition, . . . a device of Caliban"). When self-administered they could produce tears in the rectal wall, of course, but perhaps even more unsettling, they could be drawn into the intestinal canal. "I have seen more than a few dilators . . . which became lost in the performance of their duty," a physician reported, adding, unnecessarily, that such losses were "much to the distress and consternation of the patient. . . . The services of a physician will almost always be required" in such instances, he went on, "because frantic attempts to reach it [by the patient] will only cause it to travel further up the bowel." Yet matters could get worse. More than one practitioner came up against a case in which a glass expander broke while in use: "Naturally, the tedious recovery of the broken piece of glass was a matter of much mental and physical torture for the patient."[43]

The culturing of the abdomen generally, whether by dilator, vibratode, or sit-ups, might be understood as an early version of the no-pain, no-gain philosophy of muscular strengthening. There was, however, a less discomfiting approach, one that did not impose culture upon the abdomen, but rather introduced culture into it. That was one of the two major dietary prescriptions for the prevention of autointoxication that also won adherents in the early twentieth century.

7

THE CULTURED ABDOMEN: DIETARY PREVENTION

THE PERIOD OF PILLS is passing, and diet dawns instead, in hopefully hygienic hues, upon a welcoming world. . . . If human needs, in the breakfast line, can be reduced to health food and hot water, the millenium dawns broadly.

"The Spectator," 1902

THE CIVILIZED COLON is a poor cripple, maimed, misshapen, overstretched in parts, contracted in other parts, prolapsed, adherent, "kinked," infected, paralyzed, inefficient, incompetent. It is the worst abused and the most variously damaged of any organ of the body. . . . The civilized colon . . . is a Golgotha of pollution, a veritable Pandora's box of disease.

John Harvey Kellogg, 1918

One day in May, 1937, a young American woman answered her door to find a florist's delivery man there to present her with a dozen roses, and an envelope. "I am sorry," the note from her boyfriend began, "but I am sure you will understand." She didn't, of course: "She lay on the sofa and sobbed her heart away. Why was it," she cried to herself, "that she always just missed romance and marriage?" It surely wasn't her "looks and figure," which were the envy of friends. Yet she had been in "low spirits" of late, had felt "listless," "indifferent," "too tired to play up to her personality." Her eyes, in fact, had "lost their sparkle," and wrinkles were beginning to form on her face. No wonder, when she thought about it, the romance had been broken off.

Like "so many women," the ad for Kellogg's All-Bran declared, this one had failed "to realize the seriousness of common constipation." Fortunately, she had a girlfriend who was more enlightened and who "questioned her tactfully. Asked her about her habits." Thus it was discovered that the rejected woman's problem

167

was her diet, which contained insufficient bulk. "Get 'bulk' back into your daily meals," her friend advised; "correct constipation with a natural food." Start eating All-Bran for breakfast, and, the advertisement implied, it would be but a matter of time before a bridal bouquet would be in her hands, instead of "The Bouquet That Broke Her Heart."[1]

There may have been some consolation for this dejected woman in knowing that her problem was a nearly universal one in American and European society in the early twentieth century. Almost everybody needed to get bulk back into their daily meals. But that wasn't all that constipated people were missing from their diet, at least not if one believes the advertising campaigns of early-century food product manufacturers. There was, rather an extensive menu of items for people to choose from to protect themselves from intestinal toxemia. As the most popular choice, All-Bran and other breakfast cereals will be saved for last consideration. Before other choices are considered, however, one should be aware of the dramatic changes occurring in thinking about diet in general during the first third of the century. Hopes for the dietary prevention of autointoxication specifically were fueled by a broader optimism about the benefits to be derived from the scientific breakthrough hailed as "the newer nutrition."

As recently as a century before, selecting an invigorating diet had been the simplest of matters. In theory, at least, the essential food groups had numbered only three: breakfast, lunch, and dinner. Any and all items that went into those meals were supposed to contribute the same nutritive substance, a universal pabulum that physicians straightforwardly dubbed "aliment." But beginning in the mid-1800s, biochemists made steady progress in distinguishing the chemical components of foods and clarifying their roles in body functioning. By 1900, nutritionists had not only established the physiological uses of fats, carbohydrates, proteins, and several minerals but had also devised and refined methods for determining the energy values for each type of nutriment, the rates of metabolism of people engaged in different activities, and so much similar data that they were convinced they could now design ideal diets for all ages, sexes, and occupations. With good reason, they smugly referred to their science as "the new nutrition."[2]

Within 20 years, they were referring with even greater pride to a newer nutrition. During the first decade of the century, feeding experiments with animals had made it evident that diets that nutrition theory indicated ought to be entirely sufficient for health were, in fact, inadequate; they were missing something. In 1912, a Polish biochemist working in London discovered that something—actually, the first of several somethings—when he isolated thiamine, or vitamin B_1, the substance that protects against beriberi. Discoveries of other vitamins quickly followed, and it was soon apparent that a fully nutritious diet required not only the traditional macronutrients of fat, carbohydrate, and protein but also several wondrous new micronutrients. "The newer nutrition," a phrase that fairly reverberated through the dietary literature of the 1920s and '30s, expressed the boundless excitement that nutritional scientists felt over these discoveries, remarkable advances that had been made by their generation. "More actual knowledge has been acquired concerning diet in the past twenty-five years," an American physician rejoiced in 1933, "than in all the previous centuries of the life of man."[3]

New knowledge imposed new responsibilities, of course, and the newer nutritionists eagerly shouldered the burden of educating the public about the importance of expanding their eating habits to include the new nutrients. Elmer McCollum, the leader of the newer nutrition movement in the United States, estimated in the early 1920s that "at least 90 per cent" of the food eaten by most families was restricted to the old standards of white bread and butter, meat, potatoes, sugar, and coffee. Other experts and dietary surveys agreed that those were the staples of the American and British table, and joined McCollum in calling for large-scale dietary reform. Through school textbooks, popular nutrition guides, magazine articles, and newspaper releases, the principles of newer nutrition were broadcast throughout society. The public was inundated with nutrition advice, and exhorted to eat more of what McCollum called the "protective foods." "Vegetables," people were told, were "life insurance." "Children who drink milk," they were informed, "complete school two years before those who don't." And disturbing warnings were issued relating what happened to those who neglected the protective foods: in the words of a 1922 nutrition primer, "the man in the electric chair, waiting for that mysterious, invisible force to tear asunder the billion cells of his body that nature was years in building up is doomed with no more certainty than the man deprived of those mysterious substances called 'Vitamins.'" It was perhaps such images of dietary doom that motivated pupils in Fargo, North Dakota schools, who after only 2 years of newer nutrition education were eating 10 times as much spinach as before.[4]

Anyone who has struggled to get a child to give that vegetable any friendlier reception than E. B. White's "I say it's spinach, and the hell with it" will acknowledge the Fargo experiment as conclusive proof that the newer nutrition campaign did profoundly influence popular notions of diet. Perhaps it made too deep an impression: "The time may even come again," an American physician sighed in 1931, "when a six-months-old infant can nurse happily at his mother's breast without having to stop to drink orange juice and cod liver oil, and to eat spinach." The public's vitamin fixation was not solely the result of promptings by nutritionists, however; food producers and manufacturers sensed a bonanza in the newer nutrition, and quickly made the vitamin content of their fruits and vegetables the spearhead of advertising. Vitamin supplements in the form of oils and capsules became common in the 1920s, and even dog food was sold on the merits of the vitamins in each can or biscuit. "Wherever we turn," a physician grumbled in the early 1930s, "our retinas are scorched by the vitamin claims of some bread, milk or 'sunkissed' orange. Gigantic signboards proclaim the therapeutic advantage of this or that. The air is filled with radio messages in song or verse, extolling the special health giving virtues of one food or another, ad nauseum."[5]

It was not, however, just vitamins and minerals that were newly being proclaimed from billboards. Advertisements for yeast as a health food were in view everywhere people turned as well. Yeast, of course, had been one of the most commonplace items of everyday life for centuries. It made bread, it made wine, but until the early 1900s, it had no reputation for making health. With the discovery of vitamins, however, yeast manufacturers began publicizing "The New Importance of Yeast in Diet" (a booklet supplied gratis by the Fleischmann Company), extolling the virtues of vitamins A, B, and D present in "the familiar foil-wrapped cake." So eagerly was the opportunity exploited, a physician could write by 1928 that the recent promotion of yeast for health was "the most gigantic and widespread advertising ever done for such a purpose. . . . Now the sale is phenomenal." The advertising was not just gigantic, it was grossly misleading, and was frequently identified as such. In 1935, for instance, the author of an engagingly titled tirade against food faddism, *Diet and Die*, pointed to Fleischmann's yeast when he needed an example of "striking disregard for genuine scientific accuracy" in the food industry's distortion of nutritional science for profit. Three years later, the Federal Trade Commission demanded that Standard Brands, the manufacturers of Fleischmann's, cease making excessive claims for the nutritional value of yeast, as well as statements that yeast aided digestion, cleared the skin, and stopped tooth decay.[6]

There was one more advertising gambit that Fleischmann's was told to drop in 1938, its most exaggerated deception of all: that yeast was as much a laxative as a leavener, and thus the best method of avoiding autointoxication. To be fair, medical literature did contain hints that yeast was moderately helpful in correcting bowel function. But Fleischmann ads presented it as the very salvation of the race. Constipation, 1923 ads revealed, was "the greatest constant enemy of mankind today," the root cause of "wrecked bodies and ruined health"; its "total cost to human happiness can never be fully known." In one advertisement (1928), Arbuthnot Lane himself was called on to verify that "civilization's curse can be conquered" by yeast (Fig. 7-1). What Lane actually said, in an interview picked up by a number of American newspapers, was that yeast was a good source of B vitamins. But since he was the universally recognized archenemy of autointoxication, Fleischmann's needed only to place a portrait of the distinguished surgeon beside newspaper clippings of his endorsement of yeast vitamins to convey the message that yeast was the informed man's laxative: "When Sir William Arbuthnot Lane speaks the world listens!"[7]

Lillian Ramsey listened, at least. A constipated office worker from Evanston, Illinois, she became addicted to purgatives in her effort to avoid autointoxication:

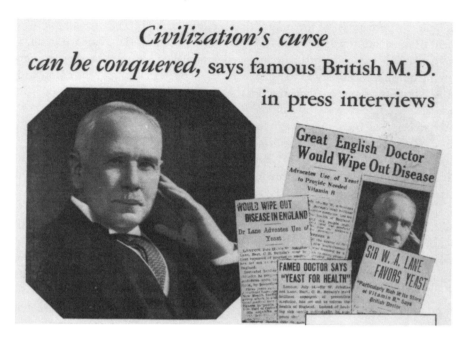

Figure 7-1. Arbuthnot Lane used to promote yeast for health [from *Literary Digest*, October 6, 1928, p. 35].

"as quickly as my sytem got accustomed to one remedy," she found, "I had to hunt a successor because it ceased to 'work'." Her husband took to ridiculing her with a new pet name, "Frenzied Medicator," until finally he couldn't take any more of Lillian's frenzy. Directing her attention to a newspaper advertisement for Fleischmann's Yeast, he presented her with two cakes of the product. "At least," he admonished, "this is *food*, not *dope*." Mrs. Ramsey tried the cakes, began eating two "yeast sandwiches" daily, and "in two months my internal economy was operating like a well-oiled motor." She lost her susceptibility to colds and drowsiness as well, and her complexion cleared. So in the end, her (and her husband's) suffering paid off, not least because her saga "of one woman's triumph over a universal menace" was accorded the $1000 first prize in the 1923 national contest for most compelling story of "What Fleischmann's Yeast has done for you."[8]

The way yeast worked for her, according to the Fleischmann rationale, was to mix with intestinal waste and both soften it and increase its bulk. In describing that action, ads made a point of explaining that "every cake of Fleischmann's fresh yeast consists of *millions of tiny living plants*."[9] In other words, the eating of yeast (whether Fleischmann's or Yeast Foam Tablets or any of the other brands that made similar claims) introduced friendly microscopic life into the colon, and in the public's perception of the matter that seeding of the bowel with a biological agent of fermention was perhaps the most persuasive piece of evidence of all. It was a plausible extension of an already well-established idea, that the key to overcoming autointoxication was to replace the usual bacterial flora of the colon with more wholesome microorganisms. That notion had been popularized during the first decade of the century by a Nobel Prize–winning scientist, Élie Metchnikoff, and had inspired yet another large category of anti-autointoxication products. In this case, the remedies were bacterial cultures for the abdomen.

Metchnikoff was born in Ukraine in 1845 and was trained in zoology at Kharkov University. Subsequently, he conducted scientific research at institutions throughout Europe, in the mid-1880s carrying out pioneering studies of the functioning of the immune system. It was for work in that field that he was awarded the Nobel Prize for medicine and physiology in 1908. By that time, Metchnikoff had become the director of the Institut Pasteur, the world-renowned medical research laboratory in Paris, and was making himself as famous with the laity as among scientists for his advocacy of a new plan for attaining health and longevity.[10]

The plan began to take shape in the late 1890s, when Metchnikoff experienced a series of physical setbacks. Only 53, he became depressed and apprehensive that he was aging prematurely, and realized how strongly he desired a long and vigorous life (this was not his first experience with depression; in younger days, he had attempted suicide on three occasions). Anxiety over aging and approaching mortality comes to everyone who lives long enough, of course, but while most people simply accept the fear of death as a natural reaction, an innate survival instinct requiring no further analysis, Metchnikoff the scientist regarded it as an anomaly that had to be explained. It struck him that humanity's aversion to aging and dying was out of step with the natural reactions to other life processes. Eating, for example, led to a feeling of satiety and a satisfied feeling of having had enough; work led to a desire for rest. But people never felt they had had enough of youth, or looked forward to the restfulness of decrepitude. That could only mean that people were growing old too soon, before a fullness of years could bring to fruition a natural, instinctive acceptance of old age and dissolution. "Our inmost convictions assure us that life is too short," Metchnikoff observed, and that seemed proof that we were not living long enough, that we were falling short of the span of life intended by nature; there, he concluded, "lies the greatest disharmony of the constitution of man."[11]

The human condition had long been addressed by the world's religions, but all faiths were inadequate, Metchnikoff objected, because they were superstition, "childish and erroneous conceptions." Philosophy he conceded to be more respectable intellectually, but metaphysics was nevertheless mired in pessimism, "resigned to the prospect of annihilation." For Metchnikoff, only science ("science is all-powerful") could provide a sound basis for optimism about life, and a prescription for holding old age at arm's length until nature was ready to accept it. Physiological science in particular provided Metchnikoff with evidence that life could be extended and death made palatable. In brief, the body aged prematurely because physical evolution worked too slowly to keep pace with cultural evolution. The disproportion was apparent, he elaborated, in the continued existence of organs that had been critical for survival at an early stage of humanity's climb up from the animal kingdom, but were useless, even harmful, in the advanced state of civilization. The vermiform appendix was one example of an obsolete and dangerous organ, the wisdom teeth another. And the colon was a third. Indeed, the large intestine was, more than any other organ, one of the body's "useless inheritances," a sack that was "superfluous."[12]

Why was the colon superfluous? Because, Metchinikoff argued, it had outlived its evolutionary survival value. The colon was well developed, he noted, only in mammals, animals that, whether as predators or prey, frequently have to move about quickly on the ground. Having to abruptly halt pursuit or flight in order to evacuate the bowel can cause an animal either to miss a meal, or to become one. The colon thus had evolved as a storage bin to hold feces until a convenient time for disposal. For urbanized humans, however, a large fecal reservoir was of no more advantage than was body hair: "Man does not secure his prey or escape from his enemies by the rapidity of his locomotion." Yet like hair, whose follicles collected microbes and could sometimes become sites of infection, the colon contained germs, many more germs than did hair follicles, and these were constantly inciting putrefaction of waste. From putrefaction, needless to say, came autointoxication: indeed, the large bowel was not just "an asylum of harmful microbes," but "the source of many poisons harmful to the body," a "source of intoxication from within." Most pertinent, "it is among such substances," the toxins generated in the bowel, "that we must look for the slow poisons which . . . produce the arterial sclerosis of old age." "Intestinal putrefaction," he put it simply, "shortens life."[13]

As a harmful vestige, the colon might be expected to slowly disappear through continued evolution. But the working out of the evolutionary process would require millenia, subjecting untold generations to unnecessary misery and untimely death. It was far preferable to accelerate evolution, and conceivably one way to accomplish that was through surgery. Even before Lane's operation became *de rigeur* among the autointoxicated higher classes, a few people had had their colons surgically removed and had continued to live comfortably enough afterwards. To Metchnikoff, they were walking proof of his theory that the large intestine "is certainly useless in the case of man" (one of his assistants went so far as to propose that "every child should have its large intestine and its appendix surgically removed when two or three years of age"). Hence, when Lane became known for his removals of the colon, Metchnikoff saw in him a kindred spirit. The two corresponded, and when professional travel brought him to London in 1904, the bacteriologist paid a surprise visit to the surgeon ("we sat discussing stasis till very late," Lane recorded). Communication continued after Metchnikoff returned home, and around 1907 he began sending two of his research assistants to London for 6 weeks every year to study Lane's surgical cases and confirm that the colon was unnecessary (one of these, a Dr. Distaso, "was careless," Lane remembered, "in that he occasionally left the excised intestine in a 'bus or train, and had great difficulty in regaining possession of it").[14]

But even when done by Lane, colectomy was a high-risk procedure and an expensive one, so it was hardly suitable as a universal solution to the problem of the superfluous bowel. Furthermore, it wasn't really necessary to remove the bowel, since the true threat to health was not the organ itself but the putrefactive microbes that inhabited it. Ultimately, it was the germs of autointoxication that had to be removed, and Metchnikoff discovered (so he believed) how to do that. He did it with milk.

Unlike most animal products (meat, for instance, or feces), milk does not readily putrefy. Rather than rotting, it turns sour, due to the action of microorganisms that degrade lactose (milk sugar) into lactic acid. Lactic acid, Metchnikoff reasoned, must inhibit the activity of putrefactive bacteria, so it followed that if lactic acid–producing microbes were introduced into the colon, autointoxication might be arrested. In sum, "the means by which the pathological symptoms may be removed from old age, and by which, in all probability, the duration of the life of man may be considerably increased," he concluded, was by transforming "the 'wild' population of the intestine into a cultured population."[15]

The most cultured of all populations, in this sense, was what was then called *Bacillus bulgaricus* (in modern terminology *Lactobacillus bulgaricus*), soon to be renowned throughout the Western world as the Bulgarian bacillus. It was the organism responsible for producing yogurt, and though other soured milk preparations (kefir and koumiss, for example) contained lactic acid–generating bacilli, Bulgarian bacilli seemed to Metchnikoff to be the cream, as it were, of microbial society. It was not just that laboratory tests identified *B. bulgaricus* as the most active producer of lactic acid; more compelling was the fact that yogurt was consumed in large quantities by the inhabitants of Bulgaria, as well as those of Georgia and other regions of Metchnikoff's native Russia. All those territories were renowned for producing people of extraordinary age (Metchnikoff himself observed a number of centenarians still laboring in the fields in Bulgaria). It was thus easy to conclude that yogurt microbes "must exercise a favorable influence in favor of longevity."[16]

Metchnikoff introduced his revolutionary ideas to the world in a lecture delivered in Manchester in 1901, then expanded upon them at length in two books: *Études sur la nature humaine* (1903, translated into English as *The Nature of Man*), and *Essais optimistes* (1907, translated as *The Prolongation of Life. Optimistic Stud-*

ies). His "Optimistic Philosophy," or, as he also called it, *orthobiosis* (true or correct way of living), was the belief that culturing the colon with lactic microbes would eliminate autointoxication, and thereby so retard aging that people would live out the number of years intended by nature—120 and more was his estimate. (The seeding of the intestine with Bulgarian bacilli had to be thorough: "We must be able," a Metchnikoff follower wrote, "to saturate the intestines from top to bottom, even its smallest recesses and corners."). Of greater import than the quantity of years, however, was their quality. By escaping premature degeneration, people would have time to grow full of life and slowly tire of existence. Then the natural instinct for death that had sunk into the psychic interior through disuse could make its way back to the surface. Age would be freed of its terrors. "It will be possible to modify old age," Metchnikoff promised; "instead of retaining its existing melancholy and repulsive character, it may become a healthy and endurable process." Then it could be appreciated that "the goal of existence [should be] the accomplishment of a complete and physiological cycle, in which occurs a normal old age ending in the loss of the instinct of life and the appearance of the instinct of death." And though it would be foolish to hope to undo the damages of centuries of autointoxication in a single generation, "each succeeding generation will get closer and closer to the solution and . . . true happiness one day will be reached by mankind." No wonder he called his scheme of thought Optimistic Philosophy.[17]

Metchnikoff, incidentally, died at the age of 71. Nevertheless, he lived to see his own natural death instinct manifest itself. When in 1913 he suffered a "cardiac crisis," he found he "felt no fear of death," but instead experienced a sense of "satiety with life." The fact that his was a "precocious" feeling of readiness for death, appearing a full half century ahead of the orthobiotic schedule, did not, however, shake his faith in his philosophy. He had led an extraordinarily intense life, (Nobel Prize winners commonly do), so had matured more rapidly than most; thereby losing his fear of dying years in advance of the norm, in the same way that "certain women cease to menstruate earlier than the great majority." He lived 3 more years. When at last the end did come, one of his final sentences was a request to a physician friend to perform an autopsy: "Look at the intestines carefully for I think there is something there now."[18]

Metchnikoff's optimism naturally inspired jests about "the modern Ponce de Leon" who searched "for the Fountain of Immortal Youth and [found] it in the Milky Whey" (Fig. 7-2). But it was not actually milk or whey or even yogurt that he proposed as the best preservative of youth. To be sure, he had found the Bulgarian bacillus in yogurt, but that and other milk preparations also contained a variety of additional species of microorganisms—"non-lactic microbes"—that could interfere with the effects of the healthful germs. It was better, therefore, to sterilize milk and then inoculate it with a pure culture of the Bulgarian bacillus.

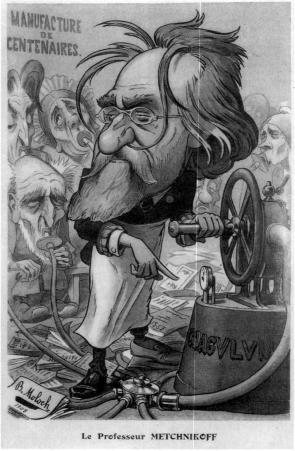

Figure 7-2. Caricature of Metchnikov's creation of centenarians through yogurt [Wellcome Institute Library,
London].

Sterile, sweetened vegetable broth worked equally well as the vehicle, and it was
even possible to dry the Bulgarian culture and use it in the form of powder or tablets. Metchnikoff's preference was for a liquid culture prepared by a Paris firm
and sold in small vials under the name Lacto Bacilline, to be taken straight or added
to boiled milk to make yogurt. He was convinced that his health had benefitted
from Lacto Bacilline, he persuaded friends to adopt the product too, and, his scientific standing being what it was, before long Paris physicians were prescribing the
sour milk regimen for patients.[19]

Patients began prescribing it for themselves even more eagerly—and not just in Paris. Metchnikoff's books were translated into English, he published articles in British and American popular magazines, and his good news about the milky way as the path to long and vigorous life was widely broadcast. *Punch*'s epic tale of "Brixton's Brave Bacterium" shows that as early as 1908 the English public was aware of the new French remedy. It seems a young man of London's Brixton neighborhood awoke one day to discover "that his interior was being violently disturbed by a gang [of germs] who are believed to have effected an entrance under cover of a pork pie of more than usual indigestibility." Pork pies of even normal digestibility can bring strong men to their knees, so it's no surprise to learn the Brixton lad was soon reduced to the very feeblest hold on life. Yet at all but the last moment, he was pulled back from the yawning grave by "the vigilance and courage of a lactic acid bacterium, who had concealed himself on the premises in some curdled milk." There had been "a desperate struggle," to say the least, but "the intruders were eventually overcome, and the bacterial benefactor, with characteristic modesty, withdrew without leaving either name or address."[20]

That sour milk bacilli were benefactors clearly was a cherished opinion among Britons and Americans by the close of the century's first decade. Curdled milk is "the fashion of the moment," a Scottish physician commented, while an English medical editor perceived the public to be "in a fit of new-found panaceal therapy" in their appetite for yogurt. Another medical commentator recalled a few years later that at that time, "one heard of nothing but the Bulgarian bacillus. The bacillus shared with Mr. Lloyd George's budget the honor of monopolizing the conversation at the dinner tables of the great. He dominated Belgravia, frolicked in Fulham, and bestrode Birmingham and the whole of the British Isles." Another practitioner reported that British patients "thought that all their diseases were curable" by lactic acid, and that one had recently informed him "that doctors would soon be a thing of the past . . . because sour milk was all-sufficient."[21]

For awhile, some doctors were only too willing to contribute to their own obsolescence by promoting sour milk preparations as therapy. As early as 1907, a French physician issued a 400-page treatise advocating the "antiputrefactive regimen" for all manner of ailments, and by the following year, British and American practitioners were making similar recommendations. A Glasgow MD, for example, proposed to readers of *The Lancet*, Britain's most prestigious medical journal, that Thomas Parr, the seventeenth century centenarian, had achieved such length of days because of the sour whey he was reputed to have consumed each day; lactic acid, he added, ought to be thought of as "nature's own intestinal germicide." That same year of 1908, the *British Medical Journal* reiterated the point, suggesting that "fighting harmful microbes with other microbes opens up great possibilities, and is in accordance with . . . the methods of Nature"; this characterization of yogurt as a form of "antibiotic" therapy, furthermore, was presented under the exuberant title "A Modern Elixir of Life." The following year, noted London gastroenterologist George Herschell devoted a short book to *Soured Milk and Pure Cultures of Lactic Acid Bacilli in the Treatment of Disease*, and in it hailed Metchnikoff's work as a "brilliant conception" for combatting autointoxication. *Soured Milk*'s first run of 8000 copies sold out in just 6 months, necessitating a considerably enlarged second edition issued later that year. Before 1909 was out, London's Royal Society of Medicine hosted a session to discuss "The Therapeutical Value of the Lactic-acid Bacillus" that revealed the Metchnikoff therapy to be widely employed in Britain. "There can be no question," a more conservative practitioner complained, "that sour milk is being . . . prescribed to patients for all manner of diseases."[22]

There was a comparable degree of professional interest in the sour milk treatment of autointoxication in America, though after only a few years it began to fade on both sides of the Atlantic. It was not just that the reality of autointoxication itself was being called into question by 1915 but that laboratory scientists had demonstrated in the early 1910s that Metchnikoff and his followers were wrong in believing the Bulgarian bacillus could establish itself as the chief component of the colonic flora (how could "a man in his position . . . have written so positively," an American physician asked about Metchnikoff, "on the basis of so little exact proof."). The bacillus does not, in fact, colonize the human intestine. Thus even if autointoxication did exist, even if it did wreak havoc with health, *B. bulgaricus* was not the way to stop it. That message was not easily conveyed to the public, however, for dissenting voices were all but drowned out by the strident promotions of a host of commercial Bulgarian bacillus products. European and American cities had been awash in sour milk since 1907 or so, opportunists having instantly seen the economic potential in Metchnikoff's optimistic philosophy. There were numerous brands of yogurt, as well as liquid versions of sour milk, broth cultures of the bacillus, malt extract cultures, dried bacilli in the form of powders and tablets to be mixed with milk, and at least one bacillus-infused chocolate cream. All were marketed with the extravagant claims usual to patent medicines. Intesti-Fermin Tablets, to pick one, claimed to "contain the finest strains of sour milk ferments of Bulgaria, where people frequently live to be 125 years of age." Another company proudly advertised that it manufactured its product in Turkey, as close to the Bulgarian source as it could get, even though the microbe could be grown in pure culture in the laboratory anywhere in the world. All such hoopla aside, most commercial preparations either did not actually contain any Bulgarian bacilli or else contained various contaminating microorganisms as well. Hence in most cases, physicians maintained, the purchasers of Bulgarian products were fools, "introspective idiots," the *Journal of the American Medical Association* called them, "who allow themselves to be treated by their lady friends."[23]

"Like other fashions soured milks wax and wane in their use in medicine," a New York physician commented in 1927. "In yesterday's fashion plates, the most figured souring germ was the Bacillus Bulgaricus [but] in today's," he elaborated, "it is the Bacillus acidophilus." *Lactobacillus acidophilus*, to give the new trendsetter its proper name, had been discovered at the beginning of the century in the digestive tract of babies fed on cow's milk. It was dubbed "acidophilus" (acid loving) because, like the Bulgarian bacillus, it could tolerate an acidic environment. Unlike the Bulgarian microbe, however, acidophilus organisms did colonize the human digestive tract, a fact demonstrated several times over by microbiologists during the 1910s. So it mattered not that the Bulgarian bacillus was nearly dead and gone; sour milk was still a golden commercial opportunity, and acidophilus preparations soon flooded the market at even higher levels than bulgaricus ones had. There were Lactophilus and Lacto-Dextrin, Optolactin and Laxatonic, Acido-Culture and Neo-Cultol; milk cultures, broth cultures, jelly cultures, powders, tablets, and chocolate-coated blocks. Euxalase combined acidophilus with biliary secretions and agar-agar in a charcoal-coated tablet. The custodians of colon laundries offered acidophilus lavage. No matter how the culture was delivered, however, the goal was the same; it was, to cite the pitch for Lederle Bacillus Acidophilus Milk, to "Exchange Germs of Decay For Those of Health." (The Bulgarian bacillus nevertheless held on valiantly. Even into the late 1920s, for example, the Yoghurt Health Laboratories of Bellingham, Washington continued to turn a profit with both yogurt and tablets of *B. bulgaricus*, as well as Anticonstipation Cookies and Physical Culture Candies, all advertised in the company newspaper *Yoghurt Health News*. Yog-a-Lax, a combination of yogurt and an unidentified laxative, was still being sold well into the 1940s, as was Insta'ghurt, an instant yogurt that was "mildly laxative.")[24]

Responding to the "exceedingly overstressed" popular interest in acidophilus therapy constituted a good portion of the workload of the American Medical Association's Bureau of Investigation during the 1920s and '30s. Gastroenterologists confirmed that the public was enthralled with acidophilus, one reporting in 1927 that he was "continuously seeing patients who have been on acidophilus milk in large daily quantities for months, or even a year or two, right up to the time of coming to me"; some "have even been having acidophilus germs injected into the bowel, yet," he found, all "still show considerable intestinal putrefaction." With most commercial preparations of acidophilus (nearly all, in fact), the germs of health did not overthrow the germs of decay. That was because most products sporting the acidophilus label did not actually contain the promised organisms. A laboratory study conducted in the 1920s determined that commercial cultures and tablets were "absolutely worthless" with regard to their acidophilus content; with even the most active preparation, "it would take one billion [tablets] to contain as many bacilli as are contained in one liter of acidophilus milk." A follow-up in-

quiry carried out several years later found live bacilli in only 13 of the 107 commercial acidophilus preparations examined.[25]

Genuine acidophilus was hardly needed, however. Ordinary milk would
work just as well if it were poured over breakfast cereal made from bran. That
was the point of an advertisement for Post's Bran Flakes in which a 10 foot–tall
menu card stood in the courtroom, flanked by two burly policemen, and was
pronounced "Indicted!" on the charge of "being responsible for a high percentage of ill health due to a definite lack of bulk food" (Fig. 7-3). The modern bill of
fare had long been recognized to be lacking in bulk. Sylvester Graham will be
recalled as one pre-twentieth-century antagonist of refined foods. But the intensified awareness of the relation of food to health that was stimulated by the newer
nutrition, combined with the phenomenal growth of the food processing industry
in the late nineteenth and early twentieth centuries, directed both scientific and
lay attention to the shortage of bulk in the modern diet to a degree not previously
approached. By the analysis that followed, constipation was rampant in modern
times because the indigestible components of foods that increased the volume of
feces and thereby encouraged regular elimination had themselves been eliminated
by evolving popular tastes and methods of food manufacture. White bread was
the most disturbing example of this trend. The steel roller milling technology
developed in the 1870s had made it possible to produce flour that was essentially
devoid of bran (the brown particles of the shell of the wheat) and that was afford-
able by all. Whiter-than-ever bread quickly became the standard loaf even among
the laboring classes, though its mineral and vitamin content was severely compromised, and its lack of bran gave it a constipating effect (at least the bolting
process used in Graham's day had allowed the smallest particles of bran to remain
in white flour). With increasing prosperity, moreover, meat and other non-bread
foods came to be eaten in larger amounts, causing the daily ingestion of bread to
decrease by 50% or more between 1870 and 1940. Some of the bread no longer
being eaten was replaced by fruits and vegetables, particularly from the 1920s on,
but a much greater share was replaced by refined sugar, which left no digestive
residue at all. Nutritionists questioned whether supplying so much of the body's
calorie needs from foods so lacking in bulk "is physiologically defensible," since
such a diet would provide inadequate stimulation to the intestines: "the digestive
organs of the genus homo," one suggested, "are not constructed for the disposal
of foods in tabloid form." Bran, which had been widely adopted as livestock food
in the late nineteenth century, promised to provide the antidote to tabloid eating.
Processed into palatable form, it could reestablish bulk in the white bread and sugar
diet.[26]

Post's Bran Flakes was one of a great swarm of breakfast cereals (and whole-
grain breads as well) that came onto the market in the early years of the century as
the best preventives of autointoxication—because they contained bran. C. W. Post,

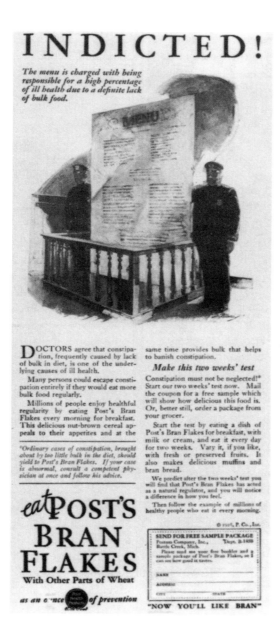

Figure 7-3. Advertisement for Post Bran Flakes,
decrying the lack of bulk in the modern diet [from
Literary Digest, March 31, 1928, p. 57].

in fact, was a signal contributor to an enthusiasm for bran foods that by the mid-1920s had attained the proportions of "The National Mania," as one health writer called it. It was, the editor of the *Journal of the American Medical Association* marvelled, a "craze [for] 'horse food'" that had "swept the country" and filled "newspapers and magazines [with] recipes for making bran biscuits, bran muffins, bran gems, bran patties and otherwise disguising this coarse and . . . unappetizing material." At the height of the craze, a rural Georgia schoolteacher even concocted a bran lemonade, the recipe for which he sent to the popular health magazine *Hygeia* in the hope that constipated children could be enticed to substitute it for soft drinks (most likely, children preferred Bran Chocolate, another Post product, "the wise selection of conscientious mothers" who wanted to keep their offspring regular without dosing them with chocolated laxatives such as Ex-Lax). With the coming of bran, there was a new optimism abroad, one that a prominent nutritionist characterized as "a hopeful feeling that eventually coarse, wheaty, nut-flavored muffins may stop the crime wave."[27]

As a promoter of bran for health, Post was second only to the most formidable reformer of American living habits of the twentieth century. What Arbuthnot Lane was to intestinal stasis in England, and Élie Metchnikoff to autointoxication in France, John Harvey Kellogg was to constipation in America. Kellogg was effectively born a health reformer. His parents were first-generation members of the Seventh Day Adventist Church, a denomination that formed in the 1840s and was committed from the start not just to spiritual purity but also to a strict code of physical hygiene virtually identical to Grahamism. Kellogg obtained a medical degree, then in 1876, at the age of 24, took over the direction of the Adventist Church's Western Health Reform Institute in Battle Creek, Michigan, church headquarters. He would remain a member in good standing of the medical profession throughout his career, earning respect particularly as a surgeon. But it was as the director of the Battle Creek Sanitarium (his new name for the Institute) and an irrepressible exponent of the virtues of "biologic living" that Kellogg was known to the world at large. He quickly built the Sanitarium (or San, as it was familiarly known) into the most famous medical and health institution in the country. By the time he passed on in 1943, Kellogg had hosted more than 300,000 patients at the San (including Rockefellers, DuPonts, and others who could afford to be cured anywhere), treating them with a mix of conventional and unorthodox therapies, and educating them in the rules of right living. Along the way, he had loosed a torrent of hygiene instruction upon the general public as well, authoring literally dozens of books (*Shall We Slay to Eat, The Evils of Fashionable Dress, Tobaccoism; or, How Tobacco Kills*), publishing articles in popular magazines and professional journals, editing his own well-subscribed journal (*Good Health*), and lecturing endlessly and everywhere. He lived to the age of 91, taking daily jogs till near the

end, "a tireless steam engine," in a contemporary's opinion, "a wonderful advertisement for his own theories."[28]

Those theories, the code of health that Kellogg called "biologic living," were
founded on vegetarianism and included close attention to exercise, fresh air, and
all the other elements of non-natural tradition. The full scope of his hygienic philosophy has been examined thoroughly elsewhere and needn't be pursued further
here. For present purposes, it is Kellogg's preoccupation with the function of
evacuation that is of interest. He believed that "most" of the more than 40,000
patients he treated at the San over one 10-year period were victims of autointoxication, and his interest in the subject required several entire books to spend itself
(*Autointoxication*, *Colon Hygiene*, *The Crippled Colon*, *The Itinerary of a Breakfast*).
He held the conviction that "world-wide autointoxication" was "the secret of nine-
tenths of all the chronic ills from which civilized human beings suffer," an affliction that potentially had "race-destroying effects," and asserted that "universal
constipation" was "the most destructive blockade that has ever opposed human
progress," and was even the source of "not a small part of our moral and social
maladies." Among the moral maladies was sexual excess. In his sex manual *Plain
Facts for Young and Old*, Kellogg argued, much as Macfadden did, that "in males,
one of the most general physical causes of sexual excitement is *constipation*." As
the rectum fills with feces, and the feces dry out, "this hardened mass presses upon
the parts most intimately concerned in the sexual act, causing excessive . . . excitement." Too frequent intimate indulgences necessarily followed, and could lead
to "most serious results," including that "horrible disease, *satyriasis*." For constipated girls, the even more horrible condition of nymphomania could result, though
usually the excitation lead only to masturbation, which was bad enough.[29]

Autointoxication was "world-wide," but only with respect to the civilized
world. It was in urbanized, industrialized countries that constipation had become
"universal," because it was there alone that the condition of "civilized colon" was
to be found. "The average colon, in civilized communities," Kellogg despaired,
"is in a desperately depraved and dangerous condition." It was "overfilled," he
explained, "distended almost to bursting . . . its tense walls crippled by the strain
to which they are subjected," and even though the abused organ persisted valiantly
in "making painful efforts to force an opening through the narrowed or even oblit-
erated passage," its possessor would "slander it by calling it lazy, and punish it by
goading and whipping it with drastic drugs." A host of factors attendant on modern life contributed to the colon's depravity, but two stood out as the worst of-
fenders: delay and diet. More often than not, Kellogg thought, urbanites postponed
answering nature's call to evacuate until some more suitable time, not realizing
that answering the call was "a sacred obligation," a duty that "no person can neglect without serious injury." If not answered, the call would soon be lost alto-

gether, and "to lose one's 'call' is almost as bad as to lose a fortune," Kellogg warned, "indeed such a loss has more than once led to loss of fortune, and to worse results." A bowel that had lost its call was, in the health crusader's imaginative terminology, a "house-broken colon," its possessor no more in command of his health than was a common dog. Just as the domesticated canine had been trained to empty its bowels at its master's rather than its own convenience, inhabitants of modern society had ceded control of their bowels to the tyrants of social convenience and modesty. "If [only] dogs were the only house-broken creatures," Kellogg speculated; "what a world of wretchedness, suffering, even crime and human wreckage would be saved" (presumably even the dire-sounding condition he called "fecal fever" would be avoided).[30]

But the primitive dog was not the ideal animal model; the chimpanzee and the ape were. It was from simians that humans had evolved, and it was to them that we had to look to rediscover our natural rhythm of evacuation. That rhythm, Kellogg learned by writing the directors of the London and the Bronx zoos, was four or more times daily. Similarly, "among primitive people . . . three evacuations are generally the habit" (this he determined from questionnaires mailed to several hundred medical missionaries around the world). Could there be any doubt, then, that the civilized person who "considers himself a model of regularity and physical rectitude if he has one bowel movement daily" was tragically deluded. "The truth is, one bowel movement a day is serious constipation."[31]

"The bowels normally move three or four times daily," Kellogg believed (that was rule one of his "practical suggestions for relief of constipation"). In the colon that had not been broken by civilization, he maintained, the ingestion of food excited peristaltic motions and brought on an evacuation after each meal. Often, the possessor of a healthy colon also enjoyed a movement soon after rising in the morning, or shortly before retiring at night (or even both). And lest a schedule of three, four, or five motions daily be mistaken for diarrhea, Kellogg hastened to assure his public that when such frequency occurred "naturally," it was not at all debilitating, "but wonderfully promotes vigor, endurance, appetite, digestion, and all that pertains to good health." Indeed, "hundreds of persons" whose colons he had restored to primitive efficiency had experienced "notable improvement in health," and had been relieved of "a great variety of . . . symptoms that form the familiar clinical picture of intestinal toxemia."[32]

How was the colon to be returned to its pristine vigor? Naturally, of course; certainly not by surgery. Kellogg knew Arbuthnot Lane, having made his acquaintance while visiting London early in the century, soon after Lane had begun his short-circuiting procedures on stasis patients. Kellogg was allowed to observe Lane in surgery, was impressed by "his admirable technic," but left feeling that what he had witnessed was more "formidable a . . . procedure" than should be needed. To his mind, there was a question as to whether "the objectionable influence of the colon was to be found in the neglect of Nature to remove a dangerous and useless portion of the anatomy which should have been left behind thousands of years ago" (Lane's and Metchnikoff's position), "or whether the real fault was to be found in the wrong use to which the colon has been put and the various abuses to which the organ has been subjected through neglect, ignorance and departures from biologic living." It was not Nature that had incapacitated the colon, but humans (nevertheless, in very obstinate cases of constipation, Kellogg himself occasionally performed short-circuits or colectomies).[33]

The way for humankind to restore nature was to replace civilized with primitive behaviors. Primitive diet, a return to vegetarianism (*The Natural Diet of Man*, another of his books called it), was the critical first step. Intestinal toxemia flourished where feces not only stagnated in the bowels but also supplied generous amounts of protein residues for the colon's putrefactive microbes to degrade into toxins. The usual diet filled the colon with "undigested and putrefying fragments of animal flesh" that decomposed into "a seething mass of corruption"; it turned the colon into "a storehouse of the most disgusting and offensive material" whose "horrible effluvium . . . taints the very springs of life." So polluted a bowel, even if moved the commonly recommended once a day, "is never emptied, and is all the time several days in arrears." It was, as Kellogg frequently described it, a "crippled colon." A vegetarian diet, on the other hand, had a relatively low protein content that provided much less fodder to the gut's greedy putrefactive germs. At the same time, its high bulk content encouraged a quick passage of waste through the canal. Vegetarianism was thus "the antitoxic diet." For any who might doubt that meat constituted a toxic diet, Kellogg related experiments he had done with "vigorous young men," enclosing them in a room with "the bowel discharges of a meat-eater." In a matter of just hours, the men all were "made very ill" by the fumes they inhaled. And only imagine, Kellogg added, "how much greater mischief" meat-based feces would create "when in the body than after removal from it."[34]

A variety of physical measures could be employed to reinforce fleshless diet and save the crippled, housebroken, civilized colon. Water was foremost. Kellogg's longest book, *Rational Hydrotherapy*, devoted more than a thousand pages to water treatments for all complaints, constipation included. Abdominal exercise followed close behind hydrotherapy, and the two were combined in his "Bath Exerciser," a dustpan-shaped scoop with handles on either side and a rubber cord mounted behind for attachment to the bathtub faucet. Purchasers intent on revitalizing their bowels would hook up the apparatus, sit in the filled tub, grip the scoop's handles, and imitate the movements of a rower. Working at a rate of 30 strokes a minute, the bath rower immersed the scoop into the water as he leaned forward, then dumped the water from the scoop onto his chest as he pulled back. After 5 minutes, "one finishes the bath with the same delightful sensation of warmth and glow which one feels after a swim in the surf" (if the bath exerciser in Fig. 7-4 is representative, it appears one could progress well beyond the state of simple glow).[35]

Colonic irrigation was also part of Kellogg's reparative repertoire, as were abdominal massage (he designed his own electric vibrator), electrotherapy, and abdominal support belts. Once restored to normalcy, the colon could be maintained by continued abdominal exercise, use of the primitive defecation posture (squatting), and chewing every bite of vegetable food thoroughly. For a period, at least, Kellogg was a devoted Fletcherite. He coined the infinitive "to fletcherize," hung a large "Fletcherize" sign at the head of the San dining room, appointed Fletcher to the staff of *Good Health* as a "Contributing Editor," and proposed that grade school instruction in "the fine art of . . . Fletcherizing" would go much farther toward halting the decline of American society than such sterile academic exercises as memorizing Greek and Latin poetry. In the end, however, he was unable to accept Fletcher's flouting of the defecation schedule set by nature. If the person who voided his bowels once a day was seriously constipated, what must be thought of the man who did so just once a week? "Horace Fletcher's Mistake," Kellogg

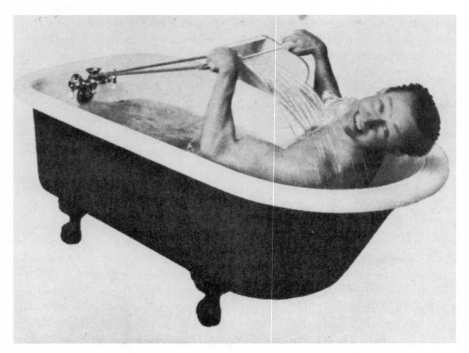

Figure 7-4. John Harvey Kellogg's Bath Exerciser [from John Harvey Kellogg, *Colon Hygiene*, p. 242].

objected, was to reject from his mouth all food material that could not be reduced to liquid by chewing, "that is, he excluded roughage entirely from his dietary" and thus "he cultivated constipation." Kellogg claimed to have "labored very earnestly with Mr. Fletcher on many occasions to convince him of his error," but with limited success. The man's disregard for frequent cleansing of his bowel was "the rock on which Fletcherism split and went to pieces," and on which Fletcher himself ran aground. "Mr. Fletcher . . . suffered greatly from chronic toxemia," Kellogg maintained; "his tongue was heavily coated and his breath was highly malodorous." Kellogg learned from Fletcher's dentist that the Great Masticator's "teeth were decaying more rapidly than in any case he had ever seen." Thus while Fletcher's death in 1919 was officially attributed to bronchitis, there was no doubt in Kellogg's mind that it was "chiefly caused, by chronic toxemia." Nor was it any wonder that many Fletcherites had consulted him, Kellogg confided, "suffering from severe constipation and resulting autointoxication."[36]

Another autointoxication theorist with whom Kellogg had a beef was Metchnikoff. He agreed wholeheartedly with the Parisian scientist that "putrefactive organisms . . . are the essential cause of old age," and in his own works forcefully recommended the introduction of lactobacilli into the intestine to displace putrefactive germs (he sometimes used Bulgarian bacilli descended from cultures obtained from Metchnikoff's laboratory). But it was necessary at the same time to cut off the supply of nourishment to the malignant organisms by removing meat from the diet. "Metchnikoff's Mistake" (the title of a full chapter in Kellogg's *Autointoxication*) had been to stop at adding yogurt and buttermilk to his meals; he should have eliminated flesh food too. As with Fletcher, Kellogg all but delighted in Metchnikoff's untimely death (from autointoxication, he was sure), explaining it with the remark he had heard from one of the assistants at the Pasteur Institute: "Metchinikoff eats a pound of meat and lets it rot in his colon and then drinks a pint of sour milk to disinfect it. I am not such a fool. I don't eat the meat."[37]

"Should the Colon Be Sacrificed," Kellogg asked in the title of one of his many articles on the subject, "or May It Be Reformed?" Lane was all too ready to sacrifice the crippled organ, and though Metchnikoff hoped to reform it, his remedial program fell far short of what was needed. For restoration to genuine "biologic rectitude" a wholly vegetable diet was required, and not just to avoid the putrefaction-prone substances of a meat diet but to provide bulk to the feces and instigate perstalsis. A bowel without bulk provided by each meal was a "paralyzed" colon, unable to push its contents forward. Bulk equated to cellulose, the indigestible material prevalent in the cell walls of plants. This unabsorbed residue from the digestive breakdown of "fruits and roots and tender shoots" (Kellogg's eulogization of natural diet) was "the physiologic laxative," stirring the colon into action by distending it. But not all cellulose was the same. However much bulk one might get from fruits and roots, there was more to be had from seaweed and grains, or more particularly, from agar-agar and bran, the two forms of cellulose Kellogg held in highest esteem.[38]

Agar-agar (commonly known to scientists simply as agar) is a gelatinous material prepared from seaweed. Its initial use in medicine was as a medium for the laboratory cultivation of microorganisms. By the early years of the twentieth century it was also being used to relieve constipation; agar absorbs considerable amounts of water, so increases the bulk of intestinal waste (autointoxicated habi-tues of Harrogate and other spas, we are told, became eloquent on "the volumi-nous well-formed satisfactions of agar-agar"). For Kellogg, who thought that virtually everybody was constipated, agar was thought of not as a laxative, as therapy for the occasional patient; rather, it was seen as a natural food, as an ele-ment of hygiene as necessary to everyone as daily bread. Daily whole-grain bread was even better, though, because it supplied bran, recognized for centuries as the stool-bulking agent *par excellence*. For Kellogg, bran was "certainly the most valu-able remedy in the treatment of constipation," and through his influence bran at-tained a preeminence in popular health philosophy and practice that Sylvester Graham could only have dreamed of. Patients at the San were served bran (a spe-cial sterilized version that Kellogg developed), and the population at large were told to include 1 to 2 tablespoons of the product with each meal (up to 2 ounces a day was Kellogg's recommendation). His readers were advised how to prepare their own sterilized bran and provided with recipes for bran bread, bran biscuits, bran mush, and bran porridge. Just to be sure the desired result was attained, Kellogg also advised that paraffin oil, the intestinal lubricant (and bulk former) popularized by Lane, be taken daily: "*Bulk and lubrication must be provided for every meal.*" A compulsive tinkerer where foods and health products were concerned, Kellogg came up with at least two improved versions of paraffin oil. Paramels was "a mineral oil that does not 'leak'," while Para-lax was a peppermint-flavored paraffin; nothing was better for the colon that was paralyzed, paradoxically, than Para-lax.[39]

People hardly had to sterilize their own bran or bake their own bran breads and biscuits. Kellogg, and a horde of imitators, saw to it that the public were sup-plied with an endless selection of already prepared bran products. The Kellogg name lives still, because of his invention of the precooked breakfast cereal. In 1877, the director of the San began offering his patients small nuggets prepared by bak-ing a mixture of Graham flour and other grains. Ever prescient, Kellogg named his new breakfast food Granola, and soon made it available commercially. A few years later, in 1895, his Battle Creek Sanitarium Food Company brought forth the first flaked cereal (Granose Flakes), and over the ensuing decade the manufac-ture of breakfast cereals turned into a booming industry. C. W. Post, an erstwhile San patient who celebrated his recovery of health by setting up his own food com-pany in Battle Creek, was one pacesetter in the rapid expansion of the cereal business, introducing Grape Nuts in 1898, then Post Toasties (originally called, none too humbly, Elijah's Manna) in 1906. The other leader of the burgeoning industry was Kellogg's own brother, Will, whose impatience with John Harvey's lack of aggressiveness as a businessman led him to open his own cereal company and introduce Kellogg's Corn Flakes to the world in 1902. It is this Kellogg's company that continues to dominate the global market.[40]

But many lesser-known names also set up shop in Battle Creek in hopes of striking gold through grain. By the end of the first decade of the twentieth century, the Michigan city was synonymous with health food, and also with hucksterism. The get-rich-quick hopes of cereal entrepreneurs were depicted only too accurately by a cartoonist of the day who surrounded the respectable-looking Battle Creek Sanitarium Food Company building with half a dozen tumbledown sheds housing such upstart businesses as "The Me-Too Battle Creek Food Company. Established Yesterday. Greatest in the World." In the middle of this tawdry scene stood a man labeled "The Public," besieged and beseeched from all sides by hawkers of "Gulpa-Hunka," "Bita-Pieca," "Have-a-Chunka," "Eat-a-Gulpa," and other cereals.[41]

Initially, the reason for gulping a hunk of any of the new breakfast foods was to build energy and strength. It was the carbohydrate and protein content of their cereals that manufacturers emphasized during the first years of this century, in line with the precepts of dietetics in the period before the advent of the newer nutrition. Thus Quaker Oats was touted as the source of "a wholesome sturdiness, a rugged health, a splendid ambition and conquering strength." Shredded Wheat's version of the conquering-strength motif drew on the prejudices of the time by picturing a marching Japanese soldier, fresh from annihilating the Russians at Tsushima (1905), alongside the statement that "the Plucky Little Jap illustrates the triumph of cereal foods in the building of a sturdy and industrious race."[42]

With the flowering of the newer nutrition, strength and energy came to be thought of as derived not simply from proteins and carbohydrates but from vitamins, too, and from bulk. When coupled with the pathological bogey of autointoxication, the newer nutrition pointed consumers toward foods that kept the bowels clear. Consequently, the bolted wheat and oats that had been the unchallenged staples of breakfast food originally, were being pushed aside by bran by 1920; toward the end of that decade, one observer noted that in just the last few years bran had "taken its place on the breakfast table of millions of Americans along with the cereals of high food value". Cereal makers would have protested such language. In their eyes, bran had high food value too, because it protected against constipation. Kellogg's All-Bran (produced by Will Kellogg's company) and Post's Bran Flakes in particular carved out large shares of the morning cereal market by threatening people with all the horrors of autointoxication if they didn't take their daily bran. "Here is what that dread disease CONSTIPATION will do if neglected," according to a 1920s advertisement for All-Bran: it will cause physical fatigue, mental lethargy, headaches, stomach disorders, bad breath, pimples, wrinkles, "AND LEAD TO OVER 40 OTHER DISEASES!" But John Harvey Kellogg lagged only a short distance behind, putting out his own large assortment of bran health foods (these were part of the "Battle Creek Diet System" that offered San-created food remedies for every ailment known). Branola, Fig and Bran Flakes, Vita-Bits, Bran Biscuit, Good Health Biscuit, Whole-wheat Cream Sticks, and, of course, Graham Crackers were just some of the cereal products distributed by the Battle Creek Sanitarium in its war against "constipation . . . the most common," according to Kellogg's ads, "and fundamentally most crippling and deadly of maladies." Hard on John Harvey's heels rolled a veritable bran wagon crammed with imitators, the masters of subtlety who manufactured DinaMite, for example, or the producers of Uncle Sam's Laxative Cereal, who tried to make dynamiting the bowels seem a patriotic duty. Bernarr Macfadden even jumped aboard, concocting a cereal he called Mealene from whole wheat and several other grains, and claiming that it not only provided bulk but also nutrients that strengthened the abdominal muscles, so as to double the attack on constipation. (Another opportunist came up with Bran-O-Lax, boluses purportedly consisting of a "heaping tablespoon of bran," but actually being made of phenolphthalein.) At least one of the early chain restaurants of the 1920s instituted the practice of providing free bowls of bran for breakfast customers.[43]

Bran appealed as the solution to autointoxication in large part because it was such an easy solution. Other preventive measures could be so irksome, so demanding of sacrifice or of effort. But bran was a convenient addition to the diet that might absolve a person of the nutritional sins committed at other meals by flushing them away. One sees here, as with vitamins, a profound reorientation in thinking about the dependence of health on food. Nineteenth-century prophets of better nutrition had renounced the common diet as a congeries of sins of commission and demanded abstention from all unwholesome fare, be it alcoholic beverage, flesh food, or stimulating spice. Only those inclined toward asceticism, naturally, answered the call. The newer nutrition's preoccupation with completeness in diet ("Not what you eat but what you don't eat—is the cause of many troubles")[44] made dietetic error a sin of omission and shifted attention away from the possible dangers of whiskey and sirloin. As long as each of the newly discovered nutrients was included in every day's menu, the optimist could reason, any potentially injurious foods would be buffered, and full health might be enjoyed without sacrifice; antidote was as preferable to abstinence as it is for smokers who switch to filtered cigarettes rather than give up their habit. The pain-free gospel of nutrition was received by the food industry with joy. Abstinence was not a product, but a food rich in vitamins, minerals, or bran, even if unappetizing, could be sold as preventive medicine. People would eat their yeast cake if they could have steak too.

Bran might likewise be substituted for the onerous duty of exercise. After renowned football coach Walter Camp's "daily dozen" setting-up exercises became a ritual many Americans aspired to practice (and a few even did), Post's Bran Flakes began to urge the public to "help your daily dozen with a teaspoon." The point was that everyone should exercise, but few had the time or the will. "If you do 'cheat' on your exercise," the 1931 ad proposed knowingly, "it's all the more important that you get a full quota of bulk in your food." Presented with the choice of push-ups or a bowl of cereal, most would opt for the latter (so a health magazine editor was perhaps not excessive in mourning the death of "the sportsman," who had "been reduced to a braneater").[45]

Bran peddlers told the tale in reverse, asserting that bran eaters were being elevated to sportsmen. Well before Wheaties began to bill itself as the "breakfast of champions" in the early 1930s, other cereal manufacturers built upon the postwar explosion of popular interest in sports and adulation of sports heroes. Time and again the bran eaters of copywriters' imagining were shown charging through defensive lines or taking Ruthian cuts at a baseball. Yet if consumers did sometimes fantasize about athletic glory, they were more seriously concerned with victory in the economic arena. The chief use of athletic iconography in cereal advertisements, therefore, was to make sport an allegory for the game of life. Indeed, the proposition that health was vital to occupational success became a commonplace throughout 1920s advertising, the portrait of the healthy and hence prosperous businessman at his desk being used by products as different as chewing gum and X-ray film. But nowhere did he appear with more regularity than in bran cereal ads. That constipation could undermine the efficiency necessary for getting ahead in business made sense to a populace conditioned to think of productivity in assembly-line terms. Food that had been processed had to pass smoothly through the body; if the intestinal conveyor stalled, the resultant backup was sure to play havoc with all the other departments of the body factory. Hence Pillsbury Health Bran could raise the banner of "Health—Your *best* business Partner." Post's Bran Flakes could describe the corporate struggle as "The Survival of the Fittest": "One of the most important allies of success is health. Guard it well, if you have your eyes fixed on the top rung of the ladder of success." According to another Post cereal advertisement, 1500 business and professional men agreed that "what a man eats when he's twenty five is more than likely to influence what he earns when he's fifty. . . . If you hope for success eat for success!"[46]

Kellogg's All-Bran explained what happened to those who ignored that advice. Men "who start in their business life with the brightest of prospects . . . energetic and tireless" suddenly "begin to slow down. They come to work tired. The ambition they once had fades away. They try to regain their grip on their work. But to no avail. Constipation has them in its grasp." One so grasped was the slouching, colorless man in a business suit that All-Bran placed next to an announcement that he had "Lost . . . another big order . . . the fourth defeat that day. All because he didn't have the energy to fight when his prospect said 'No'. Something had blunted his senses and stolen his strength. . . . That something was constipation, the world's most universal disease." The most frequently used image in this advertising genre was that of the husband setting out to work with new spring in his step, waving to his wife in the doorway, who is beaming with pride at having sent hubby off with clean bowels. Bran, women were told, is "how you can help him WIN!": "A wife, in a sense, is custodian of her husband's health. The food she selects can help him in his daily battle for success."[47]

Woman was custodian of her own health too, but in her quest for success, beauty was far more important than energy and efficiency. Beauty was also, according to cereal manufacturers, more than skin deep; it reached down to the intestines, where lurked, Post Bran Flakes warned, "cargoes of digestive waste . . . the common foe of . . . beauty." "Constipation wrecks health and happiness for thousands of women," All-Bran announced. "Some women," such as the one slumped in a chair watching two others play golf, "age so young." They may have started "out in life radiantly fresh and alive, [but] almost before you know it— their bloom and freshness have gone." They end up like the sad case who opens the chapter, being sent bouquets that break their hearts. Yet so potent was bran, it could not only maintain feminine beauty against the assaults of age, it could even endow women with the energy and drive (not to mention charm) to succeed in a man's world. In one episode of the "real life movie" series of ads run by Post's Bran Flakes in the early 1930s, Jane Talbot got off to a phenomenal start in the fashion industry, only to be stopped in her tracks by constipation. Her boss issued a "sharp reprimand," and her career seemed finished. A last-minute diagnosis of autointoxication by company Nurse Betty Lane, however, directed her to bran, Jane recovered her former zest, and she went on to realize her dream of success.[48]

An additional selling point for bran cereals was that they did the work of purgative drugs without doing the damage associated with those harsh chemicals: "laxative drugs," Kellogg estimated, "are probably responsible for more bodily injury to human beings than any other cause." But All-Bran "eliminates the evil of harmful, habit-forming patent pills" (all other bran cereals worked that theme too, Pettijohn's Bran, for example, providing "a complete release from laxatives"). Cereal, moreover, was hardly the only option to cathartics that the health food industry provided. John Harvey Kellogg's company also produced LAXA Biscuits ("crisp, crunchy biscuits of bran and agar"), Lacto-Dextrin (a preparation of Bulgarian bacilli that worked as a "refreshing colon food that . . . displaces the bad germs that destroy health"), and Psylla. The last was a preparation of psyllium, plant seeds that had been frequently used for laxation between ancient times and the nineteenth century, but that had fallen out of favor with the 1800s' enthusiasm for calomel. Appreciating the appeal of novelty, Kellogg reintroduced the seeds in two product lines, Psylla White and Psylla Black, and advertised them aggressively among physicians and pharmacists. In the late 1920s and early 1930s, Psylla was marketed in tandem with Lacto-Dextrin (in "a vast campaign," in the company's words) as a one-two punch against autointoxication. "When the Colon is Crippled What then?" a 1929 ad asked. Then, it was explained, "surely it is high time to change the intestinal flora," by removing the old flora with Psylla and implanting the new, acidophilus flora with Lacto-Dextrin (alternatively, one could take Paraffin Tablets, a blend of paraffin oil with Bulgarian bacilli). Psylla, it might be guessed, was not a stimulant laxative that worked by irritating the bowel. Rather, it acted by absorbing large quantities of water and forming bulk. Kellogg pioneered in the development of bulk laxatives, bringing out one improvement after another. In the 1930s, it was KABA, prepared from an Asian gum and such a "perfect peristaltic persuader" it could be counted on to produce the prescribed movement after every meal: "by use of KABA . . . the 'three-a-day' habit may be easily formed and with great health advantage." In the 1940s and '50s, the product was LD-LAX. Its active agent, zylin, "s-w-e-l-l-s to form a soft emollient bulkage," providing the colon "constructive help—not punishment." LD-LAX also contained an ingredient needed "to promote the growth of the master germ acidophilus," and thus displace "poison-forming germs in your colon."[49]

All-Bran, LAXA, Psylla, and the rest were all way stations on "The Road to Wellville." That phrase, anticipating the "wellness" so revered by the health promoters of the late 1900s, was actually the creation of C. W. Post rather than either of the Kelloggs (though it has lately become attached to John Harvey Kellogg because of the 1993 satirical novel *The Road to Wellville* and the less successful movie based on the book). From the beginning of his manufacture of Grape Nuts, Post supplied pamphlets with each box, explaining how the cereal directed one along the path of health. By the 1920s, "The Road to Wellville" had expanded to a booklet of nearly 100 pages, many of them given to elaboration of the theme "constipation is to be reckoned among civilization's greatest menaces," and no longer promoting Grape Nuts alone but Bran Flakes as well ("this cereal gives us a running start up the Road to Wellville every morning"). Fundamentally, what was required to get to Wellville was "efficiency." That ideal of bodily efficiency appears repeatedly in advertisements for Post's, Kellogg's, and others' cereals as the indispensable basis for health and business success. One of the many free health booklets published by the Battle Creek Sanitarium was "Eating for Efficiency." His system of "biologic living," Kellogg explained, meant not just "health" and "long life" but "efficiency." John Harvey Kellogg was one of the founders of the Health and Efficiency League of America (as was Fletcher), and one of his measures of an individual's health was a test for "colon efficiency" (essentially a determination of the time taken for a meal to pass through the digestive tract). Just as one should abide by St. Paul's dictum for spiritual health ("whatsoever ye do, do all for the glory of God"), Kellogg directed, for physical health, one must "do all for efficiency."[50]

Doubtless autointoxication seemed the menace it did to the early twentieth century in part because of the premium the era attached to the virtue of efficiency. The astonishing growth of technology in the late nineteenth century, culminating in the development of the automobile, had fostered a profound respect for smooth functioning, for the generation of maximum power with minimum waste. In the United States particularly, respect for efficiency was translated into political idealism, the Progressivism of the opening two decades of the century aiming at the elimination of waste and corruption from government and industry. Indeed, efficiency in business, government, or any other endeavor came to be seen as a virtual moral responsibility, the *sine qua non* of effective labor. The concept readily translated into physiological terms, too. The statement in Kellogg's "Eating for Efficiency" that "the body is a machine" was a commonplace (in the graphic metaphor of a 1930s' nutritionist, man is "a steam engine in breeches"). The body clearly was an intricate mechanical creation that did work and used fuel, and just as clearly, the more efficiently it did the work and burned the fuel, the healthier it would be. Thus the "efficient life" was more valued by the health-minded of the day than the "strenuous life" traditionally associated with the first Rooseveltian age. In the opinion of Luther Gulick, physical educator, founder of the YMCA, and author of a health manual titled *The Efficient Life*, "to be strenuous is no end in itself. It is only when being strenuous is an aid to efficiency that it is worth while." The equally prominent physical educator, R. Tait McKenzie, interpreted his life work as a "quest for El Dorado . . . the El Dorado of efficiency" where dwelled "the perfect man."[51]

To reach El Dorado, one had to be physiologically efficient in more ways than one, but certainly the most obvious way was to enjoy free movement of the bowels. The antonym of efficiency, after all, was waste. The body machine could hardly run smoothly if the waste products of operation were not steadily disposed of. It was not just the manufacturers of bran cereals who appreciated the power of this analogy. Constipation as the enemy of physical efficiency, and autointoxication as the consequence of inefficiency, were themes that ran through all the advertising, articles, and books of bowel health protagonists in America and Britain in the early twentieth century. As an ad for Fleischmann's Yeast phrased it, the body machine must continually expel its waste: "It can no more run efficiently with this waste piling up inside than a gasoline motor can run if you stop up the exhaust."[52] And more than ever, as the next chapter will detail, it was being recognized that the stopping up of the body's exhaust was a result of adaptation to Western civilization.

8

THE WHITE MAN'S BURDEN: CONSTIPATION AND CIVILIZATION

THE STATE OF THE ALIMENTARY CANAL of civilized man, from its opening at the mouth to its exit at the anus, is a disgrace to civilization, is a disgrace to the medical profession, is a disgrace to modern science, is a disgrace to the food chemists, who are very largely to blame for it. . . . By "improving" our natural foods, by denaturalizing them, by feeding us on devitalized, embalmed and mummified foods our food chemists have probably given a large number of diseases, among them cancer, to millions of men and women and have driven millions to an early grave. . . . Our scientific foods, our chemical foods, are a delusion and a snare."

J. Ellis Barker, 1924

TO THE NATIVE constipation is anathema.

Arbuthnot Lane, 1929

Sometime in the early 1920s, London physician A. Graham-Stewart had a 7-year-old girl brought to him for treatment. She had already been seen by several other "eminent authorities," but none had been able to relieve the bronchitis that had bothered her throughout her life. Graham-Stewart, however, immediately realized her bronchial difficulties were only a symptom of an underlying problem. He "recognized the pronounced evidences of chronic intestinal stasis," the emaciation, the stained skin, the feces that "could only be described as a 'filthy mess,' grossly offensive." X-ray examination by a colleague only confirmed the diagnosis: her intestines drooped into her pelvis, and were so kinked "that the gastric contents were imprisoned many hours."[1]

"Dr. Graham-Stewart commenced 'stasis' treatment at once," and almost as quickly the girl's symptoms began to subside. Within 3 months, in fact, "her father—who had not seen her in the meantime—could scarcely recognize her as his own child." Her weight had increased by a full 25%, her skin was no longer discolored, and she had become the very picture of robust vitality, "plump and

195

healthy-looking." The stasis treatment that had brought about this "miracle" (the evaluation of the radiologist) had run most of the gamut of nonsurgical anti-autointoxication measures, including the classic paraffin and a belt approach employed by Lane, along with abdominal exercises, daily massage, and thrice-weekly colonic lavage. But much emphasis was also placed on fresh air and sunshine (to the extent possible in the London of the early twentieth century), and on diet. Plenty of vegetables and whole-meal bread in particular were prescribed for the young patient, and in this, Graham-Stewart was following the lead of Arbuthnot Lane—the Arbuthnot Lane of the 1920s—just as fully as in relying on paraffin oil and the abdominal belt.[2]

The Lane of the '20s was still locked in combat with his mortal enemy intestinal stasis, but he fought with new weapons. Colectomy had been put aside by the end of the 1910s, as he came to appreciate that changes in diet and other living habits could remedy intestinal stasis just as surely as, and more safely and cheaply than, excision of the bowel. Part of that change of orientation was an acceptance that however regrettable the consequences of upright posture for the intestinal tract, *Homo erectus* and gravity were here to stay. But if gravity could not be countermanded, habits of eating, exercising, and defecating could be changed. It was simply a matter of getting people's attention, and educating and motivating them to live in accord with nature's guidelines. Hence in July 1925, Lane began planning, in conjunction with several others of like mind, the formation of an organization to enlighten the public in the principles of health needed for survival in the modern world. In December of that year, the New Health Society was formally announced, with Lane serving as president from headquarters at 39 Bedford Square. From then until his retirement in 1937, he labored unceasingly to engage the British populace in a close examination of their living habits, creating, he believed, a new "Health Conscience" throughout the country.[3] Further, Lane's work on behalf of new health would dramatize the differences in both habits and health between the modern people he was trying to educate and primitive (unindustrialized) races, who needed no instruction in right living. By new health, in other words, he actually had in mind a return to old health, to certain ways of life that predated urban civilization. And by concentrating attention on the relative freedom of preindustrial societies from the diseases of civilization, Lane imparted a powerful impulse to a train of hypothesis and investigation that would lead to an acceptance by many medical scientists in the late twentieth-century that autointoxication had not been a completely misguided notion after all.

Lane was 70 at the time he undertook the cause of New Health. He was still practicing surgery, and realizing considerable income therefrom, but the travel demands of the new work (he delivered addresses on health to lay audiences throughout the country) forced him to retire from the operating room. "What the public gained much more than compensated me for my financial loss," he felt, but he did suffer economic loss, and the injury was compounded by insult from the British Medical Association. Its "so-called ethical committee" (Lane's characterization) frowned upon august practitioners who stooped to giving public lectures and popularizing complex scientific issues, thereby "advertising" themselves. For his part, Lane had no higher opinion of the Association: "I knew I could count on the . . . support of the more intelligent section, but that is," he sneered, "very limited in numbers."[4]

Thus despite official professional disapprobation ("unbridled fury," in one observer's account), Lane took his tidings of new health attainable by all throughout the kingdom, and spread the news through every stratum of society. On a single day in November 1927, for instance, he gave separate presentations to the Liverpool Seamen's Friendly Society, the City of Liverpool Corporation, and finally, the Liverpool University Debating Society; at the last, he was escorted through the streets to the lecture hall by dozens of students waving loaves of whole wheat bread impaled on long sticks. Everywhere he went, apparently, people turned out in number (even "in vast numbers," according to Lane, who recalled one address at which mounted police were required to hold back the crowd that tried to force its way in even though the hall had already filled). He apparently was as enthused by the subject as his audiences, for while he had been regarded as an indifferent lecturer in his days as a Guy's surgeon, the New Health Lane positively moved listeners with "his dominating personality, his undoubted sincerity, and his mastery of decidedly picturesque English." A Harrogate journalist summarized a 1928 "Health Chat" that packed the city's Royal Hall as "an unforgettable lecture, even if it made one gasp at times." Other reporters may not actually have gasped at Lane's revelations of the dreadful effects of intestinal stasis, but they did generally find his lectures to be highly engaging and accessible to the laity—he spoke, as one put it, "straight from the shoulder." So straight was a talk given by Lane at Uxbridge in June 1927, that the vicar of a nearby church adopted the physician's remarks as the text for his next sermon.[5]

Lane and fellow society leaders offered guidance to the general public through pamphlets, newspaper articles, "summer schools," and books as well. In the years between 1927 and 1936, Lane wrote more than half a dozen books (if somewhat repetitive ones) on the full scope of healthful living: among these were *Secrets of Good Health, New Health For Everyman, Every Woman's Book of Health and Beauty*, and *The Prevention of the Diseases Peculiar to Civilization* (of this last, George Bernard Shaw is reported to have remarked that "no Bolshevist has yet written so revolutionary a pamphlet"). But still richer resources were available to those who paid a guinea (one pound and one shilling) to become active members of the New Health Society. In addition to a badge of blue, white, and gold enamel (with the words New Health Society encircling the rising sun), members received all leaflets published by the Society, admission to all lectures sponsored by the

Society, answers to their health questions from the Society's Medical and Scientific Committee (comprised of more than 40 authorities, eventually including John Harvey Kellogg), use of the Society's lending library, and a subscription to the Society's monthly journal *New Health* (edited by Lane). Members were entitled as well to attend the Society's monthly luncheon, which included vegetarian options. By the end of the first year, New Health membership stood at 2000, and branches of the Society were being opened in other British cities and even other countries. As the Society grew and gained prominence, a range of institutions (health food stores, restaurants, guest houses, spas, boarding schools) began to advertise their commitment to operate along New Health lines; some even gave discounts to Society members. Eventually, in 1933, a School of Dietetics was established at the University of London as a result of New Health Society influence.[6]

The substance of the advice provided by Lane and his Society fellows was for the most part standard hygiene counsel: exercise, fresh air, sunshine, balanced diet, and avoidance of nervous strain (the practice of "modern youth" playing loud gramophone music everywhere they went was blasted as a particularly "hideous" emotional irritant). Bowel health received special attention, purgative drugs being denounced as poisons and a range of hygienic constipation remedies, everything from bran cereal to visits to Harrogate and Cheltenham, being recommended. But New Health was hardly a narrow focus system of hygiene, or a conservative one. Among other things, it advocated enlightenment of the public about sexual matters, endorsed the contraception campaigns of Marie Stopes and Margaret Sanger (Lane personally assisted Stopes in setting up her first birth control clinic and testified on her behalf when she was arrested), granted limited approval to abortion, and countenanced the enjoyment of alcoholic beverages. Lane freely acknowledged taking a glass or two with meals, and so did his upper-crust comrades in the Society. It was easy, furthermore, to justify moderate indulgence: alcohol's "agreeable appeal to our palates [and] pleasant relaxative effects upon our nervous systems" seemed to make it evident that drink was friendly to nature if not overdone. Lane was equally friendly toward drink. Beginning in 1932, he played a leader's role in a crusade "to put the Merrie into England" by persuading the government to increase the opening hours of public houses and loosen other restrictions on the purveying of alcohol that had been imposed after World War I. The Defence of Rights and Amusements Force was primarily an objection to governmental paternalism, but Lane found a way to relate the political argument to physical health. "Can it be expected," he asked, "that a people who, in the heart of the world's greatest city, meekly agree to be thirsty only between 11.30 a.m. and 2.30 p.m. and again between 5.30 p.m. and 11 p.m. should face the realities of life?" Such questions resulted in "much abuse [being] heaped upon me" by less liberal hygienists and moralists, but Lane got revenge in the best way, by living well. At a 1937 luncheon of New Health cronies, to pick an example, the sumptuous food (dishes also rich, it was noted, in vitamins, minerals, and roughage) was accompanied by "an insinuating Léoville [and] a Pontet-Canet of respectable antecedents." (The diners congratulated themselves on their claret selections, remembering that just recently in the Médoc there had been a gathering of 14 wine-drinking couples to celebrate the 50th wedding anniversary of each.) No wonder the notoriously abstemious Bernard Shaw (participant in at least one of the New Health summer schools) had declined an invitation to a New Health Society dinner several years before on the grounds that he would be "the sole sober man present, watching you all running up doctors' bills." Nevertheless, the 400 guests who did attend seem to have comported themselves soberly enough.[7]

Bordeaux and birth control were not common ingredients in health reform programs, but there was something even newer under the New Health sun: the much more acute focus on the superior health status of the people of nonindustrialized nations. The very first article in the inaugural issue of *New Health* (January 1926) was a presentation by Lane of the Society's objectives, which began with the statement that improving the nation's health required "prevention of the diseases which are incident to civilisation." The organization's founders, Lane immediately expanded, had been "profoundly impressed by the fact" that "natives" of primitive lands were "quite free from all the diseases of the gastro-intestinal tract peculiar to civilisation." The profound fact that African and Asian "natives" (a term generally used at the time to signify what today would be called indigenous, aboriginal, or Third-World people) were healthier than European city dwellers was raised to primary significance in Lane's New Health philosophy. It would be brandished as the proof beyond challenge of the thoroughgoing malignity of intestinal stasis: "Constipation has aptly been called *the disease of diseases*, since it is the cause of all the hideous sequence of maladies peculiar to civilization."[8]

To a degree, the point was an old one. Eighteenth-century hygienists had looked to a physical golden age in the agricultural past, and nineteenth-century writers had frequently extolled the rustic as the very model of health. More recently, C. W. Post had explained why "Grandmother," our rural forebear, "needed no gymnasium or 'daily dozen' . . . did not need to know about exercise and fresh air, and vitamins and coarse foods, and where to get her iron and lime. They were all forced upon her. She couldn't escape them." She lived healthfully by necessity, by her "closeness to nature."[9] Kellogg had looked beyond grandmother, to "primitive people" who had three bowel movements a day, for his examples of closeness to nature, and well before the 1920s, Lane himself had held up "savage races" as the exemplars of how to avoid intestinal kinks.

During the 1920s, though, Lane moved beyond hypothetical propositions (savages' living habits ought to make them less susceptible to the distorting effects of gravity, for example) to solidly empirical arguments. His new line of attack was fundamentally epidemiological, marshaling evidence that the health problems he associated with constipation and civilization were rarely, if ever, found in traditional societies. This shift is significant because it was the epidemiological approach, in a much refined form, that half a century later would confirm the existence of "Western diseases" related to bowel function. Lane did not carry out the studies on primitive tribes himself; his New Health Society duties kept him in Britain (as did personal preference). But he read widely in the publications of physicians who did practice in far-flung lands, and brought together their observations of the rarity of every civilized ailment from gallstones to cancer. Though he maintained that "the diet of the natives . . . produces men of magnificent stature, capable of enduring the greatest hardship, and of a bravery which is unequalled in a state of civilisation," he did not idealize the primitive state: "I do not wish to perpetuate the myth of the noble 100-per-cent healthy savage" (thus he laughed off the idea of returning to some imagined golden age of nature, repeating the belief of nineteenth-century health reformers that the answer was not to reject civilization but to adapt it to physiological needs, to incorporate natural ways of living into civilization's superstructure). Lane knew too well that malaria, sleeping sickness, cholera, plague, and other infectious diseases ravaged nonindustrialized countries. Yet if the industrial world had succeeded in suppressing infection, it was beset by its own host of afflictions—"*filth diseases*" Lane called them, sounding like a sanitary reformer of old. These ailments that arose from the filth detained in the civilized intestine constituted the true white man's burden, a load of physical debility that advanced societies placed upon themselves by their refined manners, a mass of poisonous waste that would never be found in the bowels of a native.[10]

Foremost among the authorities Lane drew on to demonstrate the freedom of primitives from "filth diseases" was Robert McCarrison. A physician in the Indian Medical Service from 1901 to 1935, McCarrison carried out extensive field observations and laboratory research on the relations between diet and health, and was eventually knighted for his contributions to the science of nutrition. For 9 years early in the century, he was stationed in a remote area of the Himalayas, "among isolated races, far removed from the refinements of civilisation," races that were remarkable specimens of longevity, vitality, and "nervous systems of notable stability." The primitive Hunzas and other groups did require medical attention at times. Nevertheless, McCarrison reported in a 1922 paper in *The Lancet*, in nearly 4000 surgical operations he performed on them, he "never saw a case of . . . gastric or duodenal ulcer, of appendicitis, of mucous colitis, or of [intestinal] cancer." Intestinal worms were a common affliction, and there was the odd hernia, but otherwise "their consciousness of this part of their anatomy," the abdominal organs, was related only to hunger. "Amongst these people," McCarrison wrote, "the abdomen," that bane of life in the West, "was unknown." The "buoyant abdominal health" of these people, he added, "has, since my return to the West, provided a remarkable contrast with the dyspeptic and colonic lamentations of our highly civilised communities" (on returning to the West, incidentally, McCarrison joined the New Health Society).[11]

Lane quoted McCarrison's article in virtually every book he wrote for the New Health campaign. He also repeatedly cited the feeding experiments McCarrison conducted at the Nutrition Research Laboratories in Coonoor, in southern India. McCarrison suspected that the superior health of the Himalayan races was due to their diet of whole grains, dairy products, vegetables, and fruits. At Coonoor, he tested the hypothesis by raising one group of rats on the northern Indian diet of whole-wheat chapattis, milk, and raw fruits and vegetables. A second colony of rats was given rations "designed to resemble that eaten by many Western people": white bread (spread generously with jam), boiled produce ("scanty overcooked vegetables"), tinned meat, and tea (for which "the animals acquired an extraordinary liking"). After 6 months, the rats in the first colony were "well grown, sleek-coated, strong and active," while those in the second, all that invigorating tea notwithstanding, were "ill grown, poor-coated, weakly and listless." The latter group was also constipated. Postmortem examinations of the ill-grown rats uncovered injury to the entire gastrointestinal tract: "intestinal stasis is marked," McCarrison wrote of one autopsied animal, "the lower part of the bowel is filled with hard, oval, faecal masses situated one above the other [resembling] a string of beads." These experiments were repeated over a period of more than 2 years on thousands of rats, and invariably the Western-diet rats deteriorated in health, while the primitive-diet rats stayed "remarkably free of disease." McCarrison found the results to be consistent, regardless of whether guinea pigs, rabbits, pigeons, or monkeys were used in place of rats, and concluded (this in a 1931 address to the Royal College of Surgeons in London) that "it is reasonable . . . to assume that the human species is no exception to this rule, and that many of the ailments to which man is erroneously supposed to be heir are the outcome of his improper feeding." To Lane, of course, it was more than reasonable, and what made the diet improper to his mind was not so much the insufficiency of vitamins that McCarrison emphasized but the lack of bulk to stimulate the intestines.[12]

Lane called on a number of other Western-born physicians, men from both the Indian Medical Service and from stations in African and South American countries, to corroborate the low rates of European diseases among the native peoples they treated. He directed attention particularly to the exceedingly low incidence of cancer in these countries, which stood in stark contrast to the level of malignancies in Europe and America. During the early years of the century, public health programs based on the germ theory had sharply suppressed infectious diseases, allowing cancer to steadily climb up the mortality list. By the 1920s, it stood as the second-most common cause of death, and statisticians were demonstrating that it was continuing to increase at an unsettling rate. Statistical studies had also shown cancer to be an uncommon condition in undeveloped societies, with the authoritative source on cancer incidence, Frederick Hoffman's exhaustive 1915 survey *The Mortality From Cancer Throughout the World*, attributing "the rarity of cancer among native races" to the absence of conditions and habits of life "which typify our modern civilization."[13]

Only occasionally, however, had constipation specifically been identified as *the* civilized condition that produced cancer, and for the most part, the connection had been forged by disciples of Lane. London physician Alfred Jordan, for example, developed that theme in his 1920 address to the Hunterian Society (a professional group honoring the great eighteenth-century surgeon John Hunter; Jordan was the society's president that year). Reviewing the widely accepted evidence that cancer resulted from chronic irritation of body tissues, he argued that intestinal stasis constituted just such an irritation of the alimentary tract. The prevention of cancer, Jordan concluded, required the prevention of stasis. Essentially the same position was put forward by another London practitioner, Leonard Williams, in 1923, and the following year by a writer on political and economic issues, J. Ellis Barker (to be sure, Barker, Williams, and Jordan wrote extensively in support of all Lane's ideas about stasis; soon all would become founding members of the New Health Society—Barker as Secretary, Williams as a member of the Council, and Jordan as one of the Medical and Scientific Committee).[14]

Additionally, there were at least two physicians not associated with Lane who weighed in with treatises connecting cancer to constipation and other degenerate ways of Western living. Englishman Ernest Tipper's *The Cradle of the World and Cancer; a Disease of Civilization* (1927) was based on his 20 years of practicing medicine in Nigeria and seeing only 6 cases of cancer out of an estimated 300,000 patients. Struck by the simplicity of Nigerians' diet, which compared to European fare was low in meat and high in bulk, Tipper became absolutely certain (for reasons he never bothered to clarify) that "CONSTIPATION and EXCESSIVE MEAT-EATING" were the causes of cancer: "where they are present cancer is rife, where absent there is none." It would therefore behoove Europeans, who "year by year in leaps and bounds" were "becoming a more and more cancer-ridden race . . . to take," Tipper suggested, "one precious page from the Negro's book of life." He added, in language Lane would have applauded, that cancer "will not be cured in the laboratory, it will be cured in the kitchen, . . . and it will be our womenfolk who will deliver us."[15]

Constipation was also presumed to be a cause of cancer by London practitioner John Cope. Indeed, his 1932 *Cancer: Civilization: Degeneration* presumed any number of irritants to be causes: tobacco, furnace heat, false teeth, eyeglasses, glass eyes (so was it cancer that killed Monsieur Alphin?), and most of all, sexual perversion.[16] Both Tipper and Cope were eccentric, to put it kindly, and neither offered much in the way of evidence or scientific argument to back their odd conclusions. Nor did either receive much notice in serious medical literature. But one has to wonder to what extent their books inclined fellow physicians to react to any other suggestions that cancer was a product of civilization and constipation as just another bit of crackpot foolishness of the Tipper/Cope ilk.

By far the most comprehensive examination of constipation as a source of cancer was that of J. Ellis Barker, a layman (though son of a physician). *Cancer* ran to more than 400 pages and drew from both a thorough reading of medical literature and consultation with a number of experts (including McCarrison) to construct its argument that the scarcity of cancer among primitive populations was due to their freedom from intestinal stasis. Indeed, Barker determined, the "amount of testimony [that] shows conclusively that cancer is . . . brought about by chronic poisoning from the bowels" was "overwhelming." *Cancer* attracted international attention, and though written for the public, was frequently cited by medical authors through the 1930s. Rarely was Barker's case judged to be overwhelming, however. He was ridiculed by some (*Cancer* is "ludicrous," an American reviewer decided, as well as "a pernicious and harmful piece of literature"), and at best acknowledged only to have pointed out a suggestive correlation and to have proposed a possible explanation ("gives an abundance of food for thought," another American physician decided). But possibility was far from proof. Further, Barker clearly was a mouthpiece for Lane. Not only had Lane been one of the experts consulted for the book, but the surgeon was quoted repeatedly and his theories presented time and again as unassailable truth; even the introduction to the volume was written by Lane. As one offended London physician characterized it, without naming names, Barker's book was "a glaring instance" of laymen writing technical treatises "under the aegis of medical men . . . of qualified practitioners giving 'cover' to unqualified men."[17]

Lane was quite capable of speaking for himself, of course, and during his New Health era brought the stasis-cancer connection to popular attention to an extent no one had attempted before. Through public lectures, articles in *New Health* and in newspapers, and his hygiene guidebooks, he made the point over and over: significant levels of cancer were to be found only in those races that were constipated. As with Barker, this was only a suggestive correlation, a connection that needed much more extensive and sophisticated research to confirm that constipation and not some other feature(s) of civilized society was responsible. But as always, Lane spoke with certainty, and used the threat of cancer as the most compelling argument of all for reversion to the primitive regimen of bowel hygiene: "no death could be more horrible," he reminded readers, "no suffering more acute." Yet "in civilised communities" cancer was now common and was "increasing with alarming rapidity, . . . its ravages . . . extending with merciless progression." He had long been sure, it will be recalled from Chapter 3, that autointoxication lay at the root of every single case of cancer, causing it either directly (through chronic irritation of tissue) or indirectly (by undermining the ability of cells to resist other cancer stimulants). That theory of carcinogenesis was maintained without change: "the cancerous cell will only grow in a suitable soil," he wrote in 1932, "and that soil is provided by the prolonged action of toxins in the tissues." Such a conclusion was not fundamentally at odds with prevailing medical opinion. It was generally accepted that cancer resulted from chronic irritation of tissue by noxious agents of one sort or another. Several examples of chemical carcinogenesis had by then been thoroughly demonstrated (scrotal cancer from coal soot, for example, and bladder cancer from aniline dyes), so it made good medical sense that the toxins generated by intestinal stasis might cause cancer—if in fact stasis did generate absorbable toxins. That latter position was what most physicians no longer accepted. For Lane, of course, there was no doubt: cancer unquestionably "is the last chapter in the story of defective drainage of the large bowel."[18]

But if "in the chain of the diseases of civilization" cancer was still "the last link," as Lane called it, its cause was no longer the first and last kink. As Lane pondered the differences between primitive and urbanized societies, constriction of the intestinal tract lost ground in his thinking to faulty defecation posture and inadequate dietary bulk. The natural posture for the act of evacuation, the one assumed in primitive societies, was the squatting position, in which the thighs press against the abdomen and straighten the rectum for an easier passage of waste. Lane was far from alone in lamenting civilized people's abandonment of squatting in favor of the modern toilet; many writers on hygiene in the early twentieth century included the elevated toilet seat, which lifted the user out of the squatting position, among the causes of constipation. A French authority, an eminent surgeon, attributed the higher level of constipation among the British to "le water-closet à l'anglaise," and an English authority agreed: "the modern w.c. seat," the author of *The Culture of the Abdomen* opined, was designed solely for the comfort, not "the welfare of the user. . . . It were better that the contraption had killed its inventor before he launched it under humanity's buttocks." Lane frequently expressed the same sentiments, if more genteely, and designed a lowered toilet seat for personal use (as did the inventive J. H. Kellogg) (Fig. 8-1). The simpler solution, one Lane and others often recommended, was the use of a footstool in front of the toilet, the stool being about 9 inches lower than the toilet seat; if the buttocks couldn't be lowered, the thighs could be raised (enterprising businessmen quickly came forward with stools—the Hygienic Lavatory Foot Rest, for example—designed specifically for this purpose). Incidentally, at least one physician other than Lane blamed the toilet for cancer; in his 1912 *Coprostasis*, Englishman James Sawyer took note of the fact that cancer of the sigmoid and rectum "is practically unknown amongst our agricultural labourers," who, by virtue of their working in the fields, had "opportunities . . . for defaecation in the natural position . . . in exceptional prevalence."[19]

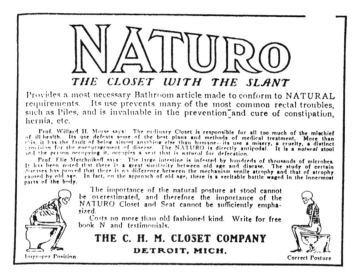

Figure 8-1. Advertisement for a toilet designed to allow natural defecation posture [from *The Naturopath and Herald of Health*, November 1908, p. 15].

It was not enough to return to the natural position, though; one had to re-store natural frequency as well. The longer waste remained in the body, the greater irritation to tissue it could cause. Lane contended that precivilized people had so little cancer in part because they defecated so often, and, like Kellogg, he labored to open his countrymen's eyes to the inadequacy of the Western standard of a single movement a day. "The ideal at which to aim," rather, was "a motion after every substantial meal" (in a New Health comrade's formulation, "the excrement should make room for the increment"). That was the norm for natives, he maintained, and Europeans should adopt it for their own; at the minimum, "in no case should less than two motions a day be accepted as adequate." Lane was nevertheless realist enough to accept that old dogs would not easily learn this new trick (most would respond, the reviewer of one of Lane's books supposed, with "let me eat unsuitable foods, and leave me to my one good action a day"). So he concentrated his efforts on convincing set-in-their-ways adults at least to rear their children on nature's schedule, aiming at making their "child's bowels act regularly after each meal as do the monkey's."[20]

The tragic reality was that civilized children were from their earliest years, to borrow a phrase from Kellogg, housebroken. Here was yet one more example of Victorian repression: indeed, "the disgusting act of defaecation" is the very first bodily activity "to be brought under the iron heel of propriety." Those were the words not of Lane but of one of his most devoted followers, Leonard Llewelyn Bulkeley Williams. Highly regarded London physician, founding member of the New Health Society, and a man who spoke in all seriousness of "the gospel according to Arbuthnot Lane," Williams was the most waggish of all the enemies of intestinal stasis. Hence, while he said nothing about bowel frequency and habits that wasn't also said by Lane, he expressed himself with such devilish cleverness that one turns to him rather than his mentor for the most engaging instruction on bringing up baby in the bathroom. On this aspect of stasis, Williams also spoke out earlier than Lane, complaining so early as 1908 and at frequent intervals thereafter that as soon as a child can be trained, its physiological cycle of multiple free movements a day "is severely battened down until it reaches the level of a grudging diurnal concession to lower things." Still more inhibition came with the tyke's graduation from chamber pot to water closet, "a change which is gravely maleficent in two important directions." First, "so strange and complicated and lonely a place does the closet seem to the childish mind, so fraught with mystery, so protected by bolts, and so gravely referred to in whispers, that Fear, the greatest of all inhibitors, is offered a free hand"; thanks to Fear, "the child quits the dread cabinet with a lie on his lips and his bowel bulging." Fear was not the only cause of bulging bowels, however. "The position which the little animal . . . is obliged to assume in this dread camera obscura" guaranteed blockage as well, for "instead of the normal crouching attitude of primitive man, he is obliged to perform the Blondin-like feat of balancing himself on a narrow ledge" (while all the time struggling to fight down the knowledge that "to fall backwards into that seemingly bottomless pit would be the end of all things").[21]

Nor were children's problems over once they matured enough to reach the floor with their feet, for on going off to school, they encountered new restraints. Teachers drummed into them that work periods must not be disrupted by the promptings of nature; "you must not give way to these feelings; you must learn to control them." And learn they did, though the control that was acquired turned out to be physiological tyranny rather than mastery. Step by deadly step, "the healthy clean-skinned adolescent" was transformed into "the sour-smelling and sour-tempered adult," an example of intestinal control in which "the tail restrains the whole dog." Lane also hammered away at this point, even providing parents with checklists to use in evaluating the lavatory provisions at schools before enrolling their children. The ratio of toilets to scholars must be determined, they were told, also the time allowed for evacuatory obligations, the encouragement given pupils to fulfill their duties, and so on. These were not trivial matters. Only when bowels were regularly emptied could brains be filled with "clean blood, and the brain cells . . . be in the best possible state of nutrition to receive and assimilate the instruction afforded by the teachers." Parents should be prepared, though, to find facilities "criminally insufficient" at many institutions; for Lane, that too common insufficiency of school life went far toward explaining the "lack of initiative and energy . . . that are so prevalent and conspicuous among the educated classes" after they graduated. Boys who are "badly drained," he aphorised, are "badly trained."[22]

That's not to say schools didn't attempt to drain their pupils. An English physician thinking back on his boarding school days in the 1930s remembered that every morning "we had to pass in line before the matron, who barked at each of us 'Been?'" The students who were "foolish enough to answer 'No' were dosed with a foul tasting draught" which he supposed was a blend of senna and rhubarb. But laxative draining was still bad draining. Natural frequency of elimination was to be insured by natural dietary bulk. Like Kellogg, Lane urged less meat and much more in the way of fruits and vegetables upon his audiences (one of his health manuals in the 1930s was titled *An Apple a Day*). Bulk in food, of course, translated eventually into bulk in waste. If there was any undeniable demonstration of the physical superiority of the native to the urbanite, it was this: the size of the stool was the measure of the man. One of the darkest areas of health ignorance among Westerners, Lane maintained, was the "very little idea" that people had of "the great quantity" of feces evacuated daily by people living in a state of nature. The only hint he offered as to how great that quantity was, however, was the intimidating fact that for gorillas the norm was 25 to 30 pounds. It was indicated that natives' output was somewhat less formidable, but just how much less readers were left to guess. Certainly they were unlikely to have been reassured of the adequacy of their own offerings by the words of Leonard Williams, who described "savage man" as a being who "has only to turn round to assure himself that the bowel is indeed empty," to know "that he is, so to speak, a free man." But whatever the approximate size of the ideal stool, Western people would do well to aim for that standard, and not for their body's sake alone. "The ocular demonstration of a really generous evacuation," Williams pointed out, "produces a most uplifting effect." The mere sight of such intestinal plenty "turns a melancholy man into a joyous one; it makes the timid courageous and the lazy energetic." To be sure, abundant stools were one of life's simpler pleasures, but "in a joyless world" they were a primal satisfaction that "should in no wise . . . be denied to anyone."[23]

For the making of a truly satisfactory stool, an apple a day and lots of other produce helped considerably. But the best results were to be achieved, in Lane's estimate every bit as much as in Kellogg's, with bran. Lane recommended bran cereals as part of the anti-stasis diet, and issues of *New Health* included advertisements for Post Bran Flakes, Kellogg's All-Bran, and like breakfast foods. Nevertheless, the magazine carried many more ads for whole wheat breads than for cereals: Granovita, "The Bread of Health"; Artox, with "every whit of the wheat"; Vita-Weat; Weetamin; even Chocker-Jack, "The Whole Cereal Chocolate Biscuit." That host of bread products was reflective of the much higher value that

Lane attached to bread as the vehicle for bran. Bread was supposed to be the staff
of life, and in its unmanipulated traditional form it was. Thus Lane listed "never
fail to include in your daily diet wholemeal bread or rye bread" as rule number
two in a list of ten "Golden Rules of Health" he compiled. Likewise, when he inaugurated a series of "Talks to Children" in *New Health*, he selected the superior
nutritiousness of whole wheat bread as the topic of his first installment. White
bread, however, was a distortion of nature's gift, "a devitalised food *par excellence*,"
a "white travesty" that, because it constituted so large a part of the average person's
diet, was destroying health throughout the industrial world. In his first presiden-
tial address to the New Health Society, Lane attributed the rise of "that dread
scourge . . . cancer" primarily to "the rapid spread of white bread." In brief, as
Lane expressed himself so succinctly on another occasion, "the whiter your bread,
the sooner you're dead." (It might be noted that Lane and his New Health co-
workers were not entirely alone in this opinion. In 1920, another British surgeon,
A. Rendle Short, presented a plausible argument that the remarkable increase in
incidence of appendicitis in Europe and North America since the 1890s was due to
lowered consumption of "the cellulose-containing foods." Others had blamed the
mysterious epidemic of inflamed appendices on everything from enameled cook-
ware to "cheap Japanese tooth-brushes" whose bristles might come loose and lodge
in the appendix; Short interpreted it as a phenomenon comparable to vitamin deficiency diseases, as a cellulose deficiency.)[24]

"The staff of life has become a delusion," Lane colleague J. Ellis Barker
warned, "and a most unsafe support to lean on." White bread was emblematic of
the devaluation of many foods through modern methods of processing and refining, a trend causing considerable worry among nutritionists by the 1920s. Much
of their concern was for the addition of compounds synthesized in the laboratories of organic chemists for the purpose of preserving, flavoring, coloring, and
otherwise altering or stabilizing food products. Such additives had been growing
in number since the later 1800s, and had been a primary target of early pure food
legislation such as America's 1906 Food and Drugs Act. But just as upsetting was
the fact that processed foods were having natural components removed from them
in even greater quantities than synthetic substances were being added. McCarrison
voiced the reservations about modern diet as well as anyone, decrying industrial
man's dissatisfaction "with the unsophisticated food made in Nature's laboratory,"
his determination instead to apply "the principles of his civilisation—the elimination of the natural and the substitution of the artificial—to the food he eats and
fluids he drinks." In one way or another, McCarrison complained, people must
have food that is "preserved, purified, polished, pickled."[25]

The preserving and polishing of food bothered McCarrison and other nutritionists mostly because of the vitamins and minerals that were lost in the process, though the elimination of bran and other forms of indigestible bulk through

processing was criticized as well. For Lane, the emphases were reversed. He regarded the deletion of vitamins and minerals as regrettable, to be sure, and he encouraged people to obtain them by eating more fruits and vegetables. But he perceived a far more serious threat in the absence of bulk in the modern diet, the bulk that was needed to forestall intestinal stasis. For Lane, full nutrition depended not just on what was digested and absorbed into the body but equally on what was not digested and passed through the body as so-called waste. To his mind, lowly roughage was an essential nutrient in as full a sense as proteins or vitamins were. He included it in his list of eight basic "classes of foods": proteins, carbohydrates, vitamins, minerals, etc.—and roughage. Roughage was a nutrient, he maintained, because it activated a physiological process critical to health, it gave "bulk to the contents of the intestines, enabling the bowel muscles to grip the contents and pass them along"[26]

On behalf of roughage, the entire New Health Society waged a "Campaign for Wholemeal Bread" through frequent articles in London's *Daily Mail* (a paper with a history of crusading for health reform) and in the publication of a 1927 "manifesto" denouncing white flour as "not a complete food for man or animal." As the Society's poster at an Ideal Home Exhibition pointed out, "You would not give your children *skimmed* milk. Why give them '*skimmed* bread'?" For that matter, why give them skimmed vegetables and fruits? The best way to counter the artificiality of the food supplied by industry, the New Health Society proposed, was for people to grow their own produce. Here some Society members veered off toward hygienic utopianism, dreaming up a "homecroft scheme of New Health housing" through which they hoped not just to restore Britons' health but also to restructure British society. Just a year after its organization, the New Health Society introduced a plan to establish Homecroft Settlements throughout Great Britain, aggregations of cottages, each with nearly a half acre of land to till, to be inhabited by working-class families wishing to live a more natural and self-sufficient life. A tool shed, chicken coops, stalls for goats: all the homecrofters' needs were to be provided, even the plumbing for transferring bowel waste to the soil to fertilize crops. "Thus the croft will be a big larder always round the house," a place where "working men . . . will grow their own food." Yet it was not only that. The croft was also a place to "cultivate independence, and stand four-square against all the chances of unemployment or civil commotion or war or any other scarcity, and set an example of how England can be fed." The example was a short-lived one. The first homecroft settlement, consisting of 10 cottages, opened in the one-time spa of Cheltenham in November 1927; but hoped-for funding from the government failed to materialize, and if there was a second settlement, its opening was not recorded.[27]

In the eyes of Lane's medical contemporaries, however, the folly of home-crofting was nothing compared to the seeming absurdity of his conviction that cancer stemmed from white bread and constipation: that "notion," Sir Thomas Horder, physician to the Prince of Wales, called it; "I will not distinguish it by the term hypothesis." Most other physicians who addressed Lane's linking of cancer to improper feeding also rejected it as unsubstantiated. Horder's statement of that majority opinion was part of the first MacAlister Lecture of the London Clinical Society, which he presented in 1927. The notion had "no established facts at all" to support it, Horder assured his audience; "we know of no single fact whatsoever concerning the causal association of diet with cancer." Nevertheless, "public apprehension" of cancer had "become seriously increased," and all, he maintained, as the result of Lane's "propaganda": of late, Horder said, patients were asking him all the time if they were giving themselves tumors through too civilized bowel habits. "Surely," he suggested with a thinly veiled swipe at the New Health Society, "surely it is time a health society arose which spread a less confusing and a more comforting gospel; it might be called the Society of Common Sense." Then concluding with an equally transparent jab at Lane, he reminded listeners how unprofessional it was for a physician "to proselytize in the name of science, instead of making it clear that what is advocated with such fervour is only a form of personal belief." A fortnight after Horder's lecture, a rebuttal of the New Health Society's anti-white bread manifesto appeared in *The Lancet* over his name, signed as well by a public health official, three professors of physiology, and a professor of agriculture. Statements that cancer resulted from white bread, all agreed, were "unwarranted"; subsequent letters from the journal's readers ran generally in support of the document.[28]

Support was still more solid in a second sampling of opinion. When Britain's National Association of Millers mailed a questionnaire to 1000 randomly selected physicians throughout the nation, soliciting their reaction to Lane's proclamation that white bread was "the curse of our civilization," 76% of the respondents denied it was a curse, 80% disagreed that white bread "was likely to lower the standard of national health," and a full 89% replied they preferred white bread themselves. Lane's reaction to the survey's findings was to dismiss it as yet another example of "the sublime ignorance" of the medical profession on questions of diet, and to characterize the whole inquiry as an "almost criminal" attempt on the part of the milling industry to confuse the public on matters of vital importance. One has to agree with the American medical commentator on this bickering between "eminent physicians" over "an apparently simple question," that it was a "spectacle" that was "not edifying for the public."[29]

Nevertheless, "it was not long," the *Journal of the American Medical Association* reported in 1927, "before the British hyperenthusiasm [i.e., Lane's, and Barker's, contention that cancer was the result of a white bread diet] infected the United States." As in Britain, physicians were largely immune to the infection. Rather, it was lay food reformers who succumbed to whole-wheat hyperenthusiasm. Well before the founding of the New Health Society, cancer had been tied to constipation and inadequate bulk in the diet by America's most vociferous antagonist of processed foods. Alfred Watterson McCann, furthermore, spoke from a considerable base of experience, having worked 5 years as an advertising manager in the food industry before being overcome by guilt over the "blind commercial enthusiasm" that had driven him into "lying about food," into "miseducating" the public, into "setting up false standards for them, . . . surrounding them with artificial compounds from which all the life and vitality had been extracted. We," he confessed, referring to himself and fellow food advertising men, had been "debauching the American people but we were satisfying our employers, and making millions of profit for them." The conscience-stricken McCann left the field of food advertising in 1912, taking up food crusading in its stead, dedicating himself to teaching Americans "the meaning of depraved foods," explaining to them "how foods are processed, bleached, colored, sifted, bolted, denatured, degerminated, demineralized, chemically treated and refined," alerting them to "the relationship of foodless food to sickness and death."[30]

McCann was scientifically unsophisticated, and favored a turgid style that owed much more to anger than to acumen ("the laws of God . . . are outraged and debauched in the food factory," he thundered in his 1918 *The Science of Eating*. There he also delivered his eulogy to the several hundred thousand American children he believed died each year from debased food: "With little knives and forks, with little baby spoons, with chubby little hands manifesting many of the outward signs of health, they dug their little graves"). All those little spoons and forks were actually metaphors for refined sugar ("sugaritis" was a national epidemic), for processed fruits and vegetables, and above all, for white bread, which had led Americans "downward into an abyss of national degeneracy." McCann worshipped bran every bit as much as Lane or Kellogg did, in great measure for all the minerals and vitamins he believed it provided the body, but also for its bulk. Though he made no direct reference to Lane, he equated autointoxication with "involuntary suicide," linked cancer to constipation and white bread, and proposed that unabsorbed bran be thought of as a nutrient because of its power to reverse the course of "modern cancer-plagued civilization."[31]

Medical orthodoxy ridiculed McCann (the *Journal of the American Medical Association* pronounced him "hopeless"), as well as all the other whole-wheat crusaders of the 1920s and '30s. There was self-appointed Professor Paul C. Bragg, for instance, who traveled the country lecturing on behalf of his National Diet and Health Association of America. At age 20, the professor told his audiences, he had been a "hopeless, helpless cripple," a pathetic ruin "given only thirty days to live." Now, just a few years later, he enjoyed resounding health, thanks to "Natural Foods," and "expect[ed] to live over 100 years" (he very nearly did. Bragg was still writing and lecturing as a "Life Extension Specialist" into the 1970s). In the

1930s, Bragg's "chief obsession" was the white bread menace, which he countered by selling his own "100 per cent bran bread" as a product that had "revolutionized the baking industry"; the American Medical Association's Bureau of Investigation suggested the people who most needed to attend his lectures were "prosecuting attorneys."[32]

Industrial giant Henry Ford was another who placed the blame for cancer on white bread. Ford, however, was notorious for holding hare-brained health beliefs, and therein lay a serious stumbling block for the champions of whole wheat bread. There were so many hare-brained ideas about diet floating about, so many misguided schemes of eating being pushed upon the public, that the virtues of whole wheat were in danger of being buried under food faddist chaff. In the early 1920s, for instance, Ford attacked chicken as unfit for human consumption; in the mid-'20s, he blessed carrots as a cure-all; and by 1930 he determined that a person should never eat before 1 pm. He could have believed all sorts of other things about food as well (in fact, he did), because American society in the 1920s and '30s was inundated with proposals for self-restoration through diet.[33]

Ironically, this smorgasbord of dubious table regimens set before the public was an outgrowth of the scientific advances accomplished by the newer nutrition. The opening of new levels of complexity in nutritional science revealed a myriad of possibilities for eccentric interpretations of the science. At the same time, newer nutritionists' exhortations to the public to pay more attention to eating backfired. The motivating assumption of nutritionists' popular education efforts was that enlightenment would overcome gullibility and superstition, would be, as it were, a vaccination against folly. To nutritionists' exasperation, education turned out to be an allergen that induced hypersensitivity to hogwash, the lay grasp of science being the sort of learning Pope had warned against. Made familiar with terms but not fully comprehending principles and mechanisms, the people became more vulnerable than ever to being misled by individuals using quasiscientific arguments to prop up schemes based on preconception or personal experience. Ill equipped to distinguish between authorities sound and spurious, the public of the 1920s and '30s drew much of their understanding of diet from misinformed reformers, haunted by the fear that "so far as diet is concerned there is not one of us who is more than one jump ahead of the hospital ambulance." The newer nutrition bred and fed the newer faddism.[34]

Hence the professional literature's hosannas to the newer nutrition were often as not accompanied by moans of disgust at the prevalence of dietary mythology among the laity. The 1935 tirade against faddism, *Diet and Die*, proposed that "no single subject, with the possible exception of religion, has had grown up around it a larger body of error, misinformation, and plain buncombe than has the subject of diet." Other books and articles echoed the protest. "America is a land of food cults," the author of *Eat, Drink and Be Wary* observed; the author of "Spinach—

for Others" scoffed at a public lost in "the Wilderness of Fad"; a third writer submitted that with respect to dietary faddism "U.S. citizens are the most credulous people on earth." But *Diet and Die*'s author turned the most telling phrase, entitling his third chapter "ODSAA," or, "One Damn System After Another."[35]

In addition, at least one of those systems (and one of the most popular ones at that) reinforced Lane's warnings about intestinal stasis. "Acidosis" was a state of nutritional imbalance conjured up by several food faddists of the 1920s, a supposed condition of excess acid circulating through the body as a result of consumption of the wrong foods. Just which foods were wrong depended on the acidosis antagonist in question, but despite all the conflicting interpretations, acidosis had become "psychically pandemic" by the 1930s; "all of us are suffering from acidosis," a writer in the *Saturday Evening Post* facetiously worried, "and so far as I can tell, everybody has suffered from acidosis since the beginning of the world." Best known of the Jeremiahs of acidosis was William Howard Hay, a Pennsylvania physician whose *Health Via Food*, a 1929 best-seller, established the idea (one that has resurfaced several times since) that proteins and carbohydrates should not be eaten at the same meal; Hay, according to the author of a 1937 chapter titled "Gullible's Travels," was "the dietary hurricane with the most victims in recent years." Fortunately, all those victims (among whom Henry Ford was counted) were provided with countless options for reversing their acidosis without undergoing the gastronomic deprivations demanded by the Hay system. Fleischmann's Yeast was promoted as an acidosis cure, as were any number of fruits and vegetables; a product called Ionite was guaranteed to "neutralise all the destructive acids in one day's foods"; even Camel cigarettes were presented as a product by whose use "alkalinity is increased." Since Hay warned that the retention of food residues in the intestines for more than 24 hours would also result in acidosis, laxative manufacturers too began to push their wares as acidosis prevention. Sal Hepatica, for instance, was pitched by radio comedian Fred Allen with the news that "when I feel logy and under the weather, I know that there are two things that usually, well, that cause it, the waste in my body and the acid in my system." Sal Hepatica, he explained, was "the mineral salt laxative that does two things, not just one. It rids the body of waste and it also combats acidity; . . . acidosis . . . and auto-intoxication are driven away." In many laxative advertisements from the late 1920s into the 1940s, it is difficult to distinguish a clear line between acidosis and auto-intoxication; the former term was more frequently used, but it was likely to be explained with theory derived from the latter.[36]

Mot people, of course, did not succumb to Hay or any other food faddist. Bran was perceived as a form of national mania not because everyone had switched to Graham bread and Bran flakes but because the promotional efforts of a handful of health reformers and food salesmen, and the declarations of praise from their converts had made whole wheat much more visible, more celebrated, than before.

Most people stopped far short of mania, though. Most agreed with the American who observed that if all the dietary schemes being pushed upon the public were true, then "the only way in which any person can save himself from a horrible illness is by ceasing to eat nearly everything to which he has hitherto been addicted and devoting the rest of his life to devouring foods that he wouldn't ordinarily eat, except on a bet." That was why people took laxatives or gobbled yeast (or smoked Camels)—to undo the effects of wrong eating rather than correct the eating. White bread was one of the wrong ways of eating that the masses did not want to give up. "The English are slow to change," a contributor to the *Times* of London pointed out in 1925; "individual voices crying in the wilderness during the last twenty or thirty years," crying about the "emasculated flour" that goes into white bread, "have made no apparent impression on the public at large."[37] Given that popular preference for white bread and the profusion of food cults in Britain as well as America, it is no surprise that Lane's promotion of whole-meal bread and other sources of dietary bulk as preventives of cancer got so lukewarm a response. To the laity as much as to physicians, his ideas looked like just one more of those damn systems that kept on coming one after another.

The people who took Lane seriously were the marketers of health products. They latched onto his connection of primitive lifestyle to freedom from cancer with as much eagerness as had been applied to every other type of warning of the dangers of constipation. In America, a Chicagoan named C. H. Woodward peddled a preparation called Whole Grain Wheat with as much "miraculous hokum," the American Medical Association judged, as "the crudest 'patent medicines'." Though nothing more than kernels of wheat packed into a can, the product was guaranteed to cure cancer, not just prevent it (equal efficacy was promised against tuberculosis, diabetes, kidney disease, goiter, obesity, emaciation, and bed-wetting). Woodward advertised coast to coast in every available medium, churned out testimonial-packed pamphlets, and issued a monthly newsletter crammed with articles such as "Civilization Versus Health," "Whole Wheat or Cancer," and "Cancer and Constipation." Berhalter's Health Foods, located in Chicago, marketed not only whole wheat bread, but whole wheat cake, whole wheat pies, and whole wheat cookies, muffins, and cupcakes.[38]

In England, the Allinson company conducted itself far more respectably, but likewise identified health with a return to the native's way of eating. T. R. Allinson was a Lancashire man trained in medicine at Edinburgh who set up in practice in London in the mid-1880s. Experience soon convinced him that hygienic living was superior to dosing with drugs, and that whole-meal bread, fruits, and vegetables comprised the ideal diet. Allinson broadcast his ideas widely (his pamphlet "The Advantages of Wholemeal Bread" sold nearly 100,000 copies), and enough of the public were favorably influenced that the Allinson Unadulterated Wholemeal Bread that he began to market in 1885 quickly became a thriving venture. This commercialism (his Natural Food Company also manufactured a coffee substitute, a baby food, and a breakfast cereal called Power) got Allinson removed from the list of registered medical practitioners, but his business continued to grow. Though Allinson died in 1918, his bread remained Britain's best-selling whole wheat loaf and was regularly advertised in the pages of *New Health* in the 1920s and '30s. The thrust of Allinson ads was that the bread was the best protection of "the family against its greatest enemy. The menace of Constipation" because it drew on preindustrial traditions. The wrap around each Allinson's loaf bore the imprint of Rembrandt's "The Mill," emblematic of the company's use of stone-grinding of grain, "after the manner of our sturdy forefathers" (customers who mailed in wrappers from a dozen loaves were sent a copy of "The Mill" suitable for framing). Allinson's Whole Wheat was a food proven beneficial by "the experience of countless ages," consumers were told; one could count on it to give "Health without Medicine" because "immemorial experience" had shown it to be "something that Nature wanted." It was the testimony of physically superior races the unindustrialized world over that, "the better the bread, the better the breed."[39]

Other manufacturers carried the theme of native as paragon of health much further. All-Bran's "what a difference there is between the active life of a savage and our modern living conditions; is there any wonder that a great majority of us suffer from constipation?" constituted a virtual leitmotiv in food advertisements of the late 1920s and '30s. Often, the savage was actually pictured in ads, not as a barbarian to rouse the reader's amusement or contempt but as a source of wisdom to be consulted. "*He* doesn't suffer from civilised teeth," Grape Nuts noted of a smiling African standing in front of his grass hut. Even enema equipment was marketed with the savage image. A 1934 ad for the Colonator featured a photograph of an African warrior as evidence of the value of "Spring-Cleaning the Colon." It was the bowel movement he had after every meal that made the warrior such "a fine specimen of one of the great primitive peoples," and with the Colonator the primitive's schedule was now attainable by anyone. Often, the savage was a cave man instead. In an ad for Fleischmann's yeast, for instance, a stylishly dressed young couple was seated in a posh restaurant, but with incongruously lethargic expressions on their faces. Their lassitude was explained by an inset in a lower corner showing a sinewy Neanderthal plucking a leafy plant to supplement the antlered carcass slung over his shoulder: "primitive man," the caption read, "easily secured the necessary food factors from his fresh meats and green leafy vegetables—modern diet too often lacks these elements." Alternatively, one might look to cave women for guidance. "The lithe forest girl of long ago," Post Bran Flakes stated, "had one 'beauty secret' that many of us moderns have forgotten." The attractive young woman in the low-cut, clinging animal skin "ate the bulk food. . . . To be slim and radiant, eat like a cave woman"[40]

Lane believed that not eating like a cave woman, and otherwise allowing autointoxication to develop, was what "precipitated" old age. He rivaled Metchnikoff in his estimate of the natural span of human life (130 years), and except for a few contusions and a fracture incurred when hit by a bus during the London blackout in 1939, Lane continued in good health until shortly before his death in 1943, at the age of 86 (when at age 70 he remarried after his first wife's death, he chose, and managed, a trip up the Amazon for the honeymoon). He grappled with intestinal stasis to the end, as late as 1941 authoring an article titled "Chronic Constipation and Self-Poisoning—A Sword of Damocles." But if Lane was virtually obsessed with autointoxication, and sometimes visionary in his expectations of a stasis-free world (he once suggested that if constipation were eliminated, "the necessity for building an increasing number of hospitals, jails and asylums will disappear simultaneously, and disease and ill health will become a thing of the past"), he nevertheless had a positive effect on the lives of many of his countrymen, and Americans as well. There was a good bit of truth in the evaluation made by McCarrison in 1956, on the centenary of Lane's birth. Lane had "led many into ways of healthful living," the renowned nutritionist stated, and done "much in helping to improve the nutritional and physical standards of the nation." A second centenary appraisal struck closer to the heart of the surgeon's career, though: "To Arbuthnot Lane the operating table was more than a workshop bench for the saving of human life and the relief of human suffering; upon it he read, as on a chart—in the maimed and toxic bodies submitted to his skill—an indictment of civilization itself, of the living conditions responsible for those dire results."[41]

9

FROM ROUGHAGE TO SOFTAGE: THE RISE OF DIETARY FIBER

ONE OF THE GRAVEST DEFECTS of the civilised diet is its lack of raw foods and ballast, or roughage. We eat over-milled cereals, chemicalised sugars, softly cooked vegetables, sloppy seasoned hashes, slushy puddings and soups, pappy porridges, sophisticated and highly-refined concocted dishes of all kinds. In such a diet there are no rough irritating substances to stimulate intestinal peristalsis.

George Dupain, 1934

In 1900, J. Ellis Barker was 30 years old and already a wreck, an object lesson in the wages of misspent youth. From early childhood, he had eaten freely of sweets and "did not pay attention to securing regular evacuations" ("I prided myself upon being able to suppress my need as long as I liked"). Consequently, he "became plagued with constipation," and resorted to the habitual taking of purgatives to keep himself open. "In course of time," inevitably, "I began to suffer from autointoxication." His digestion worsened, he developed jaundice and rheumatism, gout set in, and he lost 30 pounds in weight. All the while, he grew steadily weaker, until a mere 5-minute walk left him exhausted, and on occasion he even fainted. Neither spa treatments, massage therapy, vegetarian diet, nor Fletcherism were of any avail. Understandably, he began to have crying fits on occasion, grew ever more melancholy, and at last found himself thinking of suicide: "I was spending my days lying on the bed and on the sofa in utmost misery. . . . My presence became unpleasant to others. I became disgusting to myself."[1]

When not thinking of suicide, Barker thought of cancer, fearing that he already had a malignancy, or if not, was about to develop one. After all, for years "hard feces lacerated my bowels at the points where they were constricted by kinks," and the poisons of both autointoxication and purging drugs must have "made these lesions worse." As he thought it through, he became "convinced that I had only a few months to live," so made a last-ditch effort at survival by taking

217

"the rest cure" (one wonders what he called all those days of lying on the bed and sofa). While he rested at the nursing home, his irritating drugs were taken away from him, and "the horizontal position seemed to straighten out the kinks in my bowels" and relieve his constipation. He slowly regained weight, and finally left the home "resolved to alter my ways." The first step was to force himself to take more exercise. With that, his digestion improved, and he began eating vitamin-rich fruits and vegetables. When these agreed, he added whole-meal bread. One by one, his physical problems fell away, until by the time he helped found the New Health Society in 1925, he could boast, "I go now twice a day to that place which I used to visit often only twice a week." With his intestinal load lifted, he had far more energy and endurance, walks of 20 miles and more becoming a common weekend diversion. He felt better than he ever had, he announced at age 54; "I look the picture of health." And all because "my internal poisons have been eliminated."[2]

What had eliminated his poisons was coarse diet. Barker's daily regimen along the road to recovery included a breakfast of egg, cheese, fruit, coffee, and "coarse wholemeal bread." His lunch was comprised of more coffee, wholemeal biscuits—and "coarse porridge." For dinner, he took meat, vegetables, salad—and "coarse wholemeal bread."[3]

There was nothing particularly original about Barker's dietary program, of course; coarseness in diet had been a primary hygiene recommendation of Lane, Kellogg, and many another health reformers of the early twentieth century: "Eat with horse sense. Ask Dobbin—he knows!"[4] For Lane and Kellogg, coarseness was a compliment, an acknowledgement that the food was in its natural state, whole and wholesome, and robust enough to rouse the body's organs to vigorous activity. The coarse diet did not seem such obvious horse sense to everyone, though. To many in the medical and allied health professions, coarseness implied harshness. In their imagining of the process, the bran of whole wheat bread was an abusive ganger man who bullied the intestines into doing their labor. Just how rough roughage is, was a much debated question through the first half of the century. Out of that debate came a renewed consideration of the differences in disease patterns between industrialized and undeveloped countries and the role of roughage in keeping the latter free of the diseases of civilization. In the end, roughage would gain full acceptance into polite medical society, though under a more dignified name: dietary fiber.

Strictly speaking, the term roughage applied to the indigestible material of all plant foods, fruits and vegetables as well as grains. Much of the time it was used, however, roughage was intended to designate bran; it is still bran that one thinks of first when discussing dietary fiber, and it was the change in attitude toward bran that elevated the status of every other form of fiber. The hard shell of the wheat, bran resisted the grinding process that reduced the rest of the grain to soft powder; only partially broken down, bran's relatively large and irregularly shaped particles certainly looked like they would be rough on any mucus membrane they scraped against. In addition, people often experienced indigestion and flatulence for several days or longer after substituting whole wheat for refined wheat products. Physicians were thus disposed to think of bran as an intestinal irritant, and indeed had done so ever since Sylvester Graham's crusade to establish coarse-ground flour as the foremost health food. What had medical practitioners of the 1920s and '30s upset, however, were more recent health food campaigns. From otherwise respectable professionals such as Lane and Kellogg at the high end, to unqualified faddists such as McCann and Bragg, a horde of bran enthusiasts seemed to have overrun British and American society—and what was worse, society was answering their call.

As observed in Chapter 7, breakfast cereals were a major force in making bran the "national mania" during the 1920s. But whole wheat bread had a comparable impact, if in a less direct way. For while most people maintained a preference for the appearance and texture of the white loaf, they were constantly hearing proclamations of the superiority of brown, and the malignity of white, bread. This "propaganda" (the word used by Mayo Clinic gastroenterologist Walter Alvarez) not only frightened the laity into seeking bran in other forms, so as to offset the dangers of their white bread, it also shaped the beliefs of non-physician authority figures who had direct influence on the public's eating habits. By 1930, there was an unfortunate "tendency," many physicians agreed, for "school teachers, instructors in home economics, and amateur dietitians to prescribe rough diets for everyone." The resultant national "stampede for rabbit food," Alvarez believed, explained why so often when he looked in on hospital patients recovering from gastric surgery, patients in need of the most easily digested diet, he would find bran muffins on their lunch tray, along with raw fruit, salad, "and, I need hardly add, spinach." Absent specific menu instructions from the surgeon, the dietitian had prescribed what she thought would be best. In one case, that of a man with colon cancer, Alvarez had ordered a no-roughage diet, but the dietitian had served lettuce nonetheless; the physician concluded that the patient's death had been precipitated by the salad.[5]

Roughage was not usually lethal, but many early-century physicians did regard it as a chronic irritant that steadily eroded the vitality of the gastrointestinal system. Alvarez maintained that only those with "the digestion of an ostrich" could handle the large doses of the substance commonly being urged upon the health-conscious. An equally eminent gastroenterologist, Walter Bastedo, lamented "the coarse indigestible and fermentable messes that are so frequently swallowed," and the editor of the American Medical Association's popular health magazine warned the public directly that "whole-wheat fanatics" who blamed cancer on white bread were "violently loading" gullible people's bowels with "an irritating bulk" that would eventually injure them ("imagine . . . rubbing a piece of sandpaper over the red part of your lip," another American doctor proposed to anyone wanting a clearer idea of "the roughness of bran" with its "sharp little spicules"). In 1931, a questionnaire completed by nearly 500 physicians around the United States ("scores of the ablest medical teachers and practitioners in America") determined that though most accepted bran as an effective treatment for constipation, many were "strongly opposed to the use of bran" otherwise. Again, it was deemed too irritating, not only causing indigestion and flatulence but sometimes resulting in intestinal obstruction ("bran block," the condition was called in one clinic). Only two respondents to the questionnaire seemed "enthusiastic" about bran, and one of those was from Battle Creek.[6]

In 1936, the American Medical Association's Council on Foods reviewed the scientific literature on bran, and concluded that it was "rough, mechanically irritating food" that too many people took in excessive doses; the Council's conclusion that "the indiscriminate use of bran without the supervision of physicians . . . is undesirable" was "widely accepted." The feeling was similar in Britain, where the issue of white bread or brown was made particularly urgent by the outbreak of World War II. A shortage of wheat brought about a government requirement that millers produce only high-extraction flour (flour in which most of the bran was retained), so as to stretch the limited supply of grain. The resultant "National Loaf," the standard from 1942 to the end of the decade, stirred up a good bit of controversy among physicians, some of whom maintained that "the human alimentary tract, from the teeth to the colon, rebels against refined foodstuffs," while others, seemingly the majority, insisted that it was bran, "indigestible and an irritant," that the body rebelled against. That perception of bran was exploited, of course, by manufacturers of alternative products for bowel health. For example, the chief rival to Allinson's as a health bread in England, Hovis (from *hominis vis*, the strength of man), boasted that it was rich in wheat germ, but free of harsh bran ("which is really wood in the making"). Similarly, Heinz Rice Flakes were advertised as bran-free ("*soft and fluffy* so it cannot irritate"), and the laxative Flax-o-lin was actually designed to "heal . . . branny irritation."[7]

There were nevertheless some in the profession, not just Lane and Kellogg, who disputed the irritant interpretation of bran's action. It was not uncommon, for example, for bran to be described as "ballast" rather than roughage, suggesting the material was bulky and heavy, but not necessarily harsh. It was ballast that a contributor to the *Journal of the American Medical Association* had in mind in 1919 when he maintained that since bran absorbs water, it "becomes as soft and pliable as wet paper" when taken into the body. The rough edges of its particles are smoothed out, and instead of the "excessive irritation" commonly attributed to it, bran "produces merely a gentle titillation." As bran came into ever more common use over the course of the 1920s, the question of whether it was truly irritating or merely titillating was subjected to considerable discussion among physicians and nutritional scientists. To be sure, questions of quantity figured into the debate to a certain extent: bran's opponents focused on the eating of excessive amounts of roughage by people fearful of being overtaken by autointoxication, its supporters thought in terms of normal doses taken to compensate for the lack of bulk in the rest of the diet. But beneath the haggling over the proper quantity of bran were fundamentally differing perceptions of the material's qualitative nature. Some thought it sharp and abrasive, others believed it to be soft and soothing, disputing physicians' charges of gastrointestinal injury from bran. "Laboratory studies on both men and animals," a respected American nutritionist concluded after a thorough literature review in 1932, "have given no evidence of harmful effects." Rather, it was doctors' intuition—coarse particles of bran *ought* to be rough—that led them to imagine injury, or to wrongly attribute intestinal problems to bran. The truth, this side argued, could be determined only by experiment. Consequently, several such studies were carried out from the late 1920s into the 1940s, and the consensus that emerged was that "the effect of the rough bran . . . on the gastrointestinal mucosa has been greatly exaggerated . . . . no fear need be entertained."[8]

To consider just a few of the most thorough investigations, in 1932 two American researchers reported experiments in which human subjects had been put on diets of varying bran content, and measurements taken of their frequency of defecation and the weight of evacuations per stool and per day. Bran was determined to be superior to fruits and vegetables in relieving and preventing constipation and for increasing the frequency and size of stools. The authors of the study concluded that health demanded a certain "physiologic roughage minimum" ("90 to 100 mg. of fiber per kilogram of body weight daily") and suggested that a somewhat larger amount might be necessary to meet "the physiologic fiber optimum." Roughage was deemed a physiologic necessity, a dietary ingredient required for optimal health, and bran was recognized as the most effective substance for meeting the requirement. No evidence of harm from bran was found in the experimental subjects. The same year, nutritionists at Columbia University published findings on the effects of bran on young girls and on mature women, as well as on rats. In all three groups, bran produced more frequent defecation, as well as larger stools with a softer texture. There was no indication of intestinal injury in the human subjects, and when the rats were sacrificed and their digestive tracts examined, "in no case was there any sign of pathological lesions."[9]

In 1937, the English physician E. M. Dimock leveled another attack at the idea that bran irritated the intestine. For 5 years, he had employed bran both to cure constipation and to prevent its recurrence. "I have used it for approximately 250 patients," he reported, "old and young, in bed or at work, for those liable to peptic ulcer as well as for those with haemorrhoids, mucous colitis, and spastic colon." The only difficulties any patients had experienced—and their numbers were few—had been in chewing the bran (he gave them Kellogg's All-Bran) or in acquiring a taste for it. The "widely accepted" beliefs that bran inflamed the colon or produced obstructions, therefore, were "a bogy." And that meant the term roughage ("implies a coarse mechanical irritant") was bogus as well. "Bran forms a soft pulpy mass" in the intestines, Dimock emphasized, and those "soft moist stools . . . cannot irritate the mucous membrane"; they acted by mechanical pressure, not harsh stimulation. More than that, they were necessary for optimal health. Dimock proposed his own version of a physiologic roughage minimum, "the theory that the colon does not function normally unless it has a certain amount of cellulose residue." Similar conclusions were reached a decade later by Alexander Walker, a Scottish biochemist who had emigrated to South Africa. Examination of the stools of hundreds of subjects determined that bran not only increased the bulk of stools, it gave them a much softer consistency; when the act of evacuation was evaluated subjectively, "it is the *consistency* of the stool and not the frequency of motions that determines whether defaecation is satisfactory or otherwise." There was "no physiological basis," Walker insisted, "for this deprecation," this "alleged irritating action" of bran or whole grain bread.[10]

That roughage was necessary for intestinal health, and that bran was the best form of roughage, was borne out by still other studies that might be cited from the 1930s and '40s. The point was most successfully demonstrated, however, by another British practitioner, Surgeon Commander T. L. Cleave, Royal Navy. As early as 1930, Cleave, confronted by the problem of widespread constipation among men on shipboard, and wanting to break them of their dependence on purgatives, experimented on himself with unprocessed bran (crude bran was preferred to processed cereals because of its minimal cost, a penny a pound). Satisfied with the results, he then began ordering bran in hundredweight sacks and dispensing it from the ship's canteen, soon earning for himself the sobriquet "the bran man." The nickname was well meant, though, for "the bran was very popular with the sailors" ("even the hardiest and least imaginative tar" preferred to regulate his colon with a "natural material rather than scourge it out with unnatural . . . purgatives"). On one occasion when supplies ran out, many of the crew petitioned for the purchase of more roughage as soon as possible. (Incidentally, Sylvester Graham had backed his promotion of bran 100 years earlier with the statement that captains of whaling ships relied on whole wheat bread to stave off constipation at sea: "the coarser my ship bread," one was quoted as saying, "the healthier my crew is.")[11]

Cleave seems not to have called the medical profession's attention to his bran dosing, though, until coming across a letter in the *British Medical Journal* in 1941. A London physician had written to complain that with wartime rationing, Kellogg's All-Bran had been reclassified as a "luxury" item, and would not be available after present stock sold out. The situation was worrisome because "numerous persons" depended on the cereal to avoid constipation (it was "the only properly prepared bran at present available in England"), and would be driven to the use of purgatives without it: that "would be, I think, a great pity." But was it possible, the writer wondered, that the unprocessed bran commonly fed to farm animals might serve the purpose as well? He didn't know. M. E. Lampard, a Colchester practitioner, did know. In a response published 3 weeks later, Lampard explained he had been using crude bran on his patients and his family for several years, and "with excellent results" (so long as it was purchased from a miller; that sold by grocers was apt to contain weevils). But Cleave could speak even more authoritatively, and did in a letter 2 weeks after Lampard's. Now Senior Medical Officer on the 1500 man battleship King George V, he related that crewmen took from a teaspoon to 2 tablespoons in water, milk, or soup before each meal, and stayed completely free of constipation. Nor was there any indication of irritation of the intestinal tract; so gentle was bran, in fact, Cleave got positive results treating men with hemorrhoids with it.[12]

Cleave's modest half-page letter was a milestone in the rehabilitation of bran's reputation. Other explorations of the bran question had stopped at demonstrating its safety and its efficacy as a constipation preventive. For Cleave, however, the testing of bran triggered a process of rumination that led to the substance coming to be seen as prophylaxis for the full range of diseases of civilization, much as Arbuthnot Lane had been maintaining. The path by which bran ascended from mere battleship fodder to its late-century status as virtual fiber fetish would be a winding one, though. The first twist came with Cleave's recognition that his addition to the crews' rations had simply restored the level of roughage that had been the norm prior to the adoption of highly refined carbohydrate foods; he had, in effect, returned the crew to natural diet. There followed a deeply philosophical inquiry into the meaning of "natural," specifically into the question of the power of Nature to mold the human organism and of the physical consequences of straying from the course that Nature laid down. Ultimately, Cleave found himself drawing on evolution theory to explain modern diseases, just as Lane, Kellogg, and Metchnikoff had done.

But not until 15 years later, in an extraordinary paper published in 1956, did he present the conclusions to which these deliberations had led him. "The Neglect of Natural Principles in Current Medical Practice" opened with the statement—a most unusual, if not startling one for a medical journal article—that "Nature . . . is never wrong." That principle, Cleave submitted, was "axiomatic" if one accepted Darwinian evolution, for once any organism has "arrived" through evolution, it is perfectly adapted to its natural environment. It may succumb to predators in that environment, anything from tigers to bacteria, but death in such instances is part of the natural order; infectious diseases are therefore "natural diseases." But if an organism consciously alters its environment away from the natural, it will no longer be adapted to its surroundings and will suffer ill effects; these must be considered "the unnatural group of diseases," because they are not caused by Nature ("Nature . . . is never wrong"). Cleave had *Homo sapiens* in mind as the latter organism, of course, as the only organism that consciously acts against Nature; and the unnatural group of diseases he identified as "the majority of diseases seen in civilized countries today."[13]

The chief way in which the human species had altered its environment, Cleave went on to argue, was in its handling of food. With the discovery of fire, people had begun to cook food. But that had happened 200,000 years ago, and the human body had long since adapted to the change. Much more recently, people had begun to concentrate their food, specifically their carbohydrate foods ("all other foods [are] more or less in their natural state"), and there had been far too little time for the race to adapt to the drastically changed dietary. The hundred years that white bread and sugar had been widely consumed "counts as nothing at all . . . from an evolutionary point of view." Thus everywhere that concentration of carbohydrates had occurred, the diseases of civilization had followed. Heart disease, cancer, diabetes, peptic ulcer, dental caries, gum disease, hemmorhoids, even obesity ("no creature in the wild state is ever over-weight. They may vary in size, but never in shape") were all classified as unnatural diseases brought about by the refining of carbohydrates. So, of course, was constipation, along with its consequence "intestinal toxaemia," a condition "once so hackneyed" that now, he regretted, it had grown "rather neglected." Although he fell far short of Lane in the list of horrors he ascribed to autointoxication, Cleave did accept essentially the same theory of bacterial degradation of protein residues into toxins. Intestinal toxemia was "of paramount importance," he insisted, and "anyone who thinks it a myth" need only consider that the droppings of all animals in the wild are inoffensive in odor, while "the stools of mankind, and of the dog living under civilized conditions" (Kellogg's poor housebroken dog again) were generally "very offensive indeed." Lest the point be missed, he reminded that evolutionary adaptation had insured that "where the nose signals offensiveness, it signals danger." So just imagine, he concluded, "the consequences of the stacking of civilized Man's excretory products in a farmyard in the way that is performed with those of cattle, and then trying to explain the extraordinary difference by any argument that is not based on that of intestinal toxemia."[14]

The *Journal of the Royal Naval Medical Service*, in which Cleave's paper was published, was not a periodical regularly consulted by a majority of the profession. Likewise, "The Neglect of Natural Principles" was too vague, even mushysounding, a title to stir much interest among physicians looking for material with clear clinical relevance. Cleave's initial foray, in short, provoked little comment. Even if it had stimulated discussion, judgments would not likely have been positive. The article would have struck most as more philosophy than medicine, and as a form of naive nature worship. Cleave had actually written such things as "many of us might do well to cultivate a much greater reverence for natural principles," and "the treatments that are based on natural principles remain the same from age to age"; he had even suggested that physicians might gain insights of "considerable value from . . . naturopathists and other related cults." Readers no doubt would have agreed with his own evaluation that "it all sounds somewhat Utopian."[15] Cleave, however, was only getting started.

The stillborn 1956 article was followed by a series of short books relating first heart disease (1957), then varicose veins (1960), peptic ulcer (1962), and diabetes (1966) to twentieth-century changes in diet. But while these works continued to interpret the diseases of civilization within the context of evolutionary adaptation to refined carbohydrates, glorification of Nature's unerring wisdom was balanced with much more medical detail. In particular, statistical comparisons of the incidence of different diseases in industrial and nonindustrial societies were used to show a correlation between unrefined carbohydrate diet and freedom from "the unnatural group of diseases." Some of the statistical material was taken from medical literature, but much of it Cleave collected himself. Since undeveloped countries did not have readily available figures on morbidity and mortality rates, it was necessary to write individual physicians, an estimated several thousand in the end, and request data on the incidence of various ailments seen in their practice among both traditional and modern populations. Of greatest significance was Cleave's formulation of a unifying concept (introduced in the monograph on peptic ulcer and developed much more fully in the diabetes volume) that diabetes, ulcer, varicose veins, hemorrhoids, appendicitis, and several other conditions rife in civilized society were all manifestations of a single underlying condition, what he called "the saccharine disease."[16]

In Cleave's usage of the word, "saccharine" was pronounced to rhyme with "dine," and was not to be confused with the common synthetic sweetening agent saccharin. The saccharine disease was any ailment stemming from a diet of refined carbohydrates. It could result from the removal of protein from carbohydrate foods (he blamed peptic ulcer on this, though his rationale is peripheral to the present discussion). It could follow from the removal of cellulose and other plant fiber; constipation, hemorrhoids, and varicose veins were the injuries in that instance. It could also be caused by overconsumption of sugar, a food being eaten in much greater amounts than in previous centuries. Obesity, diabetes, and appendicitis were the most frequent consequences of sugar excess (overconsumption of sugar, furthermore, was related to elimination of fiber; bulk produces a feeling of satiety, so populations whose food was low in bulk tended to eat more of everything, sugar included). Cleave recognized that such a broad constellation of complaints might be more accurately designated "refined-carbohydrate disease," but that term was cumbersome, and the simpler label saccharine related to sugar (Latin *saccharum*), the most fully refined carbohydrate of all, and thus it most effectively symbolized the civilized practice of food processing.[17]

However one chose to describe the phenomenon, Cleave demonstrated beyond question that the complaints he called saccharine were much more frequent
among people eating refined foods than among those subsisting on natural diet.
His evidence was drawn from the reports of practitioners throughout Africa and
the Far East, and took account of racial differences between these people and
Caucasians by showing that when other races adopted European dietary ways, they
soon found themselves with European diseases as well. Tribal Zulus, for example,
who consumed sugar in the form of raw cane, almost never developed diabetes.
Town-dwelling Zulus, who had acquired the white sweet tooth and preferred refined sugar, suffered from diabetes at a rate almost equal to that of Europeans. Black
people in America, who had been using pure sugar longer than the urbanized Zulus,
now had a diabetes incidence equal to that of whites. The same pattern was shown
to apply to varicose veins and hemorrhoids, both conditions rare in Zulus who
followed traditional ways, but common in those who had moved to the city. Lane,
it might be noted, had observed the same trend, commenting in the 1930s that
"native races are imitating the more cultured ones, and it is becoming increasingly
difficult to find a people who have not become contaminated with the bad dietetic
habits of the industrial world"; though he thought in terms of intestinal toxemia
rather than saccharine disease, he would have agreed with Cleave that the ailments
due to refined carbohydrates were making a "remorseless advance." Nevertheless, the prevailing medical opinion was still that the rough diet of native races made
them less, not more, healthy. "One has but to go to the moving picture theater,"
an American physician wrote in 1956, the same year as Cleave's "Natural Principles" paper, "and see travel pictures showing Darkest Africa in order to realize
what a raw fruit and vegetable diet can do to you." Such fare was fine, he suggested, "if your ambition is to emulate the pot-bellied duskies who pop out from
the bushes in these films." But it needed to be understood that "the reason why
these African natives . . . have the peculiar pot belly is that they are so distended
with gas as a result of colitis caused by the raw fruits and vegetables. . . . In other
words, *these poor people are diseased.*"[18]

Cleave, it should be stressed, saw sugar, not white bread, as the leader of the
remorseless advance of saccharine disease. Sugar constituted "the chief problem
in the present diet," he believed, because people were eating so much more than
they had historically (consumption of sugar had risen eightfold in Britain over the
previous 150 years) and because refining processes concentrated sugar eight times
as much as it did wheat: "we therefore regard the sugar as being some eight times
as unnatural—and hence perhaps some eight times as dangerous." The starch of
refined flour, furthermore, was eventually converted to sugar in the body, so
whether one ate white bread or white sugar, the outcome was the same, a flooding of the system with the same unnatural food. Nevertheless, bran was what had
set Cleave on his course toward the saccharine disease, and bran maintained an

important place in his thinking. The bran of whole wheat flour prevented the discomforts of constipation, but further, the "colonic stasis" that inevitably followed the switch to branless bread brought on an "unnatural loading of the colon" that exerted pressure on the veins of the upper legs and the rectum and resulted in varicose veins and hemorrhoids (diverticular disease was also attributed to intestinal stasis, albeit through a different mechanism). Indeed, bran was a critical enough foodstuff for the prevention of the saccharine disease that Cleave created a "bran-plus loaf" that for a while, at least, was baked in commercial quantities by the famous London vegetarian establishment Crank's.[19]

To most of his medical colleagues, it was Cleave who appeared to be the crank. He was, first of all, something less than a household name among medical opinion-makers, having published very little outside the realm of saccharine disease theory. The theory's allegation that many conditions long regarded as distinct diseases were in truth merely different manifestations of a single, much larger disease was an oddity hard to accept. A reviewer of his volume on diabetes and the saccharine disease remarked that he had been engaged by it "because I enjoy books like *Alice in Wonderland*." Cleave's ideas were thought provoking, it was conceded, but were presented with "an evangelical fervour" that blinded the author to the many complexities of disease causation. In claiming that refined carbohydrates were "the *only* etiological factor" instead of merely *an* important factor, Cleave "overplayed [his] hand" and presented a theory that was "too simple . . . to be true," that actually "infuriates." Cleave's warnings of the dangers of saccharine ailments, furthermore, could be delivered in off-putting histrionic tones. Could not human beings eventually adapt to processed foods? Certainly, Cleave admitted, but only over "many thousands of years" and through "immense personal suffering," and who would want "to participate in this grim evolutionary event"? As his obituary notices commented, his ideas had been "too radical to attract serious attention" and had been presented "in the face of no little hostility from the medical establishment." For most of his career, he was "laughed to scorn."[20]

Yet in 1979, 4 years before his death, Cleave was honored with both the Blane Medal of the Royal Navy, for his contributions to the health of sailors, and the even more prestigious Harben Medal of the Royal Institute of Public Health (previous recipients included Pasteur, Robert Koch, and Alexander Fleming). He had gone from being "a prophet with little honor in his own Service," as one obituary described him, to being recognized as "one of the most revolutionary and farsighted medical thinkers of the present century," as another eulogist acclaimed him. The salvaging of Cleave's reputation was not so much his own doing, however, as that of the second eulogist, the internationally renowned surgeon Denis Burkitt. Under Burkitt's direction, the saccharine disease was transformed into "Western diseases," a term for the long-standing "diseases of civilization" that avoided the implication that countries that were short on cancer and diabetes were somehow uncivilized. In that same process, "roughage" became "dietary fiber." The terms fiber, indigestible fiber, and crude fiber had been used as occasional synonyms for roughage or cellulose since the early 1900s, but only in the second half of the century was fiber adopted as the standard designation for undigested dietary residues (the chemical definition of fiber was also refined during this period, and more emphasis placed on lignin and pentoses than on cellulose). Physicians and scientists attempting to gain professional acceptance of the idea that Western diseases were linked to inadequate dietary fiber saw the term as more scientific sounding than the colloquial roughage. Further, investigations of the behavior of roughage in the bowel had made it clear that the material was not rough, but rather produced a stool that was best described as soft. Thus roughage not only gave way to fiber but, among advocates of fiber for health, roughage was displaced at the informal level by "softage" (another proposal, fortunately nipped in the bud, was "cleavage," suggested in honor of Cleave's contribution).[21]

The "dietary fiber hypothesis," as it was initially known, was put forward in the 1970s, and much of it was accepted as a major addition to medicine and nutrition by the 1980s. It was a development built upon the contributions of a great number of physicians and laboratory scientists, including several of a stature rivaling Burkitt's. Yet it was Burkitt who became famous throughout Britain (not just the Royal Navy) as "the bran man." He tried to convince me that he was undeserving of so great a share of the credit for the establishment of dietary fiber as an essential component of diet. He maintained that it was Cleave who was the "genius," a man who might have worked his way to a more advanced understanding of the significance of fiber if he had not been made so defensive and intransigent by professional ridicule. Burkitt saw his own role as providing reputable backing for the idea. Cleave had no scientific standing, and could be easily dismissed. But Burkitt, thanks to work on cancer to be discussed below, held a position of authority in the profession: witness a letter to the *British Medical Journal* in 1972, from an Australian physician who began with "any proposition from Mr. Denis Burkitt must be treated with respect" (in Britain, surgeons are addressed as Mr.). Aside from being the person who forced the profession to treat fiber with respect, though, Burkitt admitted only to being just another member of "the fibre gang," as the early proponents called themselves. "I caught the last pass and fell over the line to get the try," he explained in a modernized version of the classic Newtonian comment about standing on the shoulders of giants; "but others got the ball there." The more accurate version is that others helped get the ball there, but that no one advanced it so effectively as Denis Burkitt.[22]

Born in Northern Ireland in 1911, Burkitt was drawn to the study of medicine at Trinity College, Dublin, out of a conviction that healing was God's intent for his life. Following graduation in 1935, he took up the practice of surgery in England, then volunteered for the army after war broke out. Despite having lost an eye in a childhood accident, Burkitt was accepted as a military surgeon in 1941 and, after 2 years service in England, was posted to Kenya. He would spend the next 23 years of his career in Africa, first as an army surgeon in Kenya, then, after the war, as a medical officer in the Colonial Service in Uganda. It was in the latter setting that Burkitt made his name in medicine (the first time he made it, that is), by the discovery in the late 1950s of a form of malignant lymphoma that he determined to be the most common type of childhood cancer in equatorial Africa. His follow-up studies on the geographical distribution and epidemiology of the disease resulted in it becoming known as Burkitt's lymphoma, and "Burkitt's name became a talisman in the world of cancer."[23]

Burkitt returned to England in 1966 to accept a position with the Medical Research Council in London. At that point in his career, he told me, he had had no particular interest in the relation of disease to living habits. Only weeks after assuming his new job, however, he was called by Sir Richard Doll, another eminent authority on cancer, to make the acquaintance of a retired naval physician. Burkitt had no familiarity at all with T. L. Cleave's work, but on meeting him and listening to his ideas, he felt "as if I had just climbed over the ridge of a mountain and saw a new panorama spread before me." What impressed him was not so much the specific content of the saccharine disease hypothesis as Cleave's method of analysis. Burkitt's own studies of lymphoma had involved mapping the geographical distribution of the disease (the "lymphoma belt" that spread across central Africa). He had accomplished that partly by traveling thousands of miles to collect information from hospitals, but also by sending questionnaires to physicians throughout the continent, much as Cleave had done for the diseases he studied. Likewise, Burkitt's clarification of lymphoma had involved demonstrating that tumors found in various parts of the body (jaw, thyroid, kidney, ovary, testicle) and previously diagnosed as separate cancers were, in fact, different clinical presentations of the same cancer—just as varicose veins, peptic ulcers, and diabetes were being interpreted as manifestations of the single saccharine disease. What drew Burkitt into a new area of research, then, was the possibility that seemingly unrelated ailments might have a common cause that could be discovered in the geographical distribution they shared.[24]

Burkitt knew from his years in Africa that Cleave's saccharine complaints were indeed of rare occurrence among the tribal groups of Uganda ("We taught our Ugandan doctors that they should be wary about diagnosing appendicitis in an African unless he could speak English. This was an index of his contact with Western culture!"). But to expand the picture, he tapped into the network he had already established in studying lymphoma, and prevailed on physicians at mission hospitals throughout Africa to provide him with information on the frequency of those complaints among their patients. Through the Medical Research Council, he had access to field hospitals in the rest of the nonindustrialized world ("more than two hundred hospitals in over twenty countries"). Thus within 2 years of meeting Cleave, by the use of questionnaires and personal interviews, Burkitt had collected a prodigious volume of data on the distribution of diseases in traditional populations and compiled a list even longer than Cleave's of conditions that, though common among Europeans and Americans, were rare in societies subsisting on unrefined carbohydrates.[25]

Burkitt would formulate a somewhat altered version of how refined foods related to disease, though. The first step toward revision of Cleave's ideas was taken with a 1969 submission to *The Lancet*. Published under the category heading of "Hypothesis," the article took a more methodical and tightly reasoned approach to establishing the plausibility of the idea that the processing of foods caused a range of diseases than Cleave's work had done. Its central line of argument was that the distribution of any disease, "both geographically in space and chronologically in time," was a pattern that was determined by factors in its spatial and temporal environment. Consequently, if several different diseases were always found to be present together under certain environmental conditions, one might also expect them all to be related to some common causative agent in the environment. In the instance at hand, Burkitt had determined that a number of affections of the large intestine "are universally prevalent in the so-called civilised world," but were virtually unknown in rural Africa: appendicitis, diverticular disease, colon polyps, and cancer of the colon and rectum "appear to be directly related to a Western way of life." Reasoning that intestinal disease must be related to the contents and functioning of the bowel, and that bowel content and function are related to diet, Burkitt proposed that the prevalence of such diseases in Western societies might be due to "changes in diet" in those countries, "and in particular by the removing of the unabsorbable fibre as in much modern food processing."[26]

An expanded analysis along the same lines was published in *The Lancet* a year later, attention now being called to the prevalence of diabetes and cardiovascular disease among populations using refined foods. In both papers, Burkitt suggested mechanisms by which a diet low in "indigestible fibre" might bring about colon cancer, diabetes, and heart disease. His purpose, however, was not to explain *how* lack of fiber caused disease, but to show that geographical distribution patterns demonstrated that it *did* cause disease. Subsequent publications bolstered the case with data relating additional ailments (varicose veins, hemorrhoids, gallstones) to low-fiber dietaries, and showing that that full range of diseases associated with the Western way of life had emerged as serious problems only over the last century, since the refining of carbohydrate foods had become common. "A carcass in the African bush is most easily discovered," Burkitt pointed out, by the "constantly associated telltale vultures"; in this case, the vultures were refined foods.[27]

Burkitt, like Cleave, considered one form of refinement to be more odious than all others. For him, however, it was not sugar, but bread and other cereal products from which fiber had been removed. "The relative decrease in the intake of cereal fibre" over the past century, he believed, had been a change that was "proportionately greater than the increase in the consumption of refined sugar." Further, it was the rarity of bowel diseases in traditional rural populations that impressed him most, and it was plausible that the health of the bowel might be affected by changes in the composition of its contents and the length of time of retention of those contents; fiber in particular was known to effect change in both variables. Indeed, so struck was Burkitt by fiber's ability to increase the bulk and rate of movement of feces, he went Lane one better. Instead of simply praising fiber for its enlargement and acceleration of stools, he undertook the actual measurement of fiber's effects. To be sure, he was not the first to perform such measurements. In the 1930s, Dimock had weighed stool samples as part of his study of the effects of bran, and in the next decade, South Africa's Alexander Walker had weighed the evacuations of numerous rural and urban Bantu people, as well as Caucasians, and demonstrated a correlation between stool weight and amount of fiber in the diet (rural Bantu, like other preindustrial peoples, obtained fiber primarily from grains, legumes, and tubers, all superior to fruits and vegetables as sources of fiber). Walker's investigations also included measurements of the frequency of evacuation and of "the mean time of traversal" of feces through the digestive tract. This transit time, as it would come to be called, was found to be two to three times faster in Bantu than in whites; even the slowest third of the Bantu were as quick or quicker than the fastest third of Caucasians. Nearly a third of rural Bantu met Lane's ideal of three motions daily, while less than 2% of whites managed that schedule. The bowels of the Bantu were so "facile," Walker observed, nearly 100% of their children could produce a stool within 10 minutes of request; fewer than 10% of white children could ("When we asked the White children 'Please try *now* to pass a stool for us,' promising appropriate honoraria, we were laughed out of the classroom."). Walker, incidentally, had been impressed by McCarrison's reports of superior health among Indians who did not eat a Western diet; he ended his discussion of stool weights and fiber intake with the suggestion that "the recent rise in the incidence of gastro-intestinal disorders" among town-dwelling Bantu was due to increased consumption of white bread.[28]

The stool measurements taken by Burkitt were equally extensive, and were made central components of a major transformation of understanding of how diet related to health. He began his studies on stool size and movement on his own family members in the summer of 1969, then moved on to take measurements in a variety of larger populations, everyone from English boarding school pupils to Ugandan villagers. The studies involved giving each subject 25 plastic pellets of the size of rice grains to swallow after a meal. Impregnated with barium, the pellets were opaque to X-rays, thus were easily detected after evacuation. The subject's next half dozen stools would be voided into numbered plastic bags, the time of evacuation recorded, and the stools weighed and X-rayed. The time that elapsed between the swallowing of the pellets and the evacuation of 20 of them constituted the transit time. Burkitt recruited more than 20 practitioners in several African nations, as well as in Brazil and India, to do stool weight and transit time measurements in their areas. But most of the measurements he did himself, both in England and in Africa. For a period, he hauled students' evacuations from Henley to his London office every day, and more than once in Africa drove a carload of stool bags 200 miles and more to the nearest hospital with X-ray equipment (during one of his African forays Burkitt chanced to meet Dimock, who had recently exchanged his life as a rural practitioner in England for that of a medical missionary in Uganda). Stool weights were found to vary from 2 ounces (English students and sailors) to more than a pound (African villagers); transit times ranged from more than 100 hours (English students and sailors) to less than 20 (African villagers). Even in Europeans who enjoyed a daily movement, transit times were often of the order of several days, thus confirming, Burkitt joked, that "a patient may be regular but five days late." Low stool weights and high transit times correlated, of course, with the prevalence of bowel diseases, forcing Burkitt to conclude that the movements of villagers in developing countries "are normal and that the small stiff stools and prolonged transit-times of the citizens of the Western world are abnormal." (Weighing of stools and timing of transits would henceforth be a standard part of gastroenterological research, though some medical scientists disparaged those who did such research as "fecal numerologists.")[29]

Burkitt photographed stools as well as weighing them, and as his ideas came to be broadly circulated in the 1970s, resulting in invitations to address medical audiences throughout the world, he often dramatized the significance of fiber in the diet by opening his lecture with a slide of the abundant evacuation of a rural Ugandan, followed by a slide of the paltry output of a city-dwelling Englishman. "Your chances of a long and healthy life," he told audiences, "are much more related to the amount of stool you pass than to your blood pressure or serum cholesterol levels." It was a good idea, then, for people to weigh their evacuations occasionally, to be sure they were meeting the standard. But since "most people are not prepared to do that," a simpler test was suggested. Fiber stimulates the production of gas in the bowel, some of which is trapped in the feces, making a proper stool float. Burkitt enjoined his listeners to take a look in the toilet before flushing it: "you can find out tomorrow whether you are a floater or a sinker," he pointed out, "and you will do yourself much more good by becoming and remaining a floater" than by frequently visiting the doctor. Speaking to doctors, on this occasion in the Yorkshire city of Doncaster, he suggested that "by doubling the size of Doncaster stools in the next decade you will do much more for the health of your community than if you double the number of hospital beds. And at a much lower cost."[30]

Though Burkitt postulated many benefits to becoming a floater, surely the greatest was avoidance of cancer. Lane had been certain that every type of cancer could be produced by autointoxication, but he had focused his attention on cancer of the colon, the organ most immediately exposed to any toxins generated from feces. Burkitt likewise recognized colon cancer as the most likely malignancy to result from low fecal bulk and slow transit times, and pursued the connection at length in a series of articles published in the early 1970s. The gist of his case against low fiber (the full argument is too complicated to be reviewed here) was that cancer of the colon and rectum, the second most common form of cancer in economically developed nations, was a rarity in undeveloped countries. Its incidence ranged from 51.8 per 100,000 population in Connecticut, down to 3.5 per 100,000 in Kampala, Uganda, Burkitt's former home. Furthermore, when any racial group emigrated from a region of low incidence to one of high incidence (Africans moving to America, Japanese to Hawaii and California), it acquired the rate associated with its new locale (and with a low-fiber diet) within two or three generations. It was equally telling that colon tumors most often occurred "in the areas of the bowel where the feces tend to stagnate," where "fecal arrest" was "maximum," and appeared not to occur in loops of intestine that had been surgically "short-circuited from the stream of feces" (this latter had been determined in experimental animals, not in patients of Arbuthnot Lane).[31]

These and other considerations led Burkitt to propose in a 1970 meeting of the Royal Society of Medicine, the same professional organization that had debated and rejected Lane's surgical treatment of intestinal stasis in 1913, a mechanism by which low-fiber diet might contribute to the occurrence of colon cancer (an extended version of this address was published the following year in the American journal *Cancer*). Any carcinogenic substances taken in with food would be present in more concentrated form in the colon of a person with small fecal bulk, and would stay in contact with the wall of the intestine for a longer period of time. The same principles applied to carcinogens that might actually be generated in the bowel, a more likely occurrence, he believed (relative to the surface area of intestinal wall, malignant tumors were 10,000 times more common in the large intestine than in the small, indicating carcinogenic agents were formed in the colon rather than brought to it in food). There was experimental evidence that components of bile could be degraded into cancer-causing substances through the action of intestinal bacteria and that the amount of fiber in the diet influenced bacterial populations in the gut. Reviving Cleave's observations on the inoffensiveness of animal stools, Burkitt observed that the bowel evacuations of people on high-fiber diet were also relatively nonodorous (Walker had determined this), suggesting "a lower rate of bacterial decomposition compared to that occurring in Western countries." In sum, "both bacterial activity and colonic stasis could account for the anatomical distribution of . . . malignant tumors which are found maximally in the area where fecal retention is most prolonged and bacterial action most pronounced."[32]

Burkitt's use of the term "colonic stasis" revives memories of Lane, and the attribution of cancer to carcinogens generated by intestinal bacteria sounds at first hearing like Lane's belief in the production of toxins by the germs of the gut. Lane had also maintained that the size and frequency of stools were fundamental indicators of health status. Burkitt assured me, though, that he was unaware of Lane's ideas until he was well along with the development of the dietary fiber hypothesis, and that he was not influenced by them. His hypothesis is, furthermore, quite different in detail from Lane's notions of intestinal toxemia. First, Burkitt did not suppose bowel carcinogens were absorbed into the circulatory system to wreak havoc throughout the rest of the body. In place of the one-toxin-causes-all rationale of Lane, he and fellow fiber theorists proposed specific mechanisms for each of the other diseases of civilization. Varicose veins, for example, were related to pressure on veins caused by straining at stool, the result of both low fiber–induced constipation and unnatural defecation posture; gallstones, on the other hand, were associated in part with bran's suppression of the production and/or absorption of compounds generated from bile by colonic bacteria. Nor did Burkitt blame colon cancer entirely on intestinal stasis. Rather he acknowledged that cancer was likely brought about by multiple interacting factors, of which inadequate fiber was but one: "I wouldn't even call it quite the fibre hypothesis," Burkitt said to me, "as I think it is as important to reduce fat intake as to increase fibre intake." Finally, his hypothesis had a much more substantial epidemiological, clinical, and experimental foundation than Lane's. Even so, colleagues informed him initially that he was "talking pathological rubbish" in attributing colon cancer to low fiber, and that they feared he had gone "daft."[33]

If so, Alexander Walker had gone daft too. Burkitt credited Walker with originating the idea that cancer of the colon resulted from modern diet. To be sure, Walker did submit suggestions of a dietary fiber basis for colon cancer to the *South African Medical Journal* roughly 5 months before Burkitt's presentation before the Royal Society of Medicine. Walker's paper, however, was more of an outline than Burkitt's, and was more hesitant in tone. Subsequently, the two men collaborated on several papers arguing for a causal role for low-fiber diet both in colon cancer and other diseases of civilization. Burkitt's most fruitful collaboration, however, was with an English physician he met in Uganda, Hugh Trowell. Also a medical missionary, Trowell did pioneering studies of kwashiorkor, the protein and calorie deficiency disease that plagues subsistence level populations throughout the world. It was Trowell who, in 1957, called Burkitt's attention to a child with mysterious tumors in his jaws, and started the surgeon off on his investigations of lymphoma. By that period of the mid-1950s, Trowell had become intrigued by the differences in the diseases he encountered among his African patients, and those he knew to be common in Europe. The differences in infectious diseases were easy to account for in terms of the presence of microbic agents and vectors of transmission, but there were many noninfectious illnesses, some of which were much more common in Africa than in Europe, others much less common, that eluded explanation. In 1960, 2 years after returning to England (whereupon he took holy orders and became a vicar in the Church of England), Trowell published a comprehensive survey of the incidence and geographical distribution of these ailments, *Non-Infective Disease in Africa*. In the chapter on diseases of the digestive tract, he emphasized that the various ailments of the large bowel familiar to Europeans were rare among sub-Saharan Africans, and proposed that the high fiber content of Africans' diet might be the major protective element.[34]

Once Burkitt began pursuing Cleave's saccharine hypothesis, it was virtually ordained that he and Trowell would come together again. Beginning with a 1970 meeting when both were briefly visiting Uganda, the two men cooperated on extending the analysis of fiber's role in health and constructing what would become known as the dietary fiber hypothesis (with Trowell proposing the word softage as a better term than roughage for a substance that treated the body so kindly). Their collaboration led to a 1975 edited volume, *Refined Carbohydrate Foods and Disease*, and culminated in the 1981 work *Western Diseases*. The title of the latter was a phrase the two coined to replace "diseases of civilization": it was "obnoxious," they felt, to suggest to Africans and Asians "that their communities had a low incidence of these diseases because they were uncivilized." Their list of fiber-related Western diseases was considerably shorter than what Lane and others had compiled for autointoxication, but it was striking nonetheless: dental caries, periodontal disease, appendicitis, diverticular disease, varicose veins, hemorrhoids, gallstones, kidney stones, diabetes, essential hypertension, coronary heart disease, cerebrovascular disease, colon polyps, and cancer of the colon, rectum, breast, lung, and other organs. There were still other ailments on the list, including the most basic of all: "constipation," Burkitt and Trowell wrote, "is the commonest Western disease."[35]

The "very simplicity" of the dietary fiber hypothesis, Burkitt and Trowell found, "has been offensive to some, as if complicated explanations were more likely to be valid than simple ones." But in fact, the hypothesis was not all that simple. For none of the Western diseases was lack of fiber asserted to be the single causative factor. It was deemed, rather, "to play a part," one "of differing degrees of importance in each" disease, and to operate in concert with "other environmental and genetic factors." Further, the dietary fiber hypothesis was oriented much more toward prevention than cause. Cleave had concentrated on the overconsumption of refined carbohydrate foods as the cause of the saccharine disease. Burkitt and Trowell turned that idea around by interpretating Western diseases as the result of the removal of a critical nutrient from carbohydrates; they thought in terms of

diseases of deficiency rather than excess, of ailments that could be avoided by restoring what was missing. Instead of attacking constipation as the etiological source
of civilization's diseases, as Lane and others had done, they focused on fiber as a
"protective" agent. By preventing straining at stool, softage protected against
hemorrhoids. By preventing the formation of hard fecal pellets that could block
the cavity of the appendix, softage protected against appendicitis. By reducing
absorption of cholesterol from the colon, and increasing elimination of bile acids
in the stools, fiber protected against coronary heart disease. By binding bile acids
and preventing their reabsorption to the liver, while also stimulating the production of chenodeoxycholate, fiber protected against gallstones. By increasing the
excretion of estrogen in stools, fiber might protect against breast cancer.[36]

Much of fiber's protective value was seen in connection with its relation to
dietary fat. Partly because white bread was less filling than whole wheat, twentieth-century Westerners ate more non-cereal foods than their forebears, including items high in fat. Cleave had denied that fat contributed to disease, because it
was a natural, unrefined food that the race had been eating for millenia, and thus
had long before adapted to. In the Burkitt-Trowell model, the recent increase in
fat consumption, coupled with the effects of low fiber diet on fat metabolism, was
made an important factor in several diseases. For instance, the adoption of high-
fiber diet invariably reduced a person's consumption of saturated fats and cholesterol, thus further protecting against heart disease. Lowered fat in the diet decreased
the quantity of bile secreted into the intestines, thereby lessening the amount of
bile salts that might be converted to carcinogenic substances by the colon's bacteria and thus was protective against colorectal cancer. In other ways as well, the
dietary fiber hypothesis was developed by the mid-1970s into a highly complex
and nuanced interpretation of the protective effects of fiber on physiological functioning, drawing on an exhaustive consideration of epidemiological, clinical, and
experimental data. It possessed, in short, a scientific sophistication that was well
above Cleave's work, and worlds apart from the proposals of early-century autointoxication theorists.[37]

That sophistication, combined with his formidable reputation as a cancer
researcher, put Burkitt much in demand as a speaker. During the 1970s and '80s
he traveled the world as a dietary fiber evangelist. "An evangelist," he told me,
"is somebody who proclaims good news," and he was proclaiming good news. It
was not always greeted as such, at least in the early years. A colleague of mine
who attended a Burkitt lecture in San Francisco remembers medical members of
the audience grumbling afterwards about the extravagant value attributed to bran.
Yet when he went to a health food store next day to buy some bran himself, he
was told there had been a sudden, mysterious run on the product the previous
afternoon, and the usually full barrel of bran was now empty. An English physician had the same experience, repeatedly. Whenever he spoke at any medical or-

ganization at which Burkitt had preceded him, "I would discover that his visit had two invariable effects: a record turn-out of members, followed by a local sell-out of bran." Just as Lane had impressed audiences in the 1930s with his "dominating personality," "undoubted sincerity," and "straight from the shoulder" talk, so Burkitt moved them with the "compelling power" of his "inexorable arguments," leavened with "wit and irreverence for conventional thinking" that made for "unforgettable lectures." Physicians and nutritionists were compelled as well by the volume and substance of his publications, and drawn to initiate their own investigations. By 1980, dietary fiber had become a flourishing growth industry in biomedical research, with articles on the topic appearing frequently in professional journals (more than 400 a year, as compared to 10 or so in 1970), and book-length treatments coming out on a regular basis. In 1981 an international conference on dietary fiber was held in Washington, D.C., and by the end of the decade two more international gatherings had been convened. "Interest in what used to be the disregarded cinderella nutrient," a 1986 volume on *Dietary Fiber in Human Nutrition* concluded, "has grown at a rate greater than almost any other nutrient." Roughage had found "a well-deserved niche in nutrition and medicine."[38]

The dietary fiber hypothesis was actually a number of hypotheses, each attempting to clarify the role of fiber in a specific Western disease. Inevitably, some of the postulated mechanisms had to be altered, or were completely disproven; just as Burkitt and Trowell had predicted, their hypothesis underwent a good deal of revision and modification. Nevertheless, by the close of the twentieth century, fiber had been accepted as an important component of a balanced diet, and was no longer seen as a material that roughly assaulted the bowels. "Bran and fibre" had become "household words," a British newspaper observed, crediting Burkitt for the change. His impact was summed up more fully in the obituary that appeared in *The Lancet* shortly after his death in 1993: "Thanks largely to Burkitt, the science of nutrition was galvanised into new life and people's eating habits all over the western world changed drastically—probably their bowel habits too."[39]

Certainly dietary fiber, as a softening agent that ensured easy defecation and presumably protected people against a host of ills, revived anxiety about constipation as the fundamental disease of civilization. And just as had happened with the rise of autointoxication early in the century, the triumph of dietary fiber brought forth all manner of programs and products to save society from Western diseases.

10
THE NEVER-ENDING QUEST FOR REGULARITY: CONSTIPATION IN THE LATE TWENTIETH CENTURY

EVERY HIGH SCHOOL BOY can tell you that Caesar divided all Gaul into three parts. This seemed to be a very simple and effective manner of describing the territory. Perhaps that, too, is the philosophy inspiring the medical writers who divide all human ails and ills into three parts; namely, those conditions causing constipation, those which are caused by constipation and finally constipation itself.

J. F. Montague, 1956

THE BOWEL-WISE PERSON is the one who is armed with good knowledge, practices discrimination in his eating habits and walks the path of the higher life. His days are blessed with health, vitality, optimism and the fulfillment of life's goals. He is a blessing and source of inspiration to family and associates. His cheerful disposition comes from having a vital, toxin-free body made possible by the efficient, regular and cleansing action of a loved and well-cared for bowel. Every person who desires the higher things in life must be aware of proper bowel management.

Bernard Jensen, 1981

In July 1972, a middle-aged bank executive arrived at the Mayo Clinic, in Rochester, Minnesota, seeking treatment for persistent diarrhea. For nearly 2 years, he had experienced a dozen or more loose watery stools a day, aggravated by abdominal cramps and frequent vomiting, and he had lost 100 pounds in weight. Mayo gastroenterologists performed a comprehensive physical examination, extensive laboratory tests, X-ray studies, an intestine biopsy, and finally exploratory surgery: "No intra-abdominal disease was found." Several courses of treatment were then experimented with—antibiotics, prednisone, gluten-free diet—but all were "without benefit." Consultation with several other clinic gastroenterologists led to suspicion of a pancreatic tumor, but when further exploratory surgery was proposed, the patient chose to return home. His problems continued, and in October he submitted to surgery at another hospital. No tumor was found.[1]

In January 1974, the man returned to the Mayo Clinic, still suffering from profuse diarrhea (a 24-hour stool collection weighed 10 pounds), and weak with low-serum potassium levels despite the heavy doses of potassium supplement he had been taking since his first visit. Colonoscopy, which previously had turned up nothing, this time revealed a darkening of the intestinal mucosa characteristic of heavy laxative use. Samples of the man's feces and urine were tested chemically and determined to contain phenolphthalein, but when "confronted" with this finding, "he denied laxative ingestion." He had, of course, been caught, and next day "reluctantly admitted" that for the past 4 years he had taken a dozen Ex-Lax tablets, as well as several other laxatives, daily.[2]

Laxative addiction and the resultant cathartic colon are persistent problems. Even as the enlightened twentieth century approaches its end, there are still frequent cases of colon neurosis in which fear of inner impurity has driven people to abuse their intestines with aperient drugs, impairing colon function and bringing on diarrhea that results in excessive loss of potassium. The resultant hypokalemia (potassium deficiency) causes physical weakness and mental apathy, and the heart, kidneys, and nervous system may be damaged. Occasionally, death ensues. "How many suffered and died from hypokalemia caused in this way" before the condition came to be recognized and treated, a modern physician has wondered, "nobody knows." The Mayo patient is typical as well of the difficulty of breaking habituation to artificial laxation. Though he "expressed relief that his masquerade had been uncovered," and voiced confidence he would overcome his habit, his diarrhea recurred after he left Rochester, and seriously enough to require hospitalization. His home doctor reported that the man denied he was taking laxatives again, but doubted he was telling the truth.[3]

Warnings of the dangers of self-treatment with purgative drugs abound in both medical and popular literature throughout the latter half of this century. A 1971 magazine article that offered consumers "The Straight Poop on Laxatives," for example, observed that "of every 100 Americans who dose themselves with laxatives, 99 probably shouldn't," then advised that "laxatives are easily the most dangerous over-the-counter drug on the market, as well as the most superfluous." Sentiments were the same at the professional level. A 1950s American physician denounced his country as "a great laxative nation," and identified the "great American sin" as "purgery." The following decade, the *British Medical Journal* objected that the taking of laxatives "has nowadays become such a widespread practice that it is a matter for conjecture whether constipation or catharsis constitutes the greater hazard."[4]

Actually, there is nothing to indicate the practice was any more widespread than at the beginning of the century, but surely it was widespread enough. As in the 1910s and '20s, popular magazines regularly published information pieces with titles such as "Laxatives: Overused and Undersafe." Any number of surveys of public laxative consumption were conducted in both Britain and America, and the consistent finding was that many people continued to regard purgative drugs as indispensable. Depending on the population studied, the proportion of frequent laxative users extended across a range from 5% to 80%, age being the chief determining factor. As in earlier times, infants were dosed almost universally (at a level of 79% in one British survey), subjected to a veritable "laxative onslaught" that anxious parents waged "as a kind of charm to ward off unknown hazards ahead." The onslaught slackened as babies grew into children, but still, a 1950s study found, nearly 20% of English schoolchildren were purged weekly by their parents; some were dosed daily and a few even twice a day: "The week-end appeared to be the traditional time for assaulting the bowels," this study determined, "and it was apparent that the ritual of the family purge still held sway in many homes." Once children escaped parental control, their intake of laxatives declined markedly, but eventually they became middle-aged themselves and more inclined toward their parents' ways. From midlife onward, reliance on laxatives increased steadily, until approaching 50% in women over 65. The irrational misuse of laxatives was exasperating to physicians, who could make sense of it only as a holdover from "primitive beliefs," a culturally ingrained "ritual practice." "Anthropological surveys have shown," one commented archly, "that among primitive tribes, such as the inhabitants of Nebraska farm communities, it may be the custom for every person to take a dose of laxative every day." Even if that overstated the situation, the laxative habit still constituted a significant economic phenomenon. Burkitt reported in 1984 that more than 50 million pounds were being spent annually on laxatives in Great Britain; in the United States, the figure at that time was 390 million dollars (by the late 1990s, estimates as high as 800 million dollars would be made).[5]

There were various reasons for such heroic levels of self-laxation. The Mayo Clinic patient, it turns out, dosed himself to cope with emotional pain, hoping his symptoms would gain attention from family members he felt were ignoring him. Others, including bulimics, purged as a means of weight control. But for the most part, purgation persisted as insurance against autointoxication. Among physicians, of course, the theory of self-poisoning by bowel toxins was dead by mid-century:

it "is of little more than historic interest," a British practitioner observed in 1945. It evidently remained a cherished popular belief, though, for gastroenterology texts well into the second half of the century usually included some mention of the "imaginary condition" so that doctors would know what their patients were worried about. So late as 1980, an editorial in the *British Medical Journal* remarked that "from infancy the British are brought up to regard a daily bowel action almost as a religious necessity and to believe in autointoxication from the cesspool of the unemptied colon." Six years later, a pamphlet issued by the National Institutes of Health to educate the American public about constipation began by disabusing readers of the notion that poisons generated in retained feces "are absorbed and are dangerous to health or shorten the life span"; the belief was a "common fallacy."[6]

Autointoxication did fall out of common usage as a word by mid-century, primarily because physicans no longer accepted it. "Auto-intoxication," "toxic absorption," "colonic stasis"—all "are bugaboos," an American physician wrote in 1949. That meant that laxative manufacturers generally ceased to use such words too. By mid-century, regulations governing drug labeling and advertising had been strengthened in both Great Britain and the United States to a degree that discouraged producers from issuing such grossly exaggerated warnings of danger and claims of efficacy as in the early century. At the same time, trade associations in both countries undertook internal reform, urging proprietary drug manufacturers to voluntarily refrain from distorting medical facts in their advertising. Thus once autointoxication was clearly relegated to the realm of medical bugaboo, laxative marketers sought other language to rattle consumers' nerves. Some merely became more vague, maintaining their product would "eliminate poisons" from the bowel.[7] But the stratagem that became the industry standard was to foster a fear of "irregularity," a word that was not so immediately chilling as autointoxication, certainly, but that suggested abnormality nonetheless.

"It's great to be regular," spout a beaming middle-aged couple in a 1950 Nature's Remedy ad. What made regularity great was at first telling not that much, nothing more than relief from the "headaches, bad breath and lack of pep," or from the "headachy, sluggish" feeling that dogged the bowel-clogged. Laxative advertisements in the second half of the twentieth century were tamed of their earlier extravagance (even while permeating the culture more than ever, thanks to the coming of television). No longer could manufacturers get away with calling constipation "the most formidable enemy of public health," or "the monarch of all diseases," and promise their purgative would snatch the user from the jaws of untimely death. The best that could be done overtly, at least, was to remind people of how unhappy they were when their bowels were inactive: "You feel sour, sunk and the world looks punk," was the way Carter's Little Liver Pills said it. Yet these more restrained ads were still effective. Not only would many people who felt sluggish or sour for whatever reason suppose they must need a laxative but they would also anticipate that much worse things might follow if they didn't flush their intestines. Older people, of course, would remember the ogre of autointoxication from the 1920s, but younger folks would have no trouble imagining it. The setting up of "regularity" as a golden ideal of health to which all should aspire ("What a wonderful feeling to be regular again," effused Serutan) effectively defined "irregularity" as illness, and only the most dim-witted were incapable of guessing the mechanism by which infrequency of evacuation might generate illness more serious than headaches and bad breath. "Mere contemplation of the character of the material voided," an English physician observed, "provides a specious expectation of the production and absorption of poisons through its retention." Thus even though "we are no longer threatened with the lurid horrors consequent upon intestinal stasis, it cannot be said that the bogy of autointoxication will ever be laid." Autointoxication, in brief, was a disease that need not speak its name in order to stir people to action; it was as sure to be intuited in the late twentieth century as it had been in all the centuries before, and to spur people onward in what an American health journal deplored as "the quest for regularity."[8]

Though a less outrageous distortion of accepted medical theory than the autointoxication-based laxative ads of early century, the idealization of regularity did delude and cause harm. "Regular" was likely to be interpreted as daily (public opinion surveys repeatedly found that the great majority of people believed a diurnal movement was essential, and "that serious and health-endangering consequences will occur if the bowel is not evacuated daily"). Even after the emergence of the dietary fiber hypothesis, with its encouragement to aspire to more frequent stools, prevailing medical opinion continued to hold that defecation schedules consistent with health varied considerably from individual to individual, and that anything between three movements a day and one every three days constituted "normal" regularity. Under the prodding of laxative ads, both the person who did not often have a daily stool and the person who just happened to miss a day were likely to reach for Ex-Lax or Correctol as the surest and quickest way to reestablish regularity (particularly since virtually all laxatives were promoted as "natural" substances or as mild catalysts of the natural process: "Discover Extra Gentle Ex-Lax. It's like giving nature just a gentle nudge"). From there it was only a step to taking the laxative weekly or still more often as a preventive measure to be certain that regularity was maintained. A panel appointed by America's Food and Drug Administration (FDA) in 1975 in fact concluded that "the way laxatives were being advertised tended to perpetuate, if not implant, the once-a-day idea into far too many heads." It was to forestall such abuse that government agencies charged with regulating drug advertising came to apply increasing pressure during the 1970s and '80s for manufacturers to drop references to "irregularity," as well as to stress on labels that their products were intended only "for the short-term relief of con-

INNER HYGIENE

stipation," and that "prolonged or continued use" of the preparation could result in dependency and deterioration of normal bowel function.[9]

Even if explicit references to autointoxication disappeared from laxative advertising, the theory of self-poisoning from the gut did continue to thrive in the world of alternative medicine and holistic health. "Detoxification" of the body through the use of herbal laxatives, colonic irrigations, and other "natural" remedies was, in fact, embraced by the New Age counterculture of the last third of the century as the cornerstone of physical purity. Health food stores appealed to customers for Herbal Trim N'Kleen ("Sane, Colon management") by announcing that "the average American has 5–15 pounds of excess wastes in the intestines," that the waste is "semi-permanently attached to the colon walls," and that "physical abnormalities in the colon structure like kinks" are also common. Herbal pharmacies cheered the autointoxicated masses with the promise of Intestinal Rescue, a preparation of "cleansing herbs" that "lubricates and exercises the intestines"; "in a clean body," potential rescuees were assured, "you experience more energy and motivation." A chiropractor who specialized in *Tissue Cleansing Through Bowel Management* informed readers as recently as 1981 that "autointoxication is currently the number one source of the misery and decay we are witnessing in our society and culture today."[10]

The extension of autointoxication's lease on life owed most, however, to the efforts of practitioners of naturopathy. In his 1944 *Constipation and Our Civilisation*, James Thomson, director of the Edinburgh School of Natural Therapeutics, spoke for mid-century naturopathy generally in still teaching that "auto-intoxication" produced "soured tissues" throughout the body. The natural healing system's chief journal at that time, *Nature's Path*, a publication tilted toward lay readership more than professional, regularly offered articles (some printed more than once) on constipation and its dangers: "Constipation! Auto Intoxicaton! Self Poisoning!"; "Constipation. Civilization's Curse"; "Constipation. The Greatest Menace to Beauty"; "Eliminate Constipation for All Time." In *Nature's Path*, classic autointoxication theory lived on in pristine vigor, constipation being vilified as "physical enemy No. 1" for its "fermenting, putrefying, body brew [that] perverts our judgment, stifles our morals, weakens self-control, breaks down character and stirs up trouble." The threat of body brew was made to resonate even more loudly by frequent reminders to the journal's doctor-doubting readers that the orthodox profession no longer accepted the theory: "The medical authorities say there is no such thing as 'autointoxication' caused by constipation. These terrible morning headaches must be just imagination!"[11]

To be fair, over the course of the second half of the century, such hyperbolic characterizations of constipation gradually faded from naturopathic literature. Along with other alternative systems of therapy, naturopathy undertook a process of self-improvement aimed at attaining scientific legitimacy. Mainstream medical and scientific research was carefully examined for evidence to be used to confirm (or refute) the theories and treatments previously adopted on intuitive and empirical grounds. In that way, enough "New Information to Support an Old Concept" was uncovered to justify the renewal of autointoxication under the name "bowel toxemia." The scientific literature cited as validation of bowel toxemia is too extensive to review; suffice it to say that end-of-the-century naturopathic physicians are convinced that "toxins do exist in the bowel; they are absorbed into the body; and there is considerable documentation linking them with many diseases."[12]

The naturopathic approach to preventing autointoxication/bowel toxemia remained natural living: proper diet, regular exercise, and prompt answering of nature's call. Through the middle years of the century, the naturopathic way of constipation prevention was preached most effectively by Paul Bragg, the whole wheat campaigner of the 1930s (Chapter 8) who in the next decade matured into an all-around health reformer. Bragg assisted Bernarr Macfadden with the publication of *Physical Culture* magazine, founded a food supplement company that is still doing prosperous business (under the direction of his daughter Patricia), and earned the title "Diet Advisor to Hollywood Movie Stars." Bragg even created stars, being the man who transformed Jack LaLanne from a weakling into a wonder, from a "a sickly, pimply boy" in LaLanne's words, into the first physical trainer to attract followers through television. A regular contributor to *Nature's Path* in the 1940s and '50s, Bragg warned readers "Don't Live in an Unclean Body," and provided them with Bragg Meal, a whole grain breakfast cereal, to drive uncleanness out. Bragg and other naturopaths also believed strongly in yogurt and acidophilus milk products as sustainers of intestinal health.[13]

Naturopathic practitioners continued to recommend herbal laxatives for constipation as well, though the system's signature product, Kneipp's Laxative Herbs Number Three, was rechristened in the 1940s to honor the system's founder. Dr. Benedict Lust's Herbs Number Three Pills were a "scientific blend of Herbs, Barks and Seeds" that a person could count on to "help yourself back to regularity." In addition, advertisements for any number of other gentle, natural remedies were to be found in the pages of *Nature's Path* (the gentleness of some might be called into question; the Gastro-Intestinal Cleanser available from the Glorious Health Institute in Dallas, for instance, "removes masses and strings of mucus . . . even worms and tumor-like masses"). Non-drug methods were also promoted by naturopathy. *Nature's Path* brimmed with ads for enema equipment and rectal dilators, and if one were even more adventurous, an unspecified "drugless method . . . guaranteed to clean you out" could be ordered from San Francisco's "Structor the Health Counselor" for only "25c silver."[14]

The preferred drugless method of cleaning out the bowels, however, was irrigation of the colon. "Colonic-Irrigation is the only sensible way of removing decomposed waste matter," one of the many *Nature's Path* articles on the topic maintained; "the amount of ancient sewage, which is frequently thus extricated, is beyond belief." And if one were incredulous, it was easy enough to test the statement. Naturopathic publications were filled with advertisements for mail-order irrigation equipment (including Tyrrell's J. B. L. Cascade): "enjoy the benefits of a colon purge right in your home," the manufacturer of Clark Internal Baths suggested; "do as the doctor recommends," the Thermaire Company proposed, "clean out the human death trap with high colonic irrigations at home."[15]

Under the rubric "colon therapy," irrigation would continue to be offered to naturopathic patients down to the end of the twentieth century as a means of overcoming the "intestinal dysfunction" caused by "the lifestyle . . . typical of current Western culture." One has not needed a degree in naturopathy, however, to make a living irrigating colons. Just as in the early decades of the century, irrigation has been provided by chiropractors, massage therapists, and other ancillary medical personnel, as well as by practitioners who perform colon therapy exclusively. From *Colonic Therapy. A Modern Road to Health* in 1949 ("Sudden Death Lurks in the Abnormal Colon"; "the first requisite to sanctity is to keep the intestines open"), to *Colon Health: The Key to a Vibrant Life* in 1979 ("Cause of Death?—Colon Neglect"), to *Cleansing the Body and Colon for a Happier and Healthier You* in 1996, books and pamphlets presenting irrigation as the cornerstone of health have been constantly before the public eye:

> Get your colon irrigation;
> Get that wonderful sensation
> Feeling clean inside and out.
> This should banish every doubt.
> Sing your Hallelujah song,
> Know that now it won't be long
> When aches and pains that left you aghast
> Are nightmares of the recent past.[16]

The nightmares banished by colon hydrotherapy (another synonym for colonic irrigation) are still the ravages of autointoxication. "The average colon in civilized communities," Americans have been warned as recently as 1996, "is in a desperately deprived and dangerous condition," one that results "in continued bacterial breakdown of the feces" and the release of "36 poisons" into the body. Those so poisoned are "the most miserable people on earth"; they need to ask themselves, "are you a toxic waste site?" Colon hydrotherapists also talk still of twists in the colon that call Lane's kinks to mind, and recommend yogurt be eaten after the treatment to "replenish the good bacteria." According to the International Association For Colon Hydrotherapy, there are between 5000 and 7000 colon hydrotherapists in the United States, and several hundred in the United Kingdom.[17]

Physicians report that patients frequently inquire about the value of irrigation, made curious by the heavy advertising of the procedure in every medium from newspapers to television. The doctor's answer, just as in the 1920s, is likely to be that "the much vaunted colonic irrigations are of no benefit and may be harmful or even dangerous." Indeed, more than a little harm to patients has been documented, including fatalities from such complications as infection, perforation of the bowel, and electrolyte depletion (risks increased in the 1980s with the promotion of coffee enemas as a detoxifying treatment for cancer). Even so, quackery has flourished in colon therapy as in few other fields, the purveyors of Tox-Eliminators and Detoxacolons never running short of customers. Roy DeWelles, inventor of the Detoxacolon, realized an estimated 2.5 million dollars before being convicted of fraud in 1964.[18]

Complicating the situation is the periodic appearance of favorable accounts of colon cleansing in presumably objective publications such as newspapers and magazines: "for the next half hour you bask in the most satisfying loo-going experience of your life," a London reporter confided to readers in 1991. No wonder, then, that even those who might afford any type of treatment could be converted to irrigation (Princess Diana and the Duchess of York were "always nipping into the Hale Clinic in Regent's Park for a 50 pound spot of 'hydrotherapy'"), or that they inspired imitation by many among the less affluent. It is quite clear that another London reporter's caution, "Don't do it, Di," had little effect on either the Princess or her public.[19]

However satisfying the irrigation experience may have been, the distinguishing mark of late twentieth-century interest in bowel health was the largescale adoption of fiber as daily food. Colonic irrigation's appeal was to a somewhat marginal population, the patrons of alternative therapies and health food stores who were acquainted with autointoxication theory. Dietary fiber was a mainstream idea, formulated by reputable physicians from a far more extensive clinical, experimental, and epidemiological base than autointoxication had ever had. Bran and other forms of fiber had, of course, maintained standing as health foods between the days of Kellogg and Lane and the era of Burkitt. An English physician in the 1950s, for example, was amused by how "thoroughly infatuated" people were with "the virtues of roughage"; they "go to the most absurd lengths," he marvelled, and "overload their intestines to an extent appropriate to an herbivore." But with the creation of the dietary fiber hypothesis, and the steady growth of professional support during the early 1970s, the virtues of fiber were made more apparent to society at large. Beginning with an article in the December 1974 *Reader's Digest* ("Is a Vital Ingredient Missing From Your Diet?"), followed shortly by the book *The Miracle Nutrient. How Dietary Fiber Can Save Your Life*, the European as well as American public came under a barrage of warnings that they were setting themselves up for hemorrhoids, colon cancer, and heart disease by not consuming enough fiber: "a nation of colonic cripples!" was the sad result of Western society's addiction to "fiber-depleted carbohydrates which have been pummelled, adulterated, puffed, colored, flavored, and transformed beyond all recognition." Burkitt himself made a major contribution to the burgeoning fiber awareness with a 1979 guide for the lay person, *Don't Forget Fibre in Your Diet.* Written in accessible and engaging language and filled with imaginative illustrations, the book was translated into 10 languages and sold more than 250,000 copies.[20]

There were still other popular manuals (*The Truth About Fiber in Your Food*, *The Fiber Factor*), and numerous magazine articles published in the 1970s, with no letup in the decade that followed. In 1988, for example, *The Paleolithic Prescription*, a book written by two American physicians in collaboration with an anthropologist, expanded on Cleave's thesis that modern ways of living were a harmful deviation from the ways of the Stone Age, "a mismatch, or discordance, between the genes carried forward from our environment of evolutionary adaptedness and the new environment we have 'suddenly' created." The list of bad habits was extended, sedentariness and self-abuse with tobacco and alcohol being added to refined foods as indulgences by which "we have finally estranged ourselves from the broad continuum of general mammalian experience." But a full third of the book concentrated on the question of food, exploring the content of paleolithic diet in extraordinary detail and arguing that "the nutritional environment of our past is the one our genes 'know' best; it promotes optimal operating conditions for our physiology and biochemistry." Numerous advantages were attributed to the Stone Age dietary, not the least being its much higher fiber content. Indeed, many of the diseases of civilization (afflictions accountable "for three-fourths of all deaths in the modern industrial state") were attributable to humankind's abandonment of the race's formative diet: "in the long perspective of human existence, we in the advanced nations in the twentieth century have become the soft underbelly of humanity." Among the authors' recommendations for recapturing natural health, their paleolithic prescripton, was "the more fiber the better." (Incidentally, Burkitt lent his imprimatur to the book, calling it "one of the most fascinating and convincing approaches to healthy eating that I have read for a long time.")[21]

Even greater enthusiasm for fiber was to be found in *Prevention*, the most widely read health magazine in the world. Initiated in 1950 by Jerome Rodale, the father of organic farming in America (eating organic produce, he advised, was the "first principle" for avoiding constipation), *Prevention* analyzed the latest developments in the health sciences and interpreted them for public enlightenment. Every month, a heady mix of health recommendations (some sound, some questionable) was put forth, with a share of attention going to each of the classic nonnaturals. The greatest portion, though, went to nutrition, articles on the benefits of the different vitamins and minerals appearing in virtually every issue, surrounded by advertisements for vitamins, minerals, protein supplements, lecithin, . . . and yogurt products ("yogurt may lengthen life, normalize bowel functions, protect against infection—maybe even battle cancer"). It is hardly surprising, then, that the very first presentation of the dietary fiber hypothesis for American popular consumption was a *Prevention* editorial, "Stories Your Bowels Can Tell," in January 1973. Two months later, the cover of the magazine pictured rural Africans grinding grain beside the caption "Why Primitive Food is Good Medicine"; henceforth, articles on fiber as a preventive of constipation, cancer, heart disease, and all the other Western complaints would be regular features. Not until well into the 1980s did the frequency of fiber glorification decline.[22]

Glorification is not too strong a word. Such 1970s titles as "Bran, a Blessing for the Lower You" and "Bran For What Probably Ails You" put the *Prevention* orientation in a nutshell: fiber, bran in particular, was sooner or later identified as the cure or the preventive for just about everything. "By just adding a few teaspoons of this precious substance to your diet every day," one author claimed, "chances are you can protect yourself against diverticulosis. . . . hemorrhoids, constipation, diarrhea and varicose veins . . . help cure 'em if you got 'em . . . you can lose weight and never find it again . . . strengthen your heart, relieve gallbladder problems, prevent appendicitis, even neutralize the toxic chemicals in the food you eat . . . and all for only pennies a day." Bran was insurance even against "bathroom death," the heart attack that constipates were prone to suffer when straining at stool.[23]

Medical scientists were as a rule more reserved, expressing doubt about several elements of dietary fiber theory, and finding the evidence for links between fiber and certain diseases (most notably colon cancer) inconclusive. Nevertheless, the basic principle that people would benefit by eating more fiber was widely adopted by health authorities. In 1981, the British Committee on Medical Aspects of Food Policy recommended that more fiber be incorporated into the diet, and 2 years later, the British Health Education Council proposed that average dietary fiber consumption be increased by some 50%, the largest change recommended for any one dietary component. In the United States, the 1979 *Surgeon General's Report on Health Promotion and Disease Prevention* recognized higher fiber intake as "prudent" and likely to reduce incidence of hemorrhoids and diverticular disease. It judged the evidence for prevention of colorectal cancer as "scanty at present," but in 1984, the National Cancer Institute concluded that a high-fiber, low-fat diet did appear "to protect against some cancers, particularly colorectal." A pamphlet published by the Institute that year gave considerably more space to dietary fiber than to any other risk factor in advising the public how to protect themselves from cancer and urged that "Americans increase the fiber-rich foods in their diets." In 1988, a new Surgeon General's report, this one on *Nutrition and Health*, told Americans to "increase consumption of whole grain foods and cereal products," as well as fruits and vegetables. Finally, in 1990, when the FDA mandated new labeling requirements for food manufacturers, fiber content was made one of the required nutrient categories. Still more recently, however, in January of 1999, a study that attracted widescale attention "found no association between the intake of dietary fiber and the risk of colorectal cancer." Editorial commentary on the study summed up the situation concisely: with respect to truly understanding the connection between fiber and cancer, it was submitted, "we have barely begun." (The same editorial, incidentally, noted that there is a direct correlation between sugar consumption and incidence of colorectal cancer, and pondered, "Was Cleave right?")[24]

"Roughage" remained in currency, at least within lay discourse, where it was used as often as "fiber" (and continued to be interpreted by many people as violent; "Isn't bran *scratchy?*," readers inquired of a *Prevention* editor, "won't it irritate my system?"). But by any name, the indigestible components of food soon acquired as much importance in the public's perceptions of nutrition as the digestible ones, leading to what *Psychology Today* characterized at the end of the 1980s as "fiber mania," a "high-fiber feeding frenzy." Indeed, a survey of Americans' health behavior conducted in 1984 found that a full third of respondents were eating more fiber than previously for the purpose of improving their health (for comparison, 41% were taking vitamins, 36% dieting to lose weight, and 5% following a vegetarian regimen). Much of the additional fiber was obtained from whole wheat bread and bran cereals, though there was also increased consumption of other roughage foods, including beans ("despite the well-known antisocial aspects"), which in America rose by 3 pounds per capita between 1984 and 1987. In England, even the time-hallowed mainstay of the public house, the potato crisp, was challenged, though not very seriously, by an upstart "Nature's Snack," Wholewheat Crisps that came in salt and vinegar, cheese and onion, and other traditional flavors. Popular magazines seemingly competed to come up with the grandest array of high-fiber food recipes, and the *Saturday Evening Post* actually compiled a *Fiber and Bran Better Health Cookbook*, "the most enticing cookbook of fiber and bran recipes that has ever been assembled." *The F-Plan Diet*, a volume that pushed fiber not just as healthful and enticing, but as a reducing agent, was the biggest selling book in Britain in 1982 (the paperback edition, in fact, surpassed the sales record set by *Lady Chatterly's Lover* when it was published following the famous obscenity trial in 1960). People were even instructed on how to determine their fecal transit times, and supplied with the addresses of stores from which red stool markers could be ordered. There was good reason, then, for a popular magazine to designate the colon "organ of the year" for 1986, because "practically everyone . . . is concerned about how theirs is functioning." Practically everyone included even ducks, or at least the ducks at a wildfowl sanctuary in Gloucestershire. In 1989, it was observed that the "fussy ducks" there preferred brown bread to white: "so keepers are selling bags of wholemeal loaf to visitors at 20 p a time." (Fiber frenzy was fed, incidentally, by reports in the late 1980s that oat bran lowered serum cholesterol levels; sales of oat breakfast cereals increased nearly 250% from 1988 to 1989, and all manner of other oat-derived food products flooded the market, including Otto's Original Oat Bran Beer. Enthusiasm for oat cuisine died as suddenly as it was born, however, with the 1990 publication of studies that debunked the earlier reports.)[25]

Some health experts worried that zealous fiber feeding might do more harm than good, by displacing foods providing other important nutrients. If housewives were seduced by advertisements and magazine articles to spend too much of their limited food budget on high-fiber items, a British physician worried, the family's nutritional balance would be "tipped from nutrients to fibre," and "children could well lag behind in growth." People needed to remember that in terms of building body tissue or supplying energy, fiber contributed nothing more than could be obtained from "an equal amount of finely chopped toilet paper"; in other words, while "most of what you eat turns into you, . . . dietary fibre just goes through." Fiber, like any other public frenzy, provoked humor, and in quantity. A 1987 *New Yorker* cartoon (that most sensitive barometer of shifts in America's cultural atmosphere) showed a man in bed being examined by a physician, his wife accounting for the twigs sprouting from his head by saying, "I *told* him to lay off the high-fibre diet." When Bung, the town drunk in a popular comic strip, fell ill, the doctor diagnosed fiber deficiency, and suggested the sick man eat the corks from his wine bottles before draining them. And when television comedian Bob Newhart swaggered into the bunkhouse of the ranch where he was vacationing and demanded steak for dinner, he was informed by the cowboys that Wednesday night was salad night: "We need our roughage."[26]

One of the attractions of roughage, of course, was that it was a way to better health that did not demand sacrifice. Adding a bit of bran to the diet was relatively painless, compared to cutting back on fat or sugar: "for once, medicine was saying 'do' instead of 'don't'." As has been seen, the point was not lost on food manufacturers, though one segment of the industry was particularly successful at capitalizing on it: Burkitt's "realisation of the importance of dietary fibre," an obituarist stated, "was to change the breakfast tables of the Western world." The producers of bran cereals had never stopped promoting their creations as protection against constipation without the irritating effects of laxatives. In the 1960s, All-Bran was billed as "the 'Regularity Breakfast'," and in the 1990s as "the fiber you need to help stay regular. Drug free." With the popularization of the dietary fiber hypothesis, new possibilities presented themselves. "The Inside Story" was one version of the cereal industry's interpretation of Burkitt's ideas. "When you feel fitter on the inside," All-Bran boxes sold in the United Kingdom in 1992 explained, "you feel ready for the world outside. What's the secret—the inside story that helps you feel fitter inside? It's the story of fibre." Because "people in third world countries eat two and a half times more fibre than we do in the west," breakfasters were told, "they rarely suffer from constipation, and other 'western' diseases such as piles, diverticular disease, gall stones and heart problems. . . . So start the day with the inside story!"[27]

There were worse things than piles and heart problems to worry Westerners, however. The most appealing feature of the Burkitt hypothesis in the eyes of cereal manufacturers was the linking of fiber to colorectal and other cancers; who needed autointoxication if people who didn't eat bran could be threatened with cancer? In 1984, shortly after the National Cancer Institute recognized dietary fiber as one factor in the prevention of cancer, the Kellogg Company approached the Institute with an offer to assist in publicizing the scientific findings relating diet to cancer. The Institute reviewed and approved proposed ads, and in October 1984, All-Bran began to be sold in boxes whose full back side was given to the message that the National Cancer Institute was now recommending that people avoid obesity, consume less fat and more fruits and vegetables, and "eat high fiber foods"; fortunately, "bran cereals are one of the best sources of fiber." A toll-free number through which to order the Institute's cancer prevention booklet completed the ad.[28]

The Institute's recognition of fiber as an element in cancer prevention had already been attacked by many in the research community who considered the evidence inconclusive; cooperation with a commercial concern's advertising campaign did little to lighten the criticism. The situation was complicated, moreover, by the fact that once a food was marketed with health claims attached, it became a drug in the eyes of the FDA. Drugs had to be approved for efficacy before being put on the market, and the FDA was not convinced that bran was effective in preventing cancer. On the other hand, the National Cancer Institute, a fellow federal agency, had given the ad campaign its blessing (as had the Federal Trade Commission, which regulated advertising separate from labeling and packaging), so the FDA refrained from taking action against the Kellogg Company. Uncertainty over how to deal with Kellogg's packaging claims, in fact, forced the FDA to undertake a reevaluation of policy governing health claims on food products generally, resulting in a new position of tolerating statements that provided useful health information to the public and that were not unreasonable or exaggerated interpretations of scientific opinion. Administration officials nevertheless worried that "this opens up the floodgates" for more extreme claims from other companies, and in fact Campbell's split pea soup was soon being advertised with the reminder that it contained the dietary fiber recommended by the National Cancer Institute. The ad enjoyed only a short run, being dropped abruptly when the Institute objected that the soup was still high in fat and salt, thereby neutralizing whatever benefits accrued from its fiber.[29]

The Institute did continue its support of anti-cancer messages on Kellogg's cereals ("at last," another box announced, "some news about cancer you can live with"), and sales of All-Bran and other Kellogg fiber cereals increased markedly.

Soon, of course, other cereal manufacturers were incorporating the cancer prevention theme into their advertising, with sales of high-fiber cereals generally increasing 37% within a year. The FDA, meanwhile, began to officially recognize other types of health claims on food labels: that low sodium intake decreases the risk of heart disease, for example, and that low fat consumption decreases the risk of heart disease and cancer. Finally, fiber was accepted. In 1993, the FDA adopted a policy of allowing food producers to claim that diets that are both low in fat and high in fiber may reduce the risk of some types of cancer, as well as heart disease. Such claims have been standard copy on bran cereal packages ever since.[30]

The "international symbol for the middle class," American humorist Dave Barry proposed in 1993, should be "a stick drawing of a little person trying to read the fiber content on a cereal box." High-fiber cereal became a subject for humor just as quickly as high-fiber eating in general did. A skit on the American television show Saturday Night Live in 1990, for instance, "advertised" a new breakfast food known as Colon Blow, one bowl of which was said to be equal in fiber content to 30,000 bowls of ordinary high-fiber cereal, and the effects of which were evident in its name. In *London Fields* (1989), Martin Amis created a character who kept himself going through a bout of lovesickness by "his breakfasts—his hearty bowls of Megabran," a "thick, dark, all-fibre cereal" that was so easy to digest because it had been reduced to "precisely one stage away from" intestinal waste: "Megabran was on a chemical knife-edge between cereal and human shit. . . . Everyone hated Megabran. Everyone ate it."[31]

Colon Blow and Megabran were, in effect, laxatives rather than foods, and fictional though they may have been, a legion of real-life counterparts existed. After all, whatever uncertainty there might have been about fiber's ability to protect from cancer, there was no question about its efficacy at stimulating the bowels to action. A public conditioned to equate regularity with health, and at the same time made wary of the dangers of chemical laxatives, was readily persuaded that "daily fiber therapy," as one product described itself, was a key component of health maintenance. It helped as well that bulk laxatives (psyllium, agar, and other water-absorbing fibers) were identified by medical authorities as the safest category of cathartic agents. The market niche many products carved out for themselves, however, was not "safe laxative," but "essential food supplement," easy-to-take fiber for people who didn't care for bran cereal or whole wheat bread.

John Harvey Kellogg had created the category, introducing LAXA Biscuits (bran and agar) and Psylla (psyllium seed) in the 1920s. Still sharper definition was provided in the following decade by Saraka, a product manufactured in New Jersey from the 1930s to the end of the 1950s. The bulk-forming agent in this instance was a gum, bassorin, that was reputed to absorb even more water per unit weight than agar or psyllium. To be sure their product got results, Saraka's producers added a vegetable laxative, frangula, but it was the bassorin that was the focus of advertising because it could be used to exploit both popular uneasiness about the effects of "roughage" and popular perceptions of the superior health-fulness of the primitive life. A full-page newspaper ad in 1950, for example, prom-ised to teach people "How to Learn to Live Again" by reminding them how cave men lived. They "got plenty of roughage," something that "today's scanty, hur-riedly eaten meals" did not provide. The roughage of prehistoric diets, however, was much too rough for moderns. People of the industrial age had enfeebled their intestinal apparatus with refined foods, and so needed bulk-forming fare without the "sharp particles" and "scratchy points" of bran. Saraka was not roughage, but—and this was well before Trowell would come up with the term—softage, a "soft mucilaginous mass" that "glides easily along the intestinal wall, and will not harden or clog."[32]

The same message was to be read in "The Inside Story of Constipation," a booklet mailed to thousands of consumers in 1955 in a discreet plain cover: "The contents of this envelope are of a highly intimate and personal nature. Please do not open it until you have read the accompanying letter." The inside story was told by a man identifying himself as an MD, who claimed to have traveled the world observing "the eating habits of primitive tribes" who "know little of the troubles of constipation," and to have discovered that what Westerners needed to enjoy the same freedom was not primitive roughage, but "softage" that acts with "thor-oughness" and "no griping, no urgency." Yet if Saraka was soft, it was hardly weak. Its bulk provided "intestinal exercise," making it a "diet-aid" that restores "the functional rhythm to which the intestines were accustomed, before the fast pace of modern living threw them off the track." A 1958 televison commercial presented viewers with an animated drawing of the human body in which the intestinal muscles were limp and sagging. Suddenly musculature began to undulate, then to grow taut, while a narrator explained that Saraka "rejuvenates inactive, lazy in-testinal muscles" while it also "helps clean out poison matter that often accumu-lates in a constipated system." Not surprisingly, such ads provoked the Federal Trade Commission to file charges for distortion of medical theory, but before the issue could be settled, the company went out of business.[33]

One of the rivals to whom Saraka lost was Serutan, a household word by the 1950s thanks to its sponsorship of popular television programs and relentless re-minders that the product's name was simply "Nature's" spelled backwards. Serutan was a vegetable bulk laxative that also guaranteed "smooth, soft, . . . freemoving" stools (even though it was "free from ruffage"), and presented itself as a dietary supplement. Promotional materials portrayed it as the equivalent of vitamins for the intestines: "Use it daily with confidence for as long as you desire." The bulk laxative/diet supplement field became even more crowded, of course, once dietary fiber became a phrase to conjure with in the 1970s. Colon Care, for example, of-fered 1990s consumers packets of raspberry-, pineapple-, or orange-flavored psyllium "as a food supplement and an addition to your everyday diet." But Colon Care also, manufacturer Laci Le Beau explained, "actually helps break down toxic residue" in the intestine, and "helps remove bad bacteria from the body which may be brewing many kinds of illness and disease." In short, bulk laxatives/food supplements provided another shelter for autointoxication to the end of the twentieth century. Thus FiberCleanse, a "Natural Colon Cleanser" made from psyllium husks, worked to cleanse intestines of "pounds of uneliminated feces . . . poisoning the blood stream and the entire system," according to a 1992 promotional flyer. The same was true of the Jason Winters Intestinal Cleanser, made from psyllium husks and seeds. Winters' 1996 promotional materials cited his book, *The Perfect Cleanse*, in which there were to be found such unsettling stories as that of the autopsy of a prematurely dead man that "revealed a colon that was 9 inches in diameter that had a passage through it no larger than a pencil"; another autopsied colon weighed 40 pounds, and was full of "hard and black" matter "the consistency of tire rubber." Winters warned that remnants of food could lodge in the colon and putrefy for 5 years and more, poisoning the body all the while. "A famous vegetarian told me that he was in perfect shape and needed no colon cleanser," but was persuaded to try it anyway. "Within five days he apologized to me. He just couldn't believe what he had been holding onto all these years." It was also the rule for these products to stress their botanical origins—Perdiem was a "natural vegetable laxative"—much as nineteenth-century patent medicines had maintained the superiority of vegetable purgatives over calomel and other minerals; FibreSonic combined 27 different vegetable fibers in its formulation, everything from tofu fiber to locust bean gum.[34]

In recent years, the best-selling product in the fiber supplement genre has been Metamucil, a psyllium-based preparation that purports to be "the fiber doctors recommend most to maintain regularity." Promoted as a substance that should be "taken daily as 'fiber therapy'," and even sold in fruit-flavored "Instant Mix" packets so that buyers can "have your fiber any time, anywhere," Metamucil seems to suffer from the same identity crisis as the chocolate cathartics of the 1920s: is it food? or is it a laxative? "Daily fiber therapy" suggests both. Daily fiber tempts buyers to think of it as a foodstuff, but therapy connotes the laxative action so appealing to the regular users of overt purgatives. Try to disguise itself as it may, Metamucil (and like products) is tapping directly into humanity's immortal hope that all that's needed to maintain reasonable health, no matter what forms of hygienic self-neglect one enjoys, is regular and thorough inner cleansing. Consider the aftermath of the report in 1995 that phenolphthalein had been found to produce cancer in laboratory rats. The study was criticized by some for using extraordinarily large doses of the laxative, on a strain of rats highly susceptible to tumor formation. Nevertheless, the Schering-Plough Company, manufacturers of Feen-A-Mint and Correctol, quickly reformulated their laxative preparations, substituting the compound bisacodyl for phenolphthalein, then running advertisements that attacked competitor Ex-Lax as carcinogenic. The bisacodyl formulations were less active, however, and consumers soon noticed; sales of the two Schering products dropped 27% in 1997. Were people more afraid of irregularity than of cancer? Apparently, since sales of Ex-Lax were not significantly affected. Eventually, after a 1997 report confirmed the earlier study, the manufacturers of Ex-Lax replaced the phenolphthalein in their preparations with senna. As of this writing, Ex-Lax remains the top-selling laxative in the United States, demonstrating the remarkable prescience of a 1930 advertisement: "imitations come," it observed sagely, "and imitations go, [but] Ex-Lax goes on forever."[35]

Perhaps Arbuthnot Lane does as well. "Most physicians have been consulted by the occasional patient, usually a young woman, with very severe constipation resistant to all treatment. . . . At present the most severely affected patients still require colectomy." Those sound like Lane's words, but they come instead from a late twentieth-century English surgeon, David Preston. While working in the 1970s and '80s at a London hospital that specialized in the treatment of colorectal diseases, Preston became aware of a population of patients, all female, distinguished by a history of chronic, severe constipation, and more or less "disabled" by a number of associated symptoms. All were determined to have an inordinately high transit time, but to have colons of normal size (an enlarged colon, or megacolon, had long been known to be prone to serious constipation). Subsequently, in the mid 1980s, Preston and colleagues at St. Mark's Hospital described a syndrome affecting women, typically appearing around the onset of puberty and steadily becoming "worse until [it was] often severe and disabling by the third decade." These women averaged a single bowel movement a week, achieved with the aid of laxatives (which most had been relying on for years). They complained of abdominal pain and bloating, nausea, malaise, and cold hands, and were determined to have "a high incidence of gynaecological problems": menstrual irregularity, infertility, ovarian cysts. Breast lumps and nodules were much more common than normal in these women, and a psychiatric consultant found "a very high incidence of a disturbed childhood, psychosexual problems, and personality difficulties."[36]

Such patients have been encountered before in this volume; they were the patients of Arbuthnot Lane. Preston proposed the term "idiopathic slow transit constipation" to identify the syndrome (which has since been confirmed by other clinicians), but he suggested it could equally well be called "Arbuthnot Lane's disease." Lane's disease did not, however, mean autointoxication. Though admiration was expressed for Lane's "astute clinical observations [which] appear to have been forgotten," Preston dismissed Lane's belief in intestinal toxemia as the source of a myriad of ailments, excusing it as an honest mistake resulting from the early century's limited understanding of physiology and microbiology. The cause of slow transit constipation was acknowledged to be unclear (hence "idiopathic," of

in their physical—and cultural—environment. Evolution thus could change the norms of physical functioning: for Lane, the assumption of upright posture had transformed the colon into an enemy within; for Metchnikoff, the colon had been rendered malevolent by humankind's removal from the jungle and forest; for Cleave, the refining of carbohydrate foods had done the damage. Twentieth-century health reformers strove to adapt to these changes, with surgery, yogurt, bran, and other conciliating agents. But all the while they were catching up to the changes of the past, the present was turbulent with more change that would require new adaptations. The pursuit of health has been altered, in other words, from a climb back toward an unmoving ideal state molded in distant ages, to a footrace in which the finish line is forever being moved forward, kept always just ahead of the runner's progress. Evolution works slowly, much too slowly for a person to fully adapt to a new environment before change turns it into the old environment. One strives to stay as healthy as possible, but doesn't delude oneself into thinking that full health will ever be achieved, let alone maintained for any time. In the words of Rene Dubos, "however wisely we manage our lives, we have to cope with physiological imperfection; the environment is forever changing and makes on us adaptive demands to which we cannot always respond successfully. . . . The more complete the human freedom and the more rapid the technological and social changes, the greater is the likelihood that new and unexpected causes of disease will appear." Apparently the manufacturer of a 1920s hormone preparation for the cure of intestinal stasis was right: "The happy day may come when we shall eliminate all greed, selfishness and wickedness from the world, but never this side of paradise, will we abolish constipation."[46]

References to greed and selfishness have further relevance, for in either the pre- or post-Darwinian interpretation, the pursuit of health assumes the dimensions of a moral quest. Whether trying to live up to the commandment to obey the divinely established and immutable laws of physiology, or struggling to survive in the existential battle with nature's ever-changing evolutionary demands, pursuers of health must mortify their flesh and tame their appetites, must deny pleasures and exert will power—in short, demonstrate character—to an extent unimaginable to the slothful and gluttonous. The latter have found solace of a perverse sort in the 1993 discovery of a gene predisposing to colon cancer; people can now in good conscience forego the privations of dietary restraints and regular exercise if their genes have predetermined they will develop malignancy anyway. Those who do not look to heredity to absolve themselves of hygienic duty, though, present a spectacle that is most irritating to less ardent worshipers of Hygeia; health "fanatics" are branded so not just because of the physical extremes to which they push themselves, but just as much for the moral smugness they can affect. "Hygiene," Mencken wrote, "is the corruption of medicine by morality. It is impossible to find a hygienist who does not debase his theory of the healthful with a theory of the virtuous." Because constipation results from weakness in so many areas of hygiene (diet, exercise, evacuation and repletion, passions of the mind), regularity is particularly suited to the exhibition of moral earnestness. "Pleasing our palates has become a secret vice," newspaper columnist Ellen Goodman has commented, "while fiber-fueling our colons has become a most public virtue." Similarly, fiber has been accused by a British medical editor of arousing "the same passions as teetotalism did in our Victorian ancestors," and softage advocate Hugh Trowell described as showing a "messianic fervour . . . very reminiscent of the hell-fire school of evangelists."[47] Surely it's true that "the bowel-wise person" at least thinks that she "is the one who is armed with good knowledge . . . and walks the path of the higher life." By assigning health moral as well as physical value, furthermore, proponents of bodily well-being turn the tables on civilization. Refusing to acquiesce to the notion that poor health is the price of progress, they maintain instead that good health is the only path to genuine progress, the sole foundation on which true civilization can be built.

When all is said and done, that path is still a straight and narrow one. All the environmental and social changes of the last two centuries notwithstanding, bowel wisdom has remained constant. In 1997, a newspaper health columnist answered the inquiry of a man who had been taking laxatives for 35 years and wanted to break the habit, but feared it would prove impossible for him. The correspondent was assured that he truly could free himself from aperients—but only if he added fiber to his diet, took more exercise, and visited the toilet every morning at the same time.[48] The column might as easily have been written by Dr. John Locke as by Dr. Paul Donohue.

The last word on bowel wisdom, though, was spoken by an elderly Scottish physician who practiced in London in the early nineteenth century. His name is not recorded, and we know that he existed at all only through the graces of Sir Astley Cooper, one of the most celebrated surgeons of the time (and, like Arbuthnot Lane, a practitioner at Guy's Hospital). Cooper relates that he often accompanied the old doctor on patient visits, and that it was the gentleman's habit to remind him just before they entered the sick room, "Weel, Mister Cooper, we ha' only twa things to keep in meend, and they'll searve us for here and herea'ter; one is always to have the fear of the Laird before our ees, that 'ill do for herea'ter; and the t'other is to keep your booels open, and that will do for here'."[49]

NOTES

A major source of research material was the vast collection of advertisements, labels, and packages in the American Medical Association's Historical Health Fraud and Alternative Medicine Collection in Chicago. References to these materials will be headed by AMA, followed by the box number and folder number of the item; when known, the date for the ad or label will be given in parentheses following the product name. Another valuable resource was the Patent Medicine files in the Warshaw Collection of the National Museum of American History, Smithsonian Institution; materials will be identified as Warshaw, followed by box and file number. Citations to KRF denote materials in the Kremers Reference Files, American Institute of the History of Pharmacy, University of Wisconsin. Much patent medicine advertising was consulted as well at the Royal Pharmaceutical Society, London (RPS).

PREFACE

The opening quotations are from John Smedley, *Practical Hydropathy*, 14th ed. (London: Blackwood, 1872), 261; Émile Gautier, *La Saignée Urique* (Paris: Chatelain, 1909), 18–19; and Mrs. Martha Rasmussen, letter to American Medical Association, August 10, 1932, AMA, box 156, folder 15.

    1. An Unusual Syndrome, KRF, C37 (a) VI; the original of the surgeons' inquest is reprinted in Gustave Witkowski and Augustin Cabanés, *Gayetez d'Aesculape* (Paris: Maloine, 1909), 141–143.

    2. *The New Yorker*, March 27, 1995, 65.

    3. Recent studies of the history of hygiene include Anita Fellman and Michael Fellman, *Making Sense of Self. Medical Advice Literature in Late Nineteenth-Century America* (Philadelphia: University of Pennsylvania Press, 1981); Harvey Green, *Fit for America. Health, Fitness, Sport, and American Society* (New York: Pantheon, 1986); Kathryn Grover, ed., *Fitness in American Culture. Images of Health, Sport, and the Body, 1830–1940* (Amherst, MA: University of Massachusetts Press, 1989); Bruce Haley, *The Healthy Body and Victorian Culture* (Cambridge, MA: Harvard University Press, 1978); Stephen Nissenbaum, *Sex, Diet and Debility in Jacksonian America. Sylvester Graham and Health Reform* (Westport, CT: Green-

wood, 1980); Ronald Numbers, *Prophetess of Health: A Study of Ellen G. White* (New York: Harper and Row, 1976); Hillel Schwartz, *Never Satisfied. A Cultural History of Diets, Fantasies and Fat* (New York: Free Press, 1986); James Whorton, *Crusaders for Fitness. The History of American Health Reformers* (Princeton, NJ: Princeton University Press, 1982). The only history of constipation I am aware of, and it is essentially anecdotal, is Jacques Frexinos, *Les Ventres Serrés. Histoire Naturelle et Sociale de la Constipation et des Constipes* (Paris: Pariente, 1992).

4. George Bernard Shaw, *The Complete Plays of Bernard Shaw* (London: Odhams, 1934), 10; "Periscope," *Newsweek*, March 11, 1996, 29.

5. Erik Erikson, *Young Man Luther; A Study in Psychoanalysis and History* (New York: Norton, 1958), 204–206; Lord Dawson of Penn, The colon and colitis. *British Medical Journal* (1921) ii:31–35, p. 31; James Goodhart, Round about constipation. *Lancet* (1902) ii:1241–1246, p. 1243.

6. Raymond La Charité, Rabelais: The book as therapy. In: Enid Peschl, ed., *Medicine and Literature* (New York: Neale Watson, 1980), 11–17, p. 13; Francois Rabelais, *The Works of Francis Rabelais*, Thomas Urquhart, trans. (London: Bohn, 1849), 463.

7. Investigating constipation. *British Medical Journal* (1980) i:669–670, p. 669. Also see Lynn Payer, *Medicine and Culture* (New York: Holt, 1988), 116–118; and Jonathan Miller, *The Body in Question* (New York: Random House, 1978), 44.

8. Anonymous, *Human Ordure, Botanically Considered* (London: Carpenter, 1748), 2. The work has sometimes been misattributed to Swift. See Herman Teerink, *A Bibliography of the Writings in Prose and Verse of Jonathan Swift, D.D.* (The Hague: Nijhoff, 1937), 336.

CHAPTER 1

The chapter-opening quotation is from Harmon Root, *The People's Medical Lighthouse* (New York: Ranney, 1856), 114.

1. *Dorland's Illustrated Medical Dictionary*, 28th ed. (Philadelphia: Saunders, 1994), 371.

2. Ghislain Devroede, Functions of the anorectum: Defecation and continence. In: Sidney Phillips, John Pemberton, and Roy Shorter, eds., *The Large Intestine. Physiology, Pathophysiology, and Disease* (New York: Raven Press, 1991), 115–140.

3. James Goodhart, Round about constipation. *Lancet* (1902) ii:1241–1246, p. 1245.

4. Devroede (n. 2); Michael Kamm, Pathophysiology of constipation. In: Phillips et al. (n. 2), 709–726; M. A. Eastwood and J. A. Robertson, Bulk agents in the colon. In: Luis Bustos-Fernandez, ed., *Colon. Structure and Function* (New York: Plenum Medical Books, 1983), 141–165, p. 158; William Grace, Stewart Wolf, and Harold Wolff, *The Human Colon* (New York: Hoeber, 1951); Anthony Bassler, *Diseases and Disorders of the Colon* (Springfield, IL: Thomas, 1957); Arthur Hurst, *Constipation and Allied Intestinal Disorders*, 2nd ed. (London: Frowde, 1921), 69–71.

5. John Ordronaux, trans., *Regimen Sanitatis Salernitanum* (Philadelphia: Lippincott, 1871), 163.

6. Martin Vorhaus and S. Zachary Orgel, Psychosomatic relationship to gastrointestinal diseases. *Journal of the American Medical Association* (1944) 126:225–231, p. 225; Don Tucker, Harold Sandstead, George Logan, Jr., Leslie Klevay, Janet Mahalko, LuAnn Johnson,

Linda Inman and George Inglett, Dietary fiber and personality factors as determinants of stool output. *Gastroenterology* (1981) 81:879–883, p. 882; Grace (n. 4), 213–222; Alex Comfort, *The Anxiety Makers* (London: Nelson, 1967), 114–135; Thomas Chen and Peter Chen, Intestinal autointoxication: A medical leitmotif. *Journal of Clinical Gastroenterology* (1989) 11:434–441, pp. 440–441.

7. Arthur Hurst, The unhappy colon. *Lancet* (1935) i:1483–1487, p. 1484; E. Cuyler Hammond, Some preliminary findings on physical complaints from a prospective study of 1,064,004 men and women. *American Journal of Public Health* (1964) 54:11–23; B. D. Ruben, Public perceptions of digestive health and disease. *Practical Gastroenterology*, (1986) 10:35–42; Harold Aaron, *Our Common Ailment. Constipation: Its Cause and Cure* (New York: Dodge, 1938), 23; Robert Sandler and Douglas Drossman, Bowel habits in young adults not seeking health care. *Digestive Diseases and Sciences* (1987) 32:841–845, p. 844; James Gully, *The Water-Cure in Chronic Disease* (New York: Wiley and Putnam, 1847), 251.

8. Carl Flath, *The Miracle Nutrient. How Dietary Fiber Can Save Your Life* (New York: Evans, 1975), 70.

9. Dangers of purgatives. *British Medical Journal* (1961) ii:1694–1695, p. 1694.

10. Edward Fingl, Laxatives and cathartics. In: Alfred Gilman, Louis Goodman, Steven Meyer and Kenneth Melman, eds., *Goodman and Gilman's The Pharmacological Basis of Therapeutics*, 6th ed. (New York: MacMillan, 1980), 1002–1012; Laurence Brunton, Agents affecting gastrointestinal water flux and motility. In: Joel Hardman and Lee Limbird, eds., *Goodman and Gilman's The Pharmacological Basis of Therapeutics*, 9th ed. (New York: McGraw-Hill, 1996), 917–936.

11. Gail Sekas, The use and abuse of laxatives. *Practical Gastroenterology* (1987) 11:33–39.

12. Gabriel Kune, Susan Kune, Barry Field and Lyndsey Watson, The role of chronic constipation, diarrhea, and laxative use in the etiology of large bowel cancer. *Diseases of the Colon and Rectum* (1988) 31:507–512, p. 511; Edward Johnson, *Results of Hydropathy; or, Constipation Not a Disease of the Bowels* (New York: Wiley and Putnam, 1846), 78.

13. Case reported by Dr. R. Williams. In: John Burne, *A Treatise on the Causes and Consequences of Habitual Constipation* (Philadelphia: Haswell, Barrington, and Haswell, 1840), 29–30.

14. Mary Douglas, *Purity and Danger, An Analysis of Concepts of Pollution and Taboo* (London: Routledge and Kegan Paul, 1966).

15. Terence McLaughlin, *Dirt. A Social History as Seen Through the Uses and Abuses of Dirt* (New York: Stein and Day, 1971), 2.

16. John Booty, The Anglican tradition. In: Ronald Numbers and Darryl Amundsen, eds., *Caring and Curing. Health and Medicine in the Western Religious Traditions* (New York: Macmillan, 1986), 240–270, p. 241; James Obelkovich, Proverbs and social history. In: Peter Burke and Roy Porter, eds., *The Social History of Language* (Cambridge: Cambridge University Press, 1987), 43–72, p. 51; John Cheyne, *An Essay on the Bowel Complaints of Children* (Philadelphia: Finley, 1813), 23; Dale Morse, Mary Woodbury, Kenneth Rentmeester and Darryll Farmer, Death caused by fermenting manure. *Journal of the American Medical Association* (1981) 245:63–64; Gabriel Garcia-Marquez, *Love in the Time of Cholera* (New York: Penguin, 1989), 17.

17. Bendix Ebbell, ed., *The Papyrus Ebers* (Copenhagen: Levin and Munksgaard, 1937), 30–32; Joseph Lieutaud, *Synopsis of the Practice of Medicine*, Edwin Atlee, trans. (Philadelphia: Parker, 1816), 21, 26, 29, 41, 63; Alexander Thomson, *The Family Physician* (New York: Oram, 1802), 63. Also see Cyril Bryan, *The Papyrus Ebers* (New York: Appleton, 1931). For fuller discussion of the *whdw* theory see J. Worth Estes, *The Medical Skills of Ancient Egypt* (Canton, MA: Science History Publications, 1989), 82–86, 101–107.

18. Richard Reece, *A Practical Dissertation on the Means of Obviating and Treating the Varieties of Costiveness, Which Occur at Different Periods of Life* (London: Longman, Rees, Orme, Brown and Green, 1826), 5, 101; William Hall, *Health and Disease*, 5th ed. (New York: Widdleton, 1864), 6; Burne (n. 13), 31.

19. Burne (n. 13), 22; James Thacher, *American Modern Practice* (Boston: Read, 1817), Vol. 1, 129; Anthony Carlisle, *An Essay on the Disorders of Old Age* (Philadelphia: Earle, 1819), 24; Charles Williams, *Principles of Medicine* (Philadelphia: Lea and Blanchard, 1844), 52; Edward Foote, *Plain Home Talk* (New York: Murray Hill, 1880), 44; William Hall, *The Guide-Board to Health, Peace and Competence; or, the Road to Happy Old Age*, 2nd ed. (Springfield, MA: Fisk, 1872), 139, 142.

20. Samuel Ford, ed., *The American Cyclopaedia of Domestic Medicine and Household Surgery* (Chicago: American Literary and Supply Association, 1887), Vol. 2, 482; Catharine Beecher, *Letters to the People on Health and Happiness* (New York: Harper, 1855), 73.

21. John Mennes, *Facetiae* (London: Hotten, 1817), Vol. 1, 168–169; William Alcott, Flatulence in childhood. *Library of Health and Teacher on the Human Constitution* (1842) 6:145–152; Alcott, Intestinal gases. *Teacher of Health and the Laws of the Human Constitution* (1843) 1:250–254. The most interesting discourse on the ways by which flatulence destroys health is in Joannes Fienus, *New and Needful Treatise of Spirits and Wind Offending Man's Body*, William Rowland, trans. (London: Billingsley and Blagrave, 1668).

22. Benjamin Franklin, *The Benjamin Franklin Reader*, Nathan Goodman, ed. (New York: Crowell, 1945), 739–741.

23. John Pringle, *Observations on the Diseases of the Army*, 6th ed. (London: Millar and Cadell, 1768), 84, 100–101; William Dewees, *A Practice of Physic*, 2nd ed. (Philadelphia: Carey, Lea and Blanchard, 1833), 33; Charles Williams, *Principles of Medicine* (Philadelphia: Lea and Blanchard, 1844), 382; Florence Nightingale, *Notes on Nursing* (New York: Dover, 1969), 21–22.

24. Charles E.-A. Winslow, *The Conquest of Epidemic Disease. A Chapter in the History of Ideas* (New York: Hafner, 1967), 71–74. George Rosen, *A History of Public Health* (New York: MD Publications, 1958).

25. Edwin Chadwick, *Report on the Sanitary Condition of the Labouring Population of Great Britain*, M. W. Flinn, ed. (Edinburgh: Edinburgh University Press, 1965); S. E. Finer, *The Life and Times of Edwin Chadwick* (London: Methuen, 1952).

26. Arthur Conan Doyle, *The Hound of the Baskervilles* (New York: Airmont, 1965), 120.

27. Finer (n. 25), 298; John Armstrong, *The Art of Preserving Health* (Philadelphia: Franklin, 1745), 6. For discussion of eighteenth-century consciousness of environmental filth and smells see Roy Porter, Cleaning up the great wen: Public health in eighteenth century London. In: W. F. Bynum and Roy Porter, eds., *Living and Dying in London, Medical His-*

tory, Supplement No. 11 (London: Wellcome Institute for the History of Medicine, 1991), 61–75; and Andrew Wear, Health and the environment in early modern England. In: Andrew Wear, ed., *Medicine in Society. Historical Essays* (Cambridge: Cambridge University Press, 1992), 119–148.

28. Armstrong (n. 27), 6; Chadwick (n. 25), 82, 100–101, 104, 109, 111, 119.

29. Stephen Smith, *The City That Was* (New York: Allaben, 1911), 72–76. For more on American sanitary reform see John Griscom, *The Sanitary Condition of the Laboring Population of New York* (New York: Harper, 1845).

30. John Simon, *Public Health Reports* (London: Churchill, 1887), Vol. 1, 3–5; Thomas Ewell, *The Ladies Medical Companion* (Philadelphia: Brown, 1818), 43.

31. Simon (n. 30), Vol. 1, 106–108, 113; Simon quoted in E. Royston Pike, ed., *Golden Times: Human Documents of the Victorian Age* (New York: Praeger, 1967), 297; ad for American Sugar-Coated Pills, RPS. For more on the cultural significance of the sewer in the nineteenth century see Donald Reid, *Paris Sewers and Sewermen. Realities and Representations* (Cambridge, MA: Harvard University Press, 1991).

32. George Cheyne, *An Essay on Health and Long Life* (New York: Gillespy, 1813), 24; James Agnew, *An Inaugural Dissertation on Perspiration* (Philadelphia: Carey, 1800), 44; Georges Vigarello, *The Concept of Cleanliness. Changing Attitudes in France Since the Middle Ages* (Cambridge: Cambridge University Press, 1988), 107; Lawrence Wright, *Clean and Decent. The Fascinating History of the Bathroom and the Water Closet* (New York: Viking, 1960), 114–115. For more on the history of cleanliness see Richard Bushman and Claudia Bushman, The early history of cleanliness in America. *Journal of American History* (1988) 74:1213–1238; Harold Eberlein, When society first took a bath. *Pennsylvania Magazine of History* (1943) 67:30–48; Alfred Martin, On bathing. *CIBA Symposia* (1939) 1:134–149; Virginia Smith, Cleanliness: Idea and Practice in Britain, 1770–1850 (PhD Dissertation, University of London, 1985); Marilyn Williams, *Washing the Great Unwashed. Public Baths in Urban America, 1840–1920* (Columbus: Ohio State University Press, 1991).

33. Norbert Elias, *The Civilizing Process. The History of Manners*, Edmund Jephcott, trans. (New York: Urizen Books, 1978); James Thacher, *American Modern Practice* (Boston: Read, 1817), Vol. 1, 134.

34. Bushman and Bushman (n. 32), 1228; Smith (n. 32), 133–134; Lemuel Shattuck, *Report of the Sanitary Commission of Massachusetts. 1850* (Boston: Ditton and Wentworth, 1850), 161.

35. *Les Monstres Invisibles* quoted by Vigarello (n. 32), 203; school lesson quoted by Williams (n. 32), 5.

36. Catharine Beecher, *Physiology and Calisthenics for Schools and Families* (New York: Harper, 1856), v; Elisha Bartlett, *Obedience to the Laws of Health, A Moral Duty,* (Boston: Noble, 1838), 10, 15; Elizabeth Blackwell, *The Laws of Life* (New York: Putnam, 1852), 28–29; Elizabeth Blackwell, The religion of health. In: Archibald Hunter, *Hydropathy: Its Principles and Practice* (Edinburgh: Menzies, 1881), 303–325, p. 308.

37. Bartlett (n. 36), 18; Andrew Combe, *The Physiology of Digestion*, 3rd ed. (Cooperstown, NY: Phinney, 1844), 13; Beecher (n. 20), 10.

38. A Country Clergyman, *Constipation: Its Causes and Consequences* (London: Bailliere, Tindall, and Cox, 1871), 1.

39. Country Clergyman (n. 38), 5, 7; William Hall, *The Guide-Board to Health, Peace and Competence; Or, the Road to Happy Old Age*, 2nd ed. (Springfield, MA: Fisk, 1872), 334–335; Forbes Winslow, *The Anatomy of Suicide* (Boston: Milford House, 1840), 196.

40. Quoted by Andrew McClary, Germs are everywhere: The germ threat as seen in magazine articles, 1890–1920. *Journal of American Culture* (1980) 3:33–46, p. 41.

41. Robert Hudson, Theory and therapy: Ptosis, stasis, and autointoxication. *Bulletin of the History of Medicine* (1989) 63:392–413, pp. 394–397; Charles Bouchard, *Lectures on Auto-Intoxication In Disease or Self-Poisoning of the Individual*, 2nd ed., Thomas Oliver, trans. (Philadelphia: Davis, 1906), 15, 106, 295–296; Victor Vaughan and Frederick Novy, *Ptomaines, Leucomaines, Toxins and Antitoxins*, 3rd ed. (Philadelphia: Lea, 1896), 17; T. Lauder Brunton, *An Introduction to Modern Therapeutics* (London: MacMillan, 1892), 40–65.

42. Bouchard (n. 41), 163; R. H. Dalton, The limit of human life, and how to live long. *Journal of the American Medical Association* (1893) 20:599–600, p. 600; George Cheyne, *The English Malady: Or, a Treatise of Nervous Diseases of all Kinds* (London: Strahan, 1733), 194; J. A. Irwin, *Hydrotherapy at Saratoga* (New York: Cassell, 1892), 2. For more on neurasthenia see George Beard, *A Practical Treatise on Nervous Exhaustion (Neurasthenia, Its Symptoms, Nature, Sequences, Treatment* (New York: Wood, 1880); Barbara Sicherman, The uses of a diagnosis. *Journal of the History of Medicine and allied Sciences* (1977) 32:33–54; Janet Oppenheim, *Shattered Nerves. Doctors, Patients, and Depression in Victorian England* (New York: Oxford University Press, 1991).

43. George Waring, *The Sanitary Condition of City and Country Dwelling Houses*, 2nd ed. (New York: Van Nostrand, 1898), 32, 63; Charles Chapin, *Papers of Charles V. Chapin, M.D.* (New York: Commonwealth Fund, 1934), 50. Also see James Cassedy, The flamboyant Colonel Waring: An anticontagionist holds the American stage in the age of Pasteur and Koch. *Bulletin of the History of Medicine* (1962) 36:163–176, and McClary (n. 40).

44. Marcus Hatfield, *The Physiology and Hygiene of the House in Which We Live* (New York: Chautauqua, 1887), 149–150; F. A. Hornibrook, *The Culture of the Abdomen. The Cure of Obesity and Constipation* (Garden City, NY: Doubleday, Doran, 1934), 9; *Constipation and Beecham's Pills*, 3. In: Warshaw, box 1, file 18.

CHAPTER 2

The chapter-opening quotations are from Ray Pierce, The Badge of Sympathy, ad for Pierce's Pleasant Purgative Pellets, Warshaw, box 34, file 8; and a letter from Thomas Howel to James Hamilton, Senior, June 11, 1806, citing Hamilton's brother George. In: *Letters to James Hamilton*, manuscripts collection, Royal College of Physicians of Edinburgh.

1. William Harvey, The anatomical examination of the body of Thomas Parr. In: *The Works of William Harvey*, Robert Willis, trans. (London: Johnson Reprint Corporation, 1965), 587–592. pp. 590, 592. For more details of Parr's story see John Taylor, The old, old, very old man: Or, the age and long life of Thomas Parr. In: William Thoms, *Human Longevity. Its Facts and Its Fictions* (London: Murray, 1873), 290–308 (also see pp. 85–94); William Ford, Old Parr. *Bulletin of the History of Medicine* (1950) 24:219–226; and Thomas Parr. In: Sidney Lee, ed., *Dictionary of National Biography*, Vol. 15, 364–366.

2. Lee (n. 1), 364; Harvey (n. 1), 589.

3. Thoms (n. 1), 85; Harvey (n. 1), 590–591. For an analysis of "the imposture of Old Parr," see Maurice Ernest, *The Longer Life* (London: Adam, 1938), 46–54.

4. Harvey (n. 1), 591. On the non-naturals, see Jack Berryman, The tradition of the 'six things non-natural': Exercise and medicine from Hippocrates through ante-bellum America. *Exercise and Sport Sciences Review* (1989) 17:515–559; L. J. Rather, The 'six things non-natural': A note on the origins and fate of a doctrine and a phrase. *Clio Medica* (1968) 3:337–347; Saul Jarcho, Galen's six non-naturals: A bibliographic note and translation. *Bulletin of the History of Medicine* (1970) 44:372–377; Antoinette Emch-Deriaz, The non-naturals made easy. In: Roy Porter, ed., *The Popularization of Medicine, 1650–1850* (London: Routledge, 1992), 134–159; Guenter Risse, Medicine in the age of Enlightenment. In: Andrew Wear, ed., *Medicine in Society. Historical Essays* (Cambridge: Cambridge University Press, 1992), 149–196; and Chester Burns, The non-naturals: A paradox in the Western concept of health. *Journal of Medicine and Philosophy* (1976) 1:202–211.

5. Nedra Belloc and Lester Breslow, Relationship of physical health status and health practices. *Preventive Medicine* (1972) 1:409–421, p. 415 (also see Belloc, Relationship of health practices and mortality. *Preventive Medicine* (1973) 2:67–81; and Breslow, A positive strategy for the nation's health. *Journal of the American Medical Association* (1979) 242:2093–2095).

6. John Collins Warren, *Physical Education and the Preservation of Health*, 2nd ed. (Boston: Ticknor, 1846), 31.

7. Taylor (n. 1), 300; Lois Whitney, *Primitivism and the Idea of Progress in English Popular Literature of the Eighteenth Century* (Johns Hopkins University Press: Baltimore, 1934); Charles Rosenberg, Pathologies of progress: The idea of civilization as risk. *Bulletin of the History of Medicine* (1998) 72:714–730.

8. Benjamin Waterhouse, *Cautions to Young Persons Concerning Health* (Cambridge, MA: Harvard University Press, 1805), 6.

9. Warren (n. 6), 5.

10. Poet quoted by James Ewell, *The Medical Companion* (Philadelphia: Author, 1816), 77; Thomas Trotter, *A View of the Nervous Temperament* (Troy, NY: Wright, Goodenow and Stockwell, 1808), 22, 89–90, 154; James Johnson, *The Influence of Civic Life, Sedentary Habits, and Intellectual Refinement on Human Health and Human Happiness* (Philadelphia: Hope, 1820), 47. For a thorough discussion of the eighteenth-century debate over rural versus urban health with respect to a specific city, London, see Andrew Wear, Health and the environment in early modern England. In: Andrew Wear, ed., *Medicine in Society. Historical Essays* (Cambridge: Cambridge University Press, 1992), 119–148.

11. John Burne, *A Treatise on the Causes and Consequences of Habitual Constipation* (Haswell, Barrington, and Haswell: Philadelphia, 1840); Richard Reece, *A Practical Dissertation on the Means of Obviating and Treating the Varieties of Costiveness* (Longman, Rees, Orme, Brown and Green: London, 1826); James Johnson, *The Influence of Civic Life, Sedentary Habits, and Intellectual Refinement on Human Health and Human Happiness* (Philadelphia: Hope, 1820), 18; William Kitchiner, *Directions for Invigorating and Prolonging Life; Or, The Invalid's Oracle*, 6th ed. (New York: Harper, 1831), 186; James Hamilton, *Observations on the Utility and Administration of Purgative Medicines*, 5th ed. (Philadelphia: Webster, 1818), 26.

12. John Mennes, *Facetiae* (London: Hotten, 1817), Vol. 1, 24.

13. Anonymous, *Human Ordure, Botanically Considered* (London: Carpenter, 1748), 3–15. Category two of the classification scheme was Tun-formed stools (thicker in the middle than at the extremities, and reputedly especially common among the Dutch); category three was variegated excrement, soft and marbled or striped with color (physicians' evacuations were typically of this type); category four was umbrella shaped, spreading over the ground like a full-blown rose.

14. Charles Hastings and Robert Streeten, Constipation. In: John Forbes, Alexander Tweedie, and John Conolly, eds., *The Cyclopaedia of Practical Medicine* (Philadelphia: Lea and Blanchard, 1847), Vol. 1, 477–499, p. 478; George Taylor, *Health by Exercise* (New York: Fowler and Wells, 1883), 308.

15. Clement Carylon, *Precepts for the Preservation of Health, Life, and Happiness, Medical and Moral* (London: Whittaker, 1859), 40.

16. John Abernethy, quoted in *Graham Journal of Health and Longevity* (1838) 2:130; Burne (n. 11), 112–113; Johnson (n. 11), 46–48.

17. Burne (n. 11), 110–111; A Country Clergyman, *Constipation: Its Causes and Consequences* (London: Bailliere, Tindall, and Cox, 1871), 15–16.

18. Burne (n. 11), 110; William Hall, *Health and Disease*, 5th ed. (New York: Widdleton, 1864), 49; Hall, *The Guide-Board to Health, Peace and Competence; Or, the Road to Happy Old Age*, 2nd ed. (Springfield, MA: Fisk, 1872), 141; Country Clergyman (n. 17), 5.

19. Burne (n. 11), 110–111.

20. Robley Dunglison, *The Practice of Medicine: A Treatise on Special Pathology and Therapeutics*, 2nd ed. (Philadelphia: Lea and Blanchard, 1844), Vol. 1, 152; Country Clergyman (n. 17), 11.

21. John Sinclair, *The Code of Health and Longevity* (Edinburgh: Constable, 1807), Vol. 2, 302; Thomas Cogan, *The Haven of Health* (London: Field, 1596); Thomas Elyot, *The Castell of Helth* (London: Marshe, 1572); William Bullein, *Bulleins Bulwarke of Defence Against all Sicknes Sornes and Woundes* (London: Kyngton, 1562); Virginia Smith, Prescribing the rules of health: Self-help and advice in the late eighteenth century. In: Roy Porter, ed., *Patients and Practitioners* (Cambridge University Press: Cambridge, 1985), 249–282, pp. 251–252.

22. Miles Rodgers, *Physical Education and Medical Management of Children* (Rochester, NY: Darrow, 1848), 9.

23. Martha Verbrugge, *Able-Bodied Womanhood. Personal Health and Social Change in Nineteenth-Century Boston* (New York: Oxford University Press, 1988), 36. An especially useful analysis of physiology's reflection of culture is Roger Cooter, The power of the body. In: Barry Barnes and Steven Shapin, eds., *Natural Order. Historical Studies of Scientific Culture* (Beverly Hills, CA: Sage, 1979), 73–96; also see Hillel Schwartz, *Never Satisfied. A Cultural History of Diets, Fantasies and Fat* (New York: Free Press, 1986), and Stephen Nissenbaum, *Sex, Diet, and Debility in Jacksonian America. Sylvester Graham and Health Reform* (Westport, CT: Greenwood, 1980).

24. Edward Hitchcock, *Dyspepsy Forestalled and Resisted*, 2nd ed. (Amherst, 4A: Adams, 1831), 244.

25. John Eberle, *A Treatise on the Practice of Medicine* (Philadelphia: Grigg, Elliot, 1849), 669; Edward Foote, *Plain Home Talk* (Murray Hill: New York, 1880), 386; Robley Dunglison, *On the Influence of Atmosphere and Locality; Change of Air and Climate; Seasons; Food; Cloth-*

ing; Bathing; Exercise; Sleep; Corporeal and Intellectual Pursuits, Etc. Etc. On Human Health: Constituting Elements of Hygiene (Philadelphia: Carey, Lea and Blanchard, 1835), 152; Dunglison, *Human Physiology*, 4th ed. (Lea and Philadelphia: Blanchard, 1841), Vol. 1, 564; J. N. Loughborough, *Hand Book of Health: Or, a Brief Treatise on Physiology and Hygiene* (Battle Creek, MI: Steam Press, 1868), 176; Hall, *The Guide-Board to Health* (n. 18), 47.

26. William Buchan, *Domestic Medicine* (Philadelphia: Bumstead, 1809), 417; John Ayrton Paris, *A Treatise on Diet* (London: Underwood, 1826), 170; Foote (n. 25), 387–391. For details on the history of milling and breadmaking see R. A. McCance and E. M. Widdowson, *Breads White and Brown. Their Place in Thought and Social History* (London: Pittman, 1956); H. E. Jacob, *Six Thousand Years of Bread* (New York: Doubleday, 1944); and Jacob, Bread and man. *Ciba Symposia* (December 1946) 8.

27. For a detailed discussion of Grahamism see James Whorton, *Crusaders for Fitness. The History of American Health Reformers* (Princeton, NJ: Princeton University Press, 1982), 38–131; Whorton, Patient, heal thyself: Popular health reform movements as unorthodox medicine. In: Norman Gevitz, ed., *Other Healers. Unorthodox Medicine in America* (Baltimore: Johns Hopkins University Press, 1988), 52–81; Harvey Green, *Fit For America. Health, Fitness, Sport, and American Society* (New York: Pantheon, 1986), 3–53; and Nissenbaum (n. 23).

28. Sylvester Graham, *Lectures on the Science of Human Life* (Boston: Marsh, Capen, Lyon, and Webb, 1839), Vol. 1, 552; Vol. 2, 14, 406, 423.

29. William Alcott, *Lectures on Life and Health* (Boston: Phillips, Sampson, 1853), 280–281; Alcott, Habitual constipation. *Library of Health and Teacher on the Human Constitution* (1842) 6:92–95; Alcott, Intestinal gases. *Teacher of Health and the Laws of the Human Constitution* (1843) 1:250–254, p. 253.

30. David Cambell, Bran bread legislation. *Graham Journal of Health and Longevity* (1839) 3:116–117, p. 116; M. P. M., The lay of the graham cracker. *Journal of Hygeio-Therapy* (1890) 4:59.

31. John Smith, *Fruits and Farinacea, the Proper Food of Man* (London: Churchill, 1845), 131.

32. Burne (n. 11), 15; Reece (n. 11), 12, 93; Dioclesian Lewis, *Weak Lungs, and How to Make Them Strong* (Boston: Osgood, 1871), 228; Taylor (n. 14), 170, 314; Andrew Combe, *The Physiology of Digestion*, 3rd ed. (Cooperstown, NY: Phinney, 1844), 270. For additional samples of recommendations on exercise for health maintenance see Andrew Combe, *The Principles of Physiology, Applied to the Preservation of Health*, 7th ed. (New York: Harper, 1843), 131–149; Catharine Beecher, *Calisthenic Exercises for Schools, Families and Health Establishments* (New York: Harper, 1856), particularly pp. 20–27; and Dunglison, *On the Influence of Atmosphere* (n. 25), 425–443.

33. John Locke, *Some Thoughts Concerning Education* (Cambridge: Cambridge University Press, 1902), 17–18.

34. Hitchcock (n. 24), 244 ; Burne (n. 11), 111.

35. Armand Trousseau, *Clinical Medical Lectures*, 3rd ed. (Philadelphia: Blakiston, 1882), Vol. 2, 492; Harmon Root, *The People's Medical Lighthouse* (New York: Ranney, 1856), 115; Austin Flint, *A Treatise on the Principles and Practice of Medicine*, 4th ed. (Philaelphia: Lea, 1878), 470.

36. Reece (n. 11), 16–17; Country Clergyman (n. 17), 6.

37. Charles Peale, *An Epistle to a Friend, on the Means of Preserving Health* (Philadelphia: Aitken, 1803), 3; William Bullein, *A Newe Boke of Physicke called ye Government of Health* (London: Day, 1559), 1.

38. James Adair, *An Essay on Diet and Regimen, for the Preservation of Health* (Air, Scotland: Wilson, 1799), v; Michel de Montaigne, *The Essays of Michel de Montaigne*, W. Carew Hazlitt, ed. (New York: Burt, n.d.), Vol. 1, 252–253.

39. The Garth story is told in Art Newman, *The Illustrated Treasury of Medical Curiosa* (New York: McGraw-Hill, 1988), 2.

40. Thomas Ewell, *The Ladies' Medical Companion* (Philadelphia: Brown, 1818), 44; Trousseau (n. 35), 492; Flint (n. 35), 472; Joseph Brevitt, *The Female Medical Repository* (Baltimore: Hunter and Robinson, 1810), 91; Foote (n. 25), 390.

41. Nathaniel Chapman, *Discourses on the Elements of Therapeutics and Materia Medica* (Philadelphia: Webster, 1817), Vol. 1, 218–220; Mennes (n. 12), Vol. 1, 166–169.

42. James Harvey Young, *The Toadstool Millionaires. A Social History of Patent Medicines in America Before Federal Regulation* (Princeton: Princeton University Press, NJ, 1961), 3–15.

43. Edward Ward, *The London Spy* (London: Casanova Society, 1924), 131–132; P. S. Brown, Medicines advertised in eighteenth-century bath newspapers. *Medical History* (1976) 20:152–168; Roy Porter, *Health For Sale. Quackery in England 1660–1850* (Manchester: Manchester University Press, 1989), 62–63.

44. The growth of patent medicines in the nineteenth century, and their exploitation of advertising is explored thoroughly by Young (n. 42).

45. John Gunn, *Gunn's Domestic Medicine, or Poor Man's Friend* (Knoxville: Author, 1830), 61. For more on calomel therapy in the nineteenth century see James Whorton, The purgative plan of James Hamilton, Senior: Drug therapy and pharmaceutical philosophy in the early nineteenth century. *Pharmacy in History* (1996) 38:159–174; John Haller, Samson of the materia medica: Medical theory and the use and abuse of calomel in nineteenth century America. *Pharmacy in History* (1971) 13:27–34, 67–76; and Guenter Risse, Calomel and the American medical sects during the nineteenth century. *Mayo Clinic Proceedings* (1973) 48:57–64.

46. Robert Wells, cited by Edwin Walker, The abuse of purgatives. *American Journal of Obstetrics and Diseases of Women and Children* (1906) 54:722–731, p. 724; Caleb Ticknor, *A Popular Treatise on Medical Philosophy; Or, an Exposition of Quackery and Imposture in Medicine* (New York: Gould and Newman, 1838), 209–210.

47. William Hall, *Fun Better Than Physic; Or, Everybody's Life-Preserver* (Chicago: Rand, McNally, 1882), 10; James Morison, *The Hygeist, Origin of Life and Cause of Disease* (London: Author, 1828); William Helfand, James Morison and his pills. *Transactions of the British Society for the History of Pharmacy* (1974) 1:101–135.

48. Henry Holcombe, *Patent Medicine Tax Stamps. A History of the Firms Using United States Private Die Proprietary Medicine Tax Stamps* (Lawrence, MA: Quarterman, 1979), 51; Brandreth advertisement in Gerald Carson, *One for a Man, Two for a Horse* (Garden City, NY: Doubleday, 1961), 102; pamphlet for Brandreth's Pills, Warshaw, box 4, file 22, pp. i, 3. Brandreth's career is discussed in detail by Young (n. 42), 75–89.

49. Russell Trall, A national disease. *Water-Cure Journal and Herald of Reforms* (1857) 23:16; pamphlet (n. 48), 1–4, 35, 40; Benjamin Brandreth, *The Doctrine of Purgation* (New York:

Baker and Godwin, 1871), titlepage, 5–6, 151, 183, 187; Brandreth Calendar for 1880, Warshaw, box 4, file 22; ad in Carson (n. 48), 102; William Helfand, Historical images of the drug market XXXX. *Pharmacy in History* (1993), 35:176.

50. Ma-Le-Na ad, personal collection; McLean's ad, KRF, C39; Radway's Almanac, 4, in Warshaw, box 37, file 7.

51. Beecham ad, RPS (I trust it is clear that the racist condescension of the Beecham ad reflects common Victorian attitudes, and not those of the author); Paul Theroux, *The Kingdom By the Sea* (Boston: Houghton Mifflin, 1983), 337. For a biography of Beecham, see Anne Francis, *A Guinea a Box* (London: Hale, 1968).

52. William Buchan, *Domestic Medicine* (Philadelphia: Bumstead, 1809), 107, 284; Edward Jukes, *On Indigestion and Costiveness; A Series of Hints to Both Sexes, on the Important, Safe, and Efficacious Means of Relieving Diseases of the Digestive Organs by Lavements*, 5th ed. (London: Churchill, 1833), 24–25.

53. Joel Pinney, *An Exposure of the Causes of the Present Deteriorated Condition of Health* (London: Longman, Rees, Orme, Brown, and Green, 1830), 183; William Kitchiner, *Directions for Invigorating and Prolonging Life; Or, The Invalid's Oracle*, 6th ed. (New York: Harper, 1831), 183–184; the shuttlecock passage is attributed to an unidentified physician by Joel Shew, *Hydropathy, or the Water-Cure*, 3rd ed. (New York: Fowlers and Wells, 1851), 102; Mary Gove, *Lectures to Ladies on Anatomy and Physiology* (Boston: Saxton and Pierce, 1842), 20, 24; Thomas Bull, *Hints to Mothers, for the Management of Health During the Period of Pregnancy, and in the Lying-In Room*, 3rd ed. (New York: Wiley, 1852), 72; Taylor (n. 14), 309.

CHAPTER 3

The chapter-opening quotations are from Frank Crane, The colonic. In: Charles Tyrrell, *The What, The Why, The Way of Internal Baths*, 3–4 (Warshaw, box 45, file 34); and F. A. Hornibrook, *The Culture of the Abdomen. The Cure of Obesity and Constipation* (Garden City, NY: Doubleday, Doran, 1934), 8.

1. J. Ellis Barker, *Chronic Constipation, the Most Insidious and the Most Deadly of Diseases* (London: Murray, 1927), 320–323.

2. Barker (n. 1), 323–326.

3. Barker (n. 1), 326–329.

4. Paul Woolley, Intestinal stasis and intestinal intoxications: A critical review. *Journal of Laboratory and Clinical Medicine* (1915–16) 1:45–54, p. 45; Frank Smithies, Colon filling stations. *Journal of the American Medical Association* (1926) 87:691; Charles Campbell and Alfred Detweiler, *The Lazy Colon* (New York: Educational Press, 1924), 2; Barker (n. 1), 13; Alfred Jordan, Stasis the destroyer. *Medical Journal and Record* (1925) 22:328–330, p. 330; G. Sherman Bigg, *Indigestion, Constipation and Liver Disorder* (New York: Hoeher, 1913), 85; W. Arbuthnot Lane, The sewage system of the human body. *American Medicine* (1923) 29:267–272, p. 268.

5. James Goodhart, Discussion on alimentary toxaemia. *Proceedings of the Royal Society of Medicine* (1913) 6(Suppl):294–300, p. 297.

6. Unpublished autobiography of W. Arbuthnot Lane, Wellcome Institute of the History of Medicine (the manuscript is not consecutively paginated, so specific page references cannot be given); Thomas Layton, *Sir William Arbuthnot Lane, Bt. An Enquiry into the Mind*

and Influence of a Surgeon (London: Livingston, 1956), 1; Logan Clendening, A review of the subject of chronic intestinal stasis. *Interstate Medical Journal* (1915) 22:1191–1200, pp. 1191, 1193. Among several additional sources for biographical information see William Tanner, *Sir W. Arbuthnot Lane, His Life and Work*, 2nd ed. (London: Balliere, Tyndall and Cox, 1946); Tanner, Sir W. Arbuthnot Lane, Bart., C.B., M.S., F.R.C.S. *Guy's Hospital Reports* (1945) 94:85–114; and E. G. Slesinger, Sir William Arbuthnot Lane, Bart: A tribute. *Guy's Hospital Reports* (1956) 105:261–273.

7. Autobiography of Lane (n. 6); Lane, *The Operative Treatment of Chronic Intestinal Stasis*, 4th ed. (London: Frowde, Hodder and Stoughton, 1918), 1–24, 124–201.

8. Lane, *The Operative Treatment* (n. 7), 34–37. At times, Lane suggested the first and last kink was at the point where the small intestine entered the colon: see Lane, A Clinical Lecture on Chronic Intestinal Stasis, *British Medical Journal* (1924) ii:142–143, p. 143.

9. W. Arbuthnot Lane, The sewage system of the human body. *American Medicine* (1923) 29:267–272, p. 269; Autobiography of Lane (n. 6).

10. W. Arbuthnot Lane, *The Operative Treatment of Chronic Constipation* (London: Nisbet, 1909), 36–37; Lane, Civilisation in relation to the abdominal viscera, with remarks on the corset. *The Lancet* (1909) ii:1416–1418, p. 1416. J. Lacey Smith, Sir Arbuthnot Lane, chronic intestinal stasis, and autointoxication. *Annals of Internal Medicine* (1982) 96:365–369 outlines Lane's theories and practices, as does Robert Hudson, Theory and therapy: Ptosis, stasis, and autointoxication. *Bulletin of the History of Medicine* (1989) 63:392–413.

11. Goodhart (n. 5) (on the normality of "kinks" see also Walter Alvarez, Origin of the so-called autointoxication symptoms. *Journal of the American Medical Association* (1919) 72:8–13, p. 11; W. Arbuthnot Lane, The first and last kink. *Lancet* (1925) i:1209–1210, p. 1209; Lane, The paramount importance of effective intestinal drainage in preventing ill health and disease. *American Medicine* [n.s.] (1926) 21:689–693, p. 692; Lane, An address on chronic intestinal stasis. *British Medical Journal* (1913) ii:1125–1130, p. 1125; Lane, Chronic intestinal stasis and cancer. *British Medical Journal* (1923) ii:745–747, p. 747; W. Knowsley Sibley, Discussion on alimentary toxaemia. *Proceedings of the Royal Society of Medicine* (1913) 6(Suppl):355–360, p. 359.

12. W. Arbuthnot Lane, The paramount importance (n. 11), 689–690; Lane, The sewage system (n. 9), 271.

13. Smithies (n. 4), 691; Lane, An address (n. 11), 1125–1126; Layton (n. 6), 92; Leonard Williams, The medical aspect of intestinal stasis. In: W. Arbuthnot Lane, *The Operative Treatment of Chronic Intestinal Stasis*, 4th ed. (London: Frowde, Hodder, and Stoughton, 1918), 250–263, p. 260. Tanner (n. 6), 155–187, provides a complete bibliography of Lane's papers.

14. W. Arbuthnot Lane, Cancer of the colon: Its causation and treatment, *Lancet* (1920) ii:1184–189, pp. 1184–1185; Lane, Cancer and intestinal stasis. *The Practitioner* (1924) 112:205–210, pp. 209–210.

15. Lane, Cancer of the colon (n. 14), 1185; Lane, Cancer and intestinal stasis (n. 14), 210; Lane, Chronic constipation and self-poisoning—a sword of Damocles. *Heal Thyself* (1941) 76:49–51, p. 51; Lane, Chronic intestinal stasis and cancer (n. 11), 746–747.

16. W. Arbuthnot Lane, *The Operative Treatment of Chronic Intestinal Stasis*, 4th ed. (London: Frowde, Hodder and Stoughton, 1918), 60; Lane, An address (n. 11), 1126; Lane, The sewage system (n. 9), 271; Francis Brook, Discussion on alimentary toxaemia. *Proceed-*

ings of the Royal Society of Medicine (1913) 6(Suppl):344–352, p. 345; J. F. Briscoe, Discussion of alimentary toxaemia. *Proceedings of the Royal Society of Medicine* (1913) 6(Suppl):364–367, p. 364; Lane, Civilisation (n. 10), 1418.

17. Autobiography of Lane (n. 6); W. Arbuthnot Lane, Chronic intestinal stasis: What are the indications for operative interference? *Lancet* (1919) i:333–334, p. 333; Lane, Chronic intestinal stasis and cancer (n. 11), 747; personal communication; Dinner in honor of Sir William Arbuthnot Lane. *Medical Record* (1938) 147:408–415, p. 415; Adolphe Abrahams, Chronic constipation. *The Practitioner* (1953) 170:266–272, p. 270; Malcolm Veidenheimer, Who dug your well? *Diseases of the Colon and Rectum* (1982) 25:85–89, pp. 87–88; Godfrey Taunton, Chronic intestinal stasis in children. *British Medical Journal* (1919) ii:806–809, p. 809. Paraffin oil would continue in wide use into the second half of the twentieth century, due largely to Lane's influence, but eventually would come under criticism for encouraging anal infections and perhaps contributing to gastrointestinal cancer. See George Becker, The case against mineral oil. *American Journal of Digestive Diseases* (1952) 19:344–348; J. T. Boyd and R. Doll, Gastro-intestinal cancer. *British Journal of Cancer* (1954) 8:231–237.

18. Tanner, *Sir W. Arbuthnot Lane* (n. 6), 115.

19. Surgeon readers curious about the technical specifics of Lane's procedures should consult his *The Operative Treatment of Chronic Intestinal Stasis* (n. 7), 74–83.

20. Lane, The consequences and treatment of alimentary toxaemia. *Proceedings of the Royal Society of Medicine* (1913) 6(Suppl):49–117, pp. 115–116; Lane, Cancer of the colon (n. 14), 1186; Lane, Chronic intestinal stasis: What are the indications (n. 17), 333; Lane, An address on the operative treatment of the conditions of the gastro-intestinal tract which result from chronic constipation. *Lancet* (1904) ii:1695–1699.

21. Berkeley Moynihan, Intestinal stasis. *Surgery, Gynecology and Obstetrics* (1915) 20:154–158, p. 155.

22. Lois Verbrugge, Pathways of health and death. In: Rima Apple, ed., *Women, Health, and Medicine in America* (New York: Garland, 1990), 41–79, p. 48. Richard Reece, *A Practical Dissertation on the Means of Obviating and Treating the Varieties of Costiveness* (London: Longman, Rees, Orme, Brown and Green, 1826), 1; Austin Flint, *A Treatise on the Principles and Practice of Medicine*, 4th ed. (Philadelphia: Lea, 1878), 473; John Burne, *A Treatise on the Causes and Consequences of Habitual Constipation* (Philadelphia: Haswell, Barrington, and Haswell, 1840), 25; James Hamilton, Senior, *Observations on the Utility and Administration of Purgative Medicines*, 5th ed. (Philadelphia: Webster, 1818), 65–66, 71, appendix 56–59.

23. Harold Chapple, Chronic intestinal stasis treated by short-circuiting or colectomy. *British Medical Journal* (1911) i:915–922; W. Arbuthnot Lane, The results of the operative treatment of chronic constipation. *British Medical Journal* (1908) i:126–130; Lane, An address (n. 11); Samuel Gant, *Constipation and Intestinal Obstruction (Obstipation)* (Philadelphia: Saunders, 1909), 60. For contemporary opinion about the causes of constipation in women see John Byers, The prevention of constipation in women and children. *The Practitioner* (1910) 84:553–560; and G. Ernest Herman, Constipation in women. *The Practitioner* (1910) 84:561–566.

24. N. Loughborough, *Handbook of Health: Or, a Brief Treatise on Physiology and Hygiene* (Battle Creek, MI: Steam Press, 1868), 176–177; Lane, Civilisation (n. 10), 1418; Lane, The consequences and treatment of alimentary toxaemia from a surgical point of view. *Proceedings of the Royal Society of Medicine* (1913) 6(Suppl):49–117, pp. 100–101.

25. Lane, Consequences and treatment (n. 24), 108; Harold Chapple, Some effects of chronic intestinal stasis on the female generative organs. *British Medical Journal* (1914) i:192–194, p. 193; Lane, *The Operative Treament of Chronic Intestinal Stasis*, 4th ed. (London: Frowde, Hodder and Stoughton, 1918), 66; Lane, Civilisation (n. 10), 1417–1418.

26. Lane, Consequences and treatment (n. 24), 101; Chapple (n. 25), 192.

27. Lane, Consequences and treatment (n. 24), 105; Lane, Chronic intestinal stasis. *Surgery, Gynecology and Obstetrics* (1910) 11:495–500, p. 499; Lane, Chronic intestinal stasis. *Lancet* (1912) ii:1706–1708, 1721–1724, p. 1707; Lane, An address on chronic intestinal stasis. *British Medical Journal* (1909) i:1408–1411, p. 1410; Lane, *The Operative Treatment of Chronic Constipation* (n. 10), 33.

28. Chapple (n. 23), 915; Lane, Results of the operative treatment (n. 23), 128; Lane, Civilisation (n. 10), 1418; Lane, Consequences and treatment (n. 24), 105; Lane, An address (n. 27); Lane, Chronic intestinal stasis [1912] (n. 27).

29. Lane, Results of the operative treatment (n. 23), 128–130; Lane, Chronic intestinal stasis [1912], (n. 27), 1707; Lane, Consequences and treatment (n. 24), 105; Lane, Chronic intestinal stasis [1910], (n. 27), 499.

30. H. M. W. Gray, Chronic intestinal stasis. *British Medical Journal* (1914) i:188–191, p. 191; Layton (n. 6), 122; Robert Hutchison, An address on the chronic abdomen. *British Medical Journal* (1923) i:667–669, p. 669.

31. Lane, Chronic intestinal stasis (1910), (n. 27), 499; William Hall, *Health and Disease*, 5th ed. (New York: Widdleton, 1864), 35.

32. Leonard Williams, The outwardness of chronic toxaemias. *The Medical Press* [n.s.] (1917) 103:116; Alcinous Jamison, *Intestinal Ills* (New York: Tyrrell's Hygienic Institute, 1919), vii.

33. Lane, Consequences and treatment (n. 24), 101; F. A. Hornibrook, *The Culture of the Abdomen. The Cure of Obesity and Constipation* (Garden City, NY: Doubleday, Doran, 1934), 12.

34. Letters from Margaret Taverner (2 May 1921) and Muriel Keswick (1 March 1925) to Arbuthnot Lane, Wellcome Institute for the History of Medicine.

35. Sampson Hanley quoted by Veidenheimer (n. 17), 87; Rudolph Matas, Memoirs. Sir William Arbuthnot Lane, Bart., C.B., F.R.C.S. 1856–1943. *Annals of Surgery* (1944) 119:607–612, pp. 611–612.

36. Lane, *The Operative Treatment* (n. 10), 65; William Bainbridge, Remarks on chronic intestinal stasis. *Proceedings of the Royal Society of Medicine* (1913) 6(Suppl):1129–1130; Jordan (n. 4), 329. Also see C. Fortescue Pridham, Alimentary toxaemia. *British Medical Journal* (1913) i:855 for another example of Lane's operative success.

37. I am indebted to J. J. Daws, Chief Technician in the Gordon Museum at Guy's Hospital, for directing me to George B.'s colon and retrieving information about the case. Lane, *The Operative Treatment* (n. 10), 65.

38. Bainbridge (n. 36), 1129; Walter Alvarez, *Incurable Physician. An Autobiography* (Englewood Cliffs, NJ: Prentice-Hall, 1963), 245–246; letter from Hettie Bacon to Arbuthnot Lane, July 19, 1921, Wellcome Institute for the History of Medicine.

39. Lane, An address (n. 11), 1126.

40. A discussion on alimentary toxaemia. *Proceedings of the Royal Society of Medicine* (1913) 6(Suppl):1–380.

41. W. Hale White, General survey. *Proceedings of the Royal Society of Medicine* (1913) 6(Suppl):1–10, p. 10.

42. A. Mantle, Discussion on alimentary toxaemia. *Proceedings of the Royal Society of Medicine* (1913) 6(Suppl):154–159, p. 158; W. Hale White, Summary and reply. *Proceedings of the Royal Society of Medicine* (1913) 6(Suppl):374–380, p. 380; Lane, Chronic constipation and its medical and surgical treatment. *British Medical Journal* (1905) i:700–702, p. 702.

43. Lane, The operative treatment of chronic constipation. *International Clinics* (1905) 14(iv):159–165, p. 164; Arthur Keith, Discussion on alimentary toxaemia. *Proceedings of the Royal Society of Medicine* (1913) 6(Suppl):191–195, pp. 193–194.

44. Goodhart (n. 5), 297–299. Also see James Goodhart, Discussion on chronic constipation and its treatment. *British Medical Journal* (1910) ii:1038–1046.

45. Logan Clendening, A review (n. 6), 1198.

46. Anthony Bassler, Discussion of the surgical theories of intestinal stasis. *Journal of the American Medical Association* (1914) 63:1469–1473, pp. 1469, 1471.

47. J. George Adami, An address on chronic intestinal stasis. *British Medical Journal* (1914) i:177–183, p. 179; Re-education of the intestine. *British Medical Journal* (1914) i:985; Alex Don, Alimentary toxaemia. *British Medical Journal* (1913) i:690; Paul Woolley, Intestinal stasis and intestinal intoxications: A critical review. *Journal of Laboratory and Clinical Medicine* (1915–16) 1:45–54, p. 45.

48. George Bernard Shaw, *The Complete Plays of Bernard Shaw* (London: Odhams, 1934), 509–510.

49. Hutchison (n. 30), 667–669; Walter Alvarez, Origin of the so-called autointoxication symptoms. *Journal of the American Medical Association* (1919) 72:8–13, pp. 11–12; Logan Clendening, A review of the subject of chronic intestinal stasis. *Interstate Medical Journal* (1915) 22:1191–1200, p. 1197.

50. Layton (n. 6), 97; W. Arbuthnot Lane, discussion in James Goodhart, The treatment of chronic constipation. *The Lancet* (1910) ii:468–470, pp. 469–470; Autobiography of Lane (n. 6).

51. Arthur Hurst, An address on the sins and sorrows of the colon. *British Medical Journal* (1922) i:941–943, pp. 941, 943.

52. P. Lockhart Mummery, Alimentary toxaemia from the surgical point of view. *Proceedings of the Royal Society of Medicine* (1913) 6(Suppl):181–191, p. 181; White (n. 42), 378.

53. Robert Saundby, The consequences and treatment of alimentary toxaemia from a medical point of view. *Proceedings of the Royal Society of Medicine* (1913) 6(Suppl):37–48, p. 43; F. W. Andrewes, The bacteriology of the alimentary canal. *Proceedings of the Royal Society of Medicine* (1913) 6(Suppl):11–20, p. 11.

54. Walter Alvarez, Origin of the so-called autointoxication symptoms. *Journal of the American Medical Association* (1919) 72:8–13, p. 8.

55. D. Geib and J. D. Jones, Unprecedented case of constipation. *Journal of the American Medical Association* (1902) 38:1304–1305, p. 1305; Walter Alvarez, Intestinal autointoxication. *Physiological Reviews* (1924) 4:352–393.

56. Arthur Donaldson, Relation of constipation to intestinal intoxication. *Journal of the American Medical Association* (1922) 78:884–888; Alvarez (n. 55), 379; Logan Clendening, A

review of the subject of chronic intestinal stasis. *Interstate Medical Journal* (1915) 22:1191–1200, pp. 1192–1193.

    57. Alvarez (n. 54), 8; J. George Adami, An address on chronic intestinal stasis. *British Medical Journal* (1914) i:177–183, pp. 177–178; Clendening (n. 56), p. 1192.

CHAPTER 4

The chapter-opening quotations are from James Goodhart, Discussion on chronic constipation and its treatment. *British Medical Journal* (1910) ii:1038–1046, p. 1040; and Arthur Hurst, The unhappy colon. *Lancet* (1935) i:1483–1487, p. 1483.

    1. Walter Alvarez, Origin of the so-called autointoxication symptoms. *Journal of the American Medical Association* (1919) 72:8–13, p.12.

    2. Alvarez (n. 1), 13.

    3. Alvarez (n. 1), 13.

    4. Alvarez (n. 1), 8; J. George Adami, An address on chronic intestinal stasis. *British Medical Journal* (1914) i:177–183, p. 178. Also see Adami, Autointoxication. *Journal of the American Medical Association* (1935) 104:2289.

    5. William Stemmerman, *Intestinal Management for Longer, Happier Life* (Asheville, NC: Arden, 1928), 25, 28; Charles Campbell and Albert Detweiler, *The Lazy Colon* (New York: Educational Press, 1924); William Walsh, *The Conquest of Constipation* (New York: Dutton, 1923); William Sadler, *Constipation. How to Cure Yourself* (Chicago: McClurg, 1925); Alfred Jordan, Stasis the destroyer. *Medical Journal and Record* (1925) 22:328–330; Victor Pauchet, *Le Colon Homicide*, 1922 pamphlet cited in J. Ellis Barker, *Cancer. How it is Caused; How it Can be Prevented* (Dutton: New York, 1924), 172, 434; S. E. Bilik, *The Trainer's Bible* (New York: Athletic Trainer's Supply, 1928), 88; F. A. Hornibrook, *The Culture of the Abdomen. The Cure of Obesity and Constipation* (Garden City, NY: Doubleday, Doran, 1934), 11; Leonard Williams, The medical aspects of intestinal stasis. In: W. Arbuthnot Lane, *The Operative Treatment of Chronic Intestinal Stasis*, 4th ed. (London: Frowde, Hodder, and Stoughton, 1918), 250–263, pp. 259–260; J. Ellis Barker, *Chronic Constipation. The Most Insidious and the Most Deadly of Diseases* (London: Murray, 1927).

    6. Walter Alvarez, Intestinal autointoxication. *Physiological Reviews* (1924) 4:352–393, p. 352; Benjamin Gruenberg, Motivation in health education. *American Journal of Public Health* (1933) 23:114–122, p. 116.

    7. T. Swann Harding, A purgation of purgatives. *Scientific American* (1937) 157:222–223, p. 222; Oscar Bethea, The use and abuse of purgatives. *International Medical Digest* (1934) 24:239–245, p. 240; Eno's Effervescent Salt, *American Druggist* (June 1931) 83:108; Feen-a-mint, *American Druggist* (April 1930) 81:89; Saraka booklet, AMA, box 113, folder 14; Fowler's, AMA, box 113, folder 3. For a full discussion of radio advertising in the 1920s and '30s see Peter Morell, *Poisons, Potions, and Profits. The Antidote to Radio Advertising* (New York: Knight, 1937).

    8. James Harvey Young, *The Medical Messiahs. A Social History of Health Quackery in Twentieth-Century America* (Princeton, NJ: Princeton University Press, 1967), 46–65, 113–128; J. F. Montague, *I Know Just the Thing for That* (New York: John Day, 1934), 24; Oscar Bethea, The use of cathartics. *Journal of the American Medical Association* (1936) 107:1298–1301, p. 1298.

9. T. Swann Harding, Has truth in advertising been achieved at last? *American Journal of Pharmacy* (1940) 112:325–334, p. 332; Federal Trade Commission Release: April 24, 1943 and June 2, 1943, AMA, box 342, folder 12; July 20, 1943 and December 20, 1947, AMA, box 342, folder 14; September 14, 1943 and February 2, 1948, AMA, box 246, folder 4; Stewart Chase quoted by Young (n. 8) (for a full discussion of the Wheeler-Lea Act, see Young, 296–315).

10. T. Jackson Lears, American advertising and the reconstruction of the body, 1880–1930. In: Kathryn Grover, ed., *Fitness in American Culture. Images of Health, Sport, and the Body, 1830–1940* (Amherst, MA: University of Massachusetts Press, 1989), 47–66.

11. California Fruit Bits (1934), AMA, box 246, folder 4; Hollister's Rocky Mountain Tea, AMA, box 113, folder 6.

12. Bran-Ade Helthets (1931), AMA, box 113, folder 5; Millertone (1932), AMA, folder 6; TAPS (1913), AMA, folder 3; T.A.D. (1925), AMA, folder 5; Cereal Meal (1921), AMA, folder 14; Floradex (1937), AMA, folder 6.

13. A. R. Bliss, Pharmacists should know cathartics. *Pharmaceutical Era* (1925) 60:7; J. Plesch. In: discussion of Arthur Hurst, The uses and abuses of purgatives. *Transactions of the Medical Society of London* (1939) 62:127–143, p. 142; Barker, *Chronic Constipation* (n. 5), 411.

14. *Literary Digest*, March 5, 1927, 85.

15. Steep-a-lax, *Nature's Path* (1940) 45:103; Joseph Matthews, in discussion of Edwin Walker, A further protest against the routine use of purgatives. *American Journal of Obstetrics and Diseases of Women and Children* (1911) 64:745–758, p. 753; Charles Fleming, Quackery in rural districts. *British Medical Journal* (1911) i:1246–1248.

16. Eno's, *Literary Digest*, August 8, 1925, 52, and September 26, 1925, 74; Sal Hepatica, *Time*, June 16, 1930, 32, and *Literary Digest*, April 9, 1927, 79.

17. Malena booklet, Warshaw, box 25, file 6; Friends of the Bishops' House, *Headlines Idaho Remembers* (Boise, ID: Friends of the Bishops' House, 1977), 46; Barker, *Chronic Constipation* (n. 5), 256; Walter Alvarez, *Help Your Doctor to Help You When You Have Constipation* (New York: Harper, 1942), 27. For other advertising examples, see Dr. Dunlop's Cascara Compound, Warshaw, box 6, file 11, and Doan's Regulets, Warshaw, box 11, file 6.

18. Brandreth, Warshaw, box 4, file 22, and AMA, box 113, folder 11; letter from A. E. Backman to Arthur Cramp, AMA, box 113, folder 11; Henry Holcombe, *Patent Medicine Tax Stamps. A History of the Firms Using United States Private Die Proprietary Medicine Tax Stamps* (Lawrence, MA: Quarterman, 1979), 56.

19. Nujol, *Literary Digest*: March 14, 1925, 91; February 28, 1925, 73; March 28, 1925, 73; January 5, 1924, 71; January 26, 1924, 56; and February 16, 1924, 95. Toxelin (1939), Nature's Lawlax (1928), and I-Clean-U, AMA, box 113, folder 3.

20. Vi-Lax, AMA, box 113, folder 3; Nujol, *Literary Digest*, January 5, 1924, 71; Laxative Repeaters, Warshaw, box 37, file 24; Kruschen Salts, *American Druggist*, October 1930, 102; Eno's, *American Druggist*, October 1930, 172; Arthur Hurst, *Selected Writings of Sir Arthur Hurst*, Thomas Hunt, ed. (London: Spottiswoode, Ballantyne, 1970), 166; F. Parkes Weber, Prepared bran in the prevention of constipation. *British Medical Journal* (1941) i:252–253, p. 253.

21. Move-Eze (1918), AMA, box 113, folder 4; Time Fuse Tablets (1930), AMA, box 113, folder 5; Rinoline (1928), AMA, box 113, folder 3; Ex-Lax (1938), AMA, box 246, folder 4; Boston Brown Beans (1903), KRF, file C19; Nature's Remedy, *American Druggist*, January 1931, 116; TAPS, AMA, box 113, folder 3.

22. Nujol, *American Druggist and Pharmaceutical Record,* December 1916, 9; Lacricin (1928) and Nature's Lawlax (1933), AMA, box 113, folder 3; Fruisen (1936), AMA, box 113, folder 6; Peristalso (1914), AMA, box 113, folder 4; Naturalax, *American Druggist,* October 1930, 188; Jiffy-Lax (1934), AMA, box 113, folders 3, 6.

23. Jam-O-Lax (1923), AMA, box 113, folder 4.

24. Fruisen (1936), AMA, box 113, folder 6; Lax-Krax, *Journal of the American Medical Association* (1929) 93:1008, and AMA, box 114, folder 15; Epsonade (1921), Citro-Nesia (1921), and Citrolax (1914), AMA, box 114, folder 4; Laxa Raisins, *Notices of Judgment,* 14425, 14622; Kasta Kookies (1923) and Lacricin (1928), AMA, box 113, folder 3.

25. James Whorton, The phenolphthalein follies: Purgation and the pleasure principle in the early twentieth century. *Pharmacy in History* (1993) 35:3–24; Kastor Jems (1926) and Laxybar (1930), AMA, box 113, folder 5; Cascarets, AMA, box 113, folder 6; Co-rex (1928), AMA, box 156, folder 10; Laxaphen, Phenolphthalein. *Journal of the American Medical Association* (1910) 54:1458–1459; Chu-Lax, AMA, box 246, folder 4; Tru-Lax (1929), AMA, box 246, folder 3; Tryalax, AMA, box 115, folder 19; Auto-Laks, AMA, box 113, folder 9; Brandreth's Pills (1925), AMA, box 113, folder 11; other brands cited by George Belote and Harvey Whitney, Phenolphthalein compounds. *Archives of Dermatology and Syphilology* (1937) 36:279–281; Erich Zabel, Ein Fall von Purgen-Intoxikation. *Deutsche Medizinische Wochenschrift* (1911) 37:743–744, p. 743; ad for Purgen, Royal Pharmaceutical Society; The Druggists Circular, *The Modern Materia Medica,* 2nd ed. (New York: The Druggists Circular, 1911), 19, 88, 132, 231, 318–319; Prunol (1942), AMA, box 113, folder 3; American Medical Association, *Nostrums and Quackery,* 2nd ed. (Chicago: American Medical Association, 1912), 520; Bernard Fantus, *Useful Cathartics* (Chicago: American Medical Association, 1920), 77; AMA, box 113, folders 3, 4, 5; Cathartones, folder 3; Regulax, folder 4; Biolax, folder 5 *American Druggist,* July 1927, 63.

26. Laxybar (1930) and Kastor Jems (1926), AMA, box 113, folder 5; Ex-Lax booklet (1929), AMA, box 246, folder 4; the Ex-Lax radio ad is reproduced in August 26, 1935 letter from Arthur Cramp to Charles Angoff, AMA, box 246, folder 5.

27. Ex-Lax booklet (1929), AMA, box 246, folder 4; Feen-a-mint booklet (1933), AMA, box 342, folder 12.

28. Ex-Lax booklet (1929), AMA, box 246, folder 4.

29. Belote and Whitney (n. 25), 279; *American Druggist,* 1930 Year Book and Price List, 3; *American Druggist,* June 1933, 77; files of Bureau of Investigation are in AMA, box 246, folder 6.

30. Ex-Lax sales figures are taken from ads in AMA, box 246, folder 4.

31. Manna Cake, RPS.

32. Lemuel McGee, Cathartic-conscious America. *Hygeia* (1937) 15:731–734, p. 734; A. A. Walker, Owen Wilson, and Theodore Harrell, in discussion of Lewis Elias, Practical points on purgation. *Southern Medical Journal* (1923) 16:597–602, p. 600; Lacricin, *American Druggist,* September 1928, 2. Also see Eric Pritchard, Constipation in infants. *The Practitioner* (1910) 84:583–594, p. 585.

33. William Stemmerman, *Intestinal Management for Longer, Happier Life* (Asheville, NC: Arden, 1928), 192–193; Oliver Wendell Holmes, Review of *Homeopathic Domestic Physician,*

Atlantic Monthly (1857) 1:250–252, p. 252; Glenn Sonnedecker and George Griffenhagen, A history of sugar-coated pills and tablets. *Journal of the American Pharmaceutical Association* (Practical Pharmacy Edition) (1957) 18:486–488.

34. Ex-Lax pamphlets, Warshaw, box 9, folder 25; and AMA, box 246, folder 5.

35. Co-Rex (1928), AMA, box 156, folder 10; Feen-a-mint (1928), AMA, box 342, folder 12.

36. Feen-a-mint (1934), AMA, box 342, folder 12; Ex-Lax, *Life*, April 19, 1937, 46; Ex-Lax (1929), AMA, box 246, folder 4, and *Life*, March 22, 1937, 38.

37. H. F. Gillette, Accidental overdose of phenolphthalein. *Journal of the American Medical Association* (1908) 51:1782; October 5, 1933 letter from R. H. Warner to AMA, box 113, folder 6; 37; Montague Cleeves, Poisoning by Ex-Lax tablets. *Journal of the American Medical Association* (1932) 99:654; June 18, 1932 letter from Montague Cleeves to AMA, box 246, folder 12. There was a far more serious problem with a smaller group of laxatives, those that included strychnine in the formula in order to stimulate the intestinal muscles. At least a dozen deaths a year were attributed to strychnine laxative overdose, often from mailed samples, during the 1920s. See Everett Brown, Deaths from laxative tablets containing strychnine. *Journal of the American Medical Association* (1915) 64:1781–1782; John Aikman, Strychnine poisoning in children. *Journal of the American Medical Association* (1930) 95:1661–1665.

38. What do you think 2362 kiddies told us? *Junior Life* article, AMA, box 246, folder 4.

39. Hillel Schwartz, *Never Satisfied. A Cultural History of Diets, Fantasies and Fat* (New York: Free Press, 1986), 110–111, 183; Arthur Cramp, ed., *Nostrums and Quackery* (Chicago: American Medical Association, 1921), 680–682.

40. Kruschen Salts ads in *American Druggist*, August 1930, 86; *American Druggist*, February 1932, 131; *American Druggist*, March 1931, 142; *Vogue*, June 15, 1933, 68; *American Druggist*, May 1933, 123; *American Druggist*, October 1930, 102; *American Druggist*, December 1931, 73; W. M. Coplin, A basis for the prevention of cancer. *Journal of the American Medical Association* (1922) 78:1523–1529, p. 1526.

41. Beecham's Help to Scholars, advertising booklet, Warshaw, box 1, folder 18; Nujol, *Good Housekeeping*, January 1922, 127, and *Literary Digest*, February 16, 1924, 95; Sal Hepatica, AMA, box 768, folder 13; Dr. Tutt's Manual, Warshaw, box 45, file 31.

42. Sal Hepatica, *Literary Digest*, April 9, 1927, 79; Nujol, *Literary Digest*, November 8, 1924, 73.

43. *American Druggist*, January 1928, 69; Feen-a-mint (1928), AMA, box 342, folder 12. Numerous other ploys were used to sell laxatives. Purgatives were combined with the recently introduced wonder drug aspirin (CathAspirin, Asper-Lax, Laxa-Pirin), for example, and with the even more recent wonder, vitamins (Vi-Lax): CathAspirin, *Pharmaceutical Era*, July 3, 1926, 31; Asper-Lax, *Pharmaceutical Era*, April 1929, 100; Laxa-Pirin, AMA, box 113, folder 4; Vi-Lax, AMA, box 113, folder 3.

44. Letter of August 10, 1932, from Martha Rasmussen to the American Medical Association, AMA, box 156, folder 15.

45. For reduced wholesale prices and other promotional strategies, see Feen-a-mint reception. *The Druggists Circular*, December 1925, 50; Cascarets, *The Apothecary*, June 1920, 38; Sal Hepatica, *Pharmaceutical Era*, July 3, 1926, 3.

46. *American Druggist,* March 1933, 83; *American Druggist,* October 1931, 190; *American Druggist,* March 1930, 188; *American Druggist,* June 1931, 138; *American Druggist,* December 1933, 90; *American Druggist,* June 1933, 134.

47. The Feen-a-mint stock offer is made in the letter from Health Products Corporation to Dr. Alex Thomson, November 30, 1923, AMA, box 342, folder 13; James Goodhart, Round about constipation. *Lancet* (1902) ii:1241–1246, p. 1246.

48. Walker (n. 15), 746, 752–756; L. J. Witts, Ritual purgation in modern medicine. *Lancet* (1937) i:427–430. A 1933 survey determined that purgatives had come to be prescribed less frequently than in the past, but they still were being administered much more often than necessary. See E. N. Gathercoal, *The Prescripton Ingredient Survey* (American Pharmaceutical Association: Chicago, 1933), 172.

49. Manfred Kraemer, Laxatives and bowel consciousness—A clinical study. *American Journal of Digestive Diseases and Nutrition* (1937–8) 5:9–12, p. 12; T. L. Hardy, Order and disorder in the large intestine. *The Lancet* (1945) i:519–524, 553–559, p. 553; P. J. Cammidge, *The Faeces of Children and Adults* (New York: Wood, 1914), 434; A. A. Walker. In: discussion of Elias (n. 32), 600; Harding (n. 7), 222. Clearly many people abused phenolphthalein. A study performed in the late 1930s, for example, determined that nearly 20% of the patients who visited a gastroenterologic clinic had been taking phenolphthalein daily for at least 2 months (and some for as long as 2 years). Nearly all were suffering from colitis, yet all recovered on discontinuing their laxative habit. See Horace Soper, Phenolphthalein. *American Journal of Digestive Diseases* (1938) 5:297.

50. James Goodhart, The treatment of chronic constipation. *The Lancet* (1910) ii:468–470, p. 468; McGee (n. 32), 734; Bernard Fantus, *Useful Cathartics* (Chicago: American Medical Association, 1920), 77; Hurst (n. 13), 131; Kraemer (n. 49), 11.

51. March 5, 1931 letter from Josephine Patterson to AMA, box 113, folder 5; Elias (n. 32), 598; John Bower, The mortality of acute appendicitis. *Journal of the American Medical Association* (1932) 99:1765–1768, p. 1768. Physicians too were sometimes guilty of prescribing purgatives in cases of appendicitis. See M. C. Harris, Dangers from indiscriminate use of cathartics in acute intestinal conditions. *Journal of the American Medical Association* (1905) 44:622–624, p. 624.

52. Edward Emery, The significance of so-called constipation. *Medical Clinics of North America* (1927) 10:1345–1352, p. 1347; Alvarez (n. 17), 33–34.

53. Alvarez (n. 17), 21; Montague (n. 8), 3.

Chapter 5

The chapter opening quotations are from Dioclesian Lewis, *Our Digestion; Or, My Jolly Friend's Secret* (Philadelphia: McLean, 1872), 167; and Charles Tyrrell, *The Royal Road to Health, Or the Secret of Health Without Drugs,* 250th ed. (New York: Tyrrell Hygienic Institute, 1920), 23–24, 34–35.

1. Letter from Andrew Vena to American Medical Association, September 30, 1931, AMA, box 868, folder 5. Michaela Sullivan-Fowler, Doubtful theories, drastic therapies: Autointoxication and faddism in the late nineteenth and early twentieth centuries. *Journal of the History of Medicine and Allied Sciences* (1995) 50:364–390, gives a good bit of attention to the J. B. L. Cascade and its manufacturer Charles Tyrrell.

2. Vena (n. 1).

3. Vena (n. 1).

4. Letters from American Medical Association to Ulysses Smith, August 2, 1935, AMA, box 868, folder 5, and to J. Stuart Hamilton, November 16, 1916, AMA, box 868, folder 4.

5. Tobias Venner, *The Baths of Bathe* (London: Moore, 1628) (the baths of Bath have been tested more recently and determined to have approximately the same effect as tap water; see J. P. O'Hare, A. Heywood, C. Summerhayes, G. Lunn, J. M. Evans, G. Walters, R. J. M. Corrall and P.A. Dieppe, Observations on the effects of immersion in bath spa water. *British Medical Journal* (1985) 291:1747–1751.

6. Noel Coley, 'Cures without care.' 'Chymical physicians' and mineral waters in seventeenth-century English medicine. *Medical History* (1979) 23:191–214; Phyllis Hembry, *The English Spa 1560–1815. A Social History* (London: Athlone, 1990), 43. Also see Allen Debus, *The Chemical Philosophy: Paracelsian Science and Medicine in the Sixteenth and Seventeenth Centuries* (New York: Science History, 1977), Vol. 1, 109–112; Debus, *The English Paracelsians* (London: Oldbourne, 1965), 158–165; and F. N. L. Poynter, A seventeenth-century medical controversy. Robert Wittie versus William Simpson. In: E. Ashworth Underwood, ed., *Science, Medicine and History* (London: Oxford University Press, 1953), Vol. 1, 72–81.

7. William Addison, *English Spas* (London: Batsford, 1951), 14–15; Hembry (n. 6), 45; John Mennes, *Facetiae* (London: Hotten, 1817), Vol. 1, 22–24.

8. Charles Trench, *The Royal Malady* (New York: Harcourt, Brace and World, 1964), 4–7; Ida Macalpine and Richard Hunter, *George III and the Mad-Business* (London: Allen Lane, 1969), 4–11; Alexander Thomson, *The Family Physician* (New York: Oram, 1802), 369–372; 9; [Giles Grinagain], "The Rapid Effects of the Cheltenham Waters," Cheltenham Art Gallery and Museums.

9. S. W. Fores, Effects of the Cheltenham waters. Cheltenham Art Gallery and Museums; T. D. Fosbroke, *A Picturesque and Topographical Account of Cheltenham and Its Vicinity* (Cheltenham: Harper, 1826), 168. Cartoonish depictions of the operation of spa waters were common throughout the nineteenth century, and those produced at Continental watering places could be considerably more blunt. See Jacques Frexinos, *L'Art de Purger. Histoire Générale et Anecdotique des Laxatifs* (Paris: Pariente, 1997), 135–159.

10. S. Y. Griffith, *New Historical Description of Cheltenham* (Cheltenham: Author, 1826), 35, 38; Alfred Landseer, *A Panoramic Sketch of Cheltenham and its Environs*, 2nd ed. (London: Longman, 1829), 7; Gwen Hart, *A History of Cheltenham*, 2nd ed. (Gloucester, England: Alan Sutton, 1981), 183–184. For more on Cheltenham's rise to fashionable status see Hart, 115–183; H. Davies, *The Stranger's Guide Through Cheltenham* (Cheltenham: Davies, 1832), 6–28; Frederick Alderson, *The Inland Spas and Resorts of Britain* (David and Charles: Newton Abbot, 1973), 66–71; Hembry (n. 6), 179–201.

11. T. F. Dibdin, *The History of Cheltenham and its Environs* (Cheltenham: Ruff, 1803), 70–71; G. A. Williams, *The New Guide to Cheltenham* (Cheltenham: Bettison, 1820), 71–84. For more on the spa schedule see John Lee, *A New Guide to Cheltenham and Its Environs* (Cheltenham: Author, 1834), 99–100, and G. A. Williams, *Williams' New Guide to Cheltenham* (Cheltenham: Author, 1824), 22. On Saratoga, see Henry Sigerist, The early medical history of Saratoga Springs. *Bulletin of the History of Medicine* (1943) 13:540–584; Joseph Wechsberg, *The Lost World of the Great Spas* (New York: Harper and Row, 1979), 180–197.

12. Arthur Hurst, An address on the sins and sorrows of the colon. *British Medical Journal* (1922) i:941–943, pp. 942–943.

13. Celia Fiennes, *The Journeys of Celia Fiennes*, Christopher Morris, ed. (London: Cresset, 1947), 80; Tobias Smollett, *Works of Tobias Smollett* (New York: Routledge, n.d.), Vol. 1, 382–383.

14. Malcolm Neesam, *Exclusively Harrogate* (Otley, England: Smith Settle, 1989), 13, 38; Alderson (n. 10), 73–80.

15. Alderson (n. 10), 82; S. P. B. Mais, *Harrogate. The Spa in a Holiday Environment*, (no city, publisher, or date given; apparently 1910s), 5, 11; Anonymous, *A Pictorial and Descriptive Guide to Harrogate*, 8th ed. (London: Ward, Locke, 1909), 10; Harrogate Medical Society, *A Brief Account of the Nature of Spa Treatment* (Harrogate: Harrogate Medical Society, ca. 1920), 18–29; personal communication from Sheila Moore, MD, of Harrogate; Walter McClellan, *Hydrotherapeutic Measures in Hepatic, Gallbladder and Biliary Tract Diseases* (Saratoga, NY: Saratoga Spa, 1935), 12.

16. W. Kerr Russell, *Colonic Irrigation* (Edinburgh: Livingstone, 1932), 16, 19–20; Russell, Colonic lavage, fallacies and facts. *British Journal of Physical Medicine* (1933) 8:24–26, p. 25.

17. Leonard Williams, The spa treatment of chronic constipation. *Practitioner* (1910) 84:662–670, p. 665; Hurst (n. 12), 943; A. Mantle, Discussion on alimentary toxaemia. *Proceedings of the Royal Society of Medicine* (1913) 6(Suppl):154–159, p. 154.

18. Harrogate Medical Society (n. 15), 30–31; Hermann Weber and F. Parkes Weber, *Climatotherapy and Balneotherapy* (London: Smith, Elder, 1907), 548; H. Douglas Wilson, Discussion on alimentary toxaemia. *Proceedings of the Royal Society of Medicine* (1913) 6:340–344.

19. Anonymous (n. 15), 13; Mais (n. 15), 10; A Resident Doctor, *What to Eat When Spawing at Harrogate* (Harrogate: Author, 1903); Anonymous, *The Harrogate Cure* (no city, publisher, or date; at Harrogate Public Library), 36.

20. Williams (n. 17), 662–663; Samuel Gant, *Constipation and Intestinal Obstruction (Obstipation)* (Philadelphia: Saunders, 1909), 312.

21. Harrogate Medical Society (n. 15), 30, 47; minutes of April 23, 1945 meeting of Wells and Baths Committee of Harrogate. In: possession of Sheila Moore, MD.

22. Leonard Williams, The medical aspect of intestinal stasis. In: W. Arbuthnot Lane, *The Operative Treatment of Chronic intestinal stasis*, 4th ed. (London: Frowde, Hodder, and Stoughton, 1918), 250–263, p. 263; Arthur Hurst, The unhappy colon. *Lancet* (1935) i:1483–1487, p. 1485; papers of Harrogate Medical Society. In: possession of Sheila Moore, MD.

23. George Bernard Shaw, Doctors' Delusions. In: *The Collected Works of Bernard Shaw* (New York: Wise, 1932), Vol. 22, 3–170, pp. 51–52 ; John Carroll, Have spas an essential place in the national economy. *New York State Journal of Medicine* (1940) 40:23–28, p. 27; Albert Wallace, The modern health resort. *Journal of the American Medical Association* (1936) 107:419–421; Bernard Jennings, *A History of Harrogate and Knaresborough*, (no city or publisher, 1969), 445; Neesam (n. 14), i; J. A. Patmore, *An Atlas of Harrogate* (Harrogate: Corporation of Harrogate, 1963), 32; David Cantor, The contradictions of specialization: Rheumatism and the decline of the spa in inter-war Britain. In: Roy Porter, ed., *The Medical History of Spas and Waters*, Medical History Supplement No. 10 (London: Wellcome Institute for the History of Medicine, 1990), 127–144.

24. Aquaperia, *The Chemist and Druggist,* January 30, 1915, 79; Bernard Fantus, Our insufficiently appreciated american spas and health resorts. *Journal of the American Medical Association* (1938) 110:40–42, p. 41. Also see The propaganda for reform. *Journal of the American Medical Association* (1913) 60:1013–1014, p. 1013; James Crook, *The Mineral Waters of the United States and Their Therapeutic Uses* (New York: Lea, 1899), 34.

25. Carlsbad (1913), AMA, box 513, folder 13 (for other foreign mineral water ads, see KRF, C 39 (c) II).

26. Arthur Hurst, *Constipation and Allied Intestinal Disorders,* 2nd ed. (London: Frowde, 1921), 389–390; Sal Hepatica, AMA, box 768, folder 13.

27. Arthur Cramp, ed., *Nostrums and Quackery* (Chicago: American Medical Association, 1936), 73–77; ads in AMA, box 511, folders 4, 5; Theodora Andrews and Varro Tyler, 'Taking the Waters' in Indiana. *Pharmacy in History* (1993) 35:55–64, pp. 55–58.

28. Andrews and Tyler (n. 27), 59–61; letters from Pluto Water, AMA, box 514, folder 14.

29. Andrews and Tyler (n. 27), 57; Pluto Water, AMA, box 515, folder 1; and box 514, folder 14.

30. Andrews and Tyler (n. 27), 61.

31. Ads in AMA, box 511, folders 5, 8; box 512, folder 16; and box 515, folder 15.

32. Nigel Tallis, Portraits of Peter Squire. *Pharmaceutical Journal* (1988) 24:375–376, p. 375. For information on the history of the enema, see Julius Friedenwald and Samuel Morrison, The history of the enema, with some notes on related procedures. *Bulletin of the History of Medicine* (1940) 8:68–114, 239–276; J. F. Montague, History and appraisal of the enema. *Medical Record* (1934) 139:91–93, 142–145, 194–195, 245–247, 297–299, 458–460; and William Lieberman, The history of the enema. *Ciba Symposia* (February, 1944) 5.

33. George Taylor, *Health by Exercise* (New York: Fowler and Wells, 1883), 309–310; J. H. Tilden, *Constipation. A New Reading on the Subject* (Denver: Author, 1923), 86.

34. Charles Tyrrell, *The Royal Road to Health,* 94th ed. (New York: Author, 1913), 56–57; Tyrrell, Professor Tyrrell's celebrated cascade treatment, pamphlet, Warshaw, box 45, file 34.

35. Who's Who in New York, AMA, box 868, folder 3; Charles Tyrrell, *The What, The Why, The Way of Internal Baths,* 2, Warshaw, box 45, file 34; Charles Tyrrell, *Professor Chas. A. Tyrrell's Wonderful J. B. L. Cascade Treatment* (New York: Tyrrell, 1897), no pagination; Tyrrell, *The Royal Road* (n. 34), 66; A. Wilford Hall, *Dr. A. Wilford Hall's Hygienic Treatment for the Cure of Disease, Preservation of Health, and the Promotion of Longevity* (New York: Author, 1889).

36. Who's Who in New York (n. 35); Tyrrell, *The Royal Road* (n. 34), 46, 48–49, 227.

37. Tyrrell, *Professor Chas. A. Tyrrell's* (n. 35).

38. Tyrrell, *Professor's Chas. A. Tyrrell's* (n. 35); letter from Tyrrell's Hygienic Institute to J. A. Yunker, May 21, 1935, AMA, box 868, folder 5.

39. Letter (n. 38); Tyrrell, *The What, The Why* (n. 35), 30.

40. Tyrrell, *Professor Chas. A. Tyrrell's* (n. 35); Illustrations of the J. B. L. Cascade, AMA, box 868, folder 1; testimonial, AMA, box 867, folder 10; ad for Cascade, *Health* (June 1906) 56, advertising section.

41. Tyrrell, *Professor Chas. A. Tyrrell's* (n. 35); pamphlet from Tyrrell's Hygienic Institute, Warshaw, box 45, file 33; Tyrrell, *The Royal Road* (n. 34), 226; Arthur Cramp, ed., *Nostrums and Quackery* (Chicago: American Medical Association, 1921), 703.

42. Pamphlet, Warshaw, box 45, file 34; Tyrrell, *The Royal Road* (n. 34), 228; Tyrrell ad, AMA, box 867, folder 10; Cramp (n. 41), 697–698; J. B. L. Products of Quality, pamphlet, AMA, box 868, folder 5.

43. Tyrrell Hygienic Club pamphlet, Warshaw, box 45, file 34; Tyrrell ad, *American Druggist*, September 1928, 60–61; *American Druggist*, March 1928, 60.

44. Letters from Tyrrell's Hygienic Institute to J. A. Yunker, May 7, 1935, May 21, 1935, and June 18, 1935, AMA, box 868, folder 5.

45. Cramp (n. 41), 705; William Stemmerman, *Intestinal Management for Longer, Happier Life* (Asheville, NC: Arden, 1928), 119; Sullivan-Fowler (n. 1), 390; letter from H. Clay Horner to AMA, November 20, 1918, AMA, box 868, folder 4.

46. Davol, *Pharmaceutical Era*, September 1927, 1; Hunt's, AMA, box 867, folder 9; Eager Intestine Cleanser, *Brain and Brawn* (May 1914) 2:iv; Williams' Alimentary Douche, AMA, box 0236, folder 1; letters from Cramp to North Carolina druggist, July 2, 1913, AMA, box 0236, folder 1, and to Albert Haas, May 13, 1935, AMA, box 0235, folder 11.

47. Alcinous Jamison, pamphlet on *Intestinal Irrigation*, KRF, C37(a), VI; Jamison, *Intestinal Ills* (New York: Tyrrell's Hygienic Institute, 1919), xv–xvi.

48. Jamison pamphlet (n. 47).

49. Montague (n. 32), 143; John Lichty, The present consideration and care of the colon. *Journal of the American Medical Association* (1931) 96:649–653, p. 653.

50. Frank Krusen, Colonic irrigation. *Journal of the American Medical Association* (1936) 106:118–121, p. 118; Walter Bastedo, Colon irrigations. Their administration, therapeutic application and dangers. *Journal of the American Medical Association* (1932) 98:734–736, p. 734.

51. Krusen (n. 50), 119; James Wiltsie, *Chronic Intestinal Toxemia and Its Treatment*, (Baltimore: Wood, 1938), 106–132; Oscar Schellberg, *Lectures on Colonic Therapy* (New York: Oboschell Corporation, 1930); W. Kerr Russell, *Colonic Irrigation* (Edinburgh: Livingstone, 1932); Julius Friedenwald and Samuel Morrison, Value, limitations, indications and technic of colonic irrigations. *Medical Clinics of North America*, May 1935, 1611–1629, p. 1613; Harold Marshall, The place of colon therapy in the mentally ill. *Medical Record* (1936) 144:8–11, p. 9.

52. Stemmerman (n. 45), 123–124; Walter Bastedo, Colon irrigations. *New England Journal of Medicine* (1928) 199:865–866, p. 865; Gant (n. 20), 231.

53. James Wiltsie, Colonic therapy: A method of special drainage. *Archives of Physical Therapy* (1931) 12:292–295, p. 294; Irrigating the colon. *Journal of the American Medical Association* (1927) 89:1804; Frank Smithies, Colon filling stations. *Journal of the American Medical Association* (1926) 87:691; Bastedo (n. 50), 734; W. Kerr Russell, Colonic lavage, fallacies and facts. *British Journal of Physical Medicine* (1933) 8:24–26, p. 24.

54. Bastedo (n. 50), 736; Bastedo (n. 52), 866; Horace Soper, Colon irrigations. *Journal of the American Medical Association* (1932) 98:1677–1678; Wiltsie (n. 51), 1, 2, 4; John Dewis, The misuse of cathartics and laxatives. *Boston Medical and Surgical Journal* (1925) 193:152–157, p. 154.

55. Bastedo (n. 50), 736; Krusen (n. 50), 118, 120; Stemmerman (n. 45), 118; Lichty (n. 49), 650, 652. Also see Friedenwald and Morrison (n. 51), 1617.

56. Correspondence and advertisements, AMA, box 156, folders 8, 12, and 15; Smithies (n. 53), 691.

CHAPTER 6

The chapter-opening quotations are from Leonard Williams, The medical aspect of intestinal stasis. In: W. Arbuthnot Lane, *The Operative Treatment of Chronic intestinal stasis*, 4th ed. (London: Frowde, Hodder, and Stoughton, 1918), 250–263, pp. 256–258, and Williams cited by William Lieberman, History of the enema. *Ciba Symposia* (February 1944) 5:1709; and Charles Campbell and Albert Detweiler, *The Lazy Colon* (New York: Educational Press, 1924), 188.

1. The Radical Cure, pamphlet for Dr. Young's Rectal Dilators, KRF, C39 (k), 50.
2. The Radical Cure (n. 1), 37–39, 51.
3. The Radical Cure (n. 1), 39, 51, 62–64.
4. The Radical Cure (n. 1), 50–51.
5. The Radical Cure (n. 1), 9.
6. F. A. Hornibrook, *The Culture of the Abdomen. The Cure of Obesity and Constipation* (Garden City, NY: Doubleday, Doran, 1934), 24–25, 41.
7. J. F. Montague, *I Know Just the Thing For That* (New York: John Day, 1934), 155; Charles Campbell and Albert Detweiler, *The Lazy Colon* (New York: Educational Press, 1924), 161; Hornibrook (n. 6).
8. James Whorton, *Crusaders for Fitness. The History of American Health Reformers* (Princeton, NJ: Princeton University Press, 1982), 296–303. Also see William Hunt, *Body Love: The Amazing Career of Bernarr Macfadden* (Bowling Green, OH: Bowling Green State University Popular Press, 1989), and Robert Ernst, *Weakness is a Crime: The Life of Bernarr Macfadden* (Syracuse, NY: Syracuse University Press, 1991).
9. Bernarr Macfadden, *Vitality Supreme* (New York: Physical Culture, 1923), ix, 83; Mary Macfadden and Emile Gauvreau, *Dumbbells and Carrot Strips. The Story of Bernarr Macfadden* (New York: Holt, 1953).
10. Bernarr Macfadden, *Constipation. Its Cause, Effect and Treatment* (Macfadden: New York, 1924); Macfadden, *Macfadden's Encyclopedia of Physical Culture* (New York: Physical Culture, 1914), Vol. 5, 2448.
11. Macfadden (n. 9), 69–76, 80, 179–180; Macfadden, *Constipation. Its Cause, Effect and Treatment* (New York: Macfadden, 1924), 194–236; Macfadden, *Macfadden's Physical Training* (New York: Macfadden, 1900), 120; Macfadden, *Macfadden's Encyclopedia* (n. 10), Vol. 4, 1958–1962.
12. Campbell and Detweiler (n. 7), 186–188; G. Sherman Bigg, *Indigestion, Constipation and Liver Disorder* (New York: Hoeher, 1913), 108; Samuel Gant, *Constipation and Intestinal Obstruction (Obstipation)* (Philadelphia: Saunders, 1909), 221; H. Illoway, *Constipation in Adults and Children* (New York: MacMillan, 1897), 197; Hornibrook (n. 7), 81–97; Maxalding, *New Health* (December 1927) 2:13, and *New Health* (December 1929) 4:40; Cascarets, *Cosmopolitan Magazine* (1905–6) 40:486; Oscar Bethea, The use and abuse of purgatives. *International Medical Digest* (1934) 24:239–245, pp. 242–243.
13. George Taylor, *Health by Exercise* (New York: Fowler and Wells, 1883), xiv; Douglas Graham, *A Treatise on Massage*, 3rd ed. (Philadelphia: Lippincott, 1902), 17–48; Joseph Schreiber, *A Manual of Treatment by Massage and Methodical Muscle Exercise*, Walter Mendelson, trans. (Philadelphia: Lea, 1887), 17–30; Hartvig Nissen, *Practical Massage and Corrective Exercises*, 5th ed. (Philadelphia: Davis, 1929), 17–27.

14. Mary Mulliner, *Mechanotherapy. A Textbook for Students* (Philadelphia: Lea and Febiger, 1929), 24–36; Mary McMillan, *Massage and Therapeutic Exercise*, 3rd ed. (Philadelphia: Saunders, 1932), 17–41; J. George Adami, An address on chronic intestinal stasis. *British Medical Journal* (1914) i:177–183, p. 179.

15. Thomas Dowse, Mechano-therapeutics for constipation. *The Practitioner* (1910) 84:719–733, p. 728; James Mennell, *Massage. Its Principles and Practice*, 2nd ed. (Philadelphia: Blakiston, 1920), 400.

16. Mennell (n. 15), 404–406; Mulliner (n. 14), 188; Illoway (n. 12), 203–242; R. Tait McKenzie, *Exercise in Education and Medicine*, 3rd ed. (Philadelphia: Saunders, 1923), 495–497.

17. William Stemmerman, *Intestinal Management for Longer, Happier Life* (Asheville, NC: Arden, 1928), 141, 154–155; Bernarr Macfadden, *Virile Powers of Superb Manhood. How Developed; How Lost; How Regained* (London: Macfadden, 1900), 173–174; Macfadden (n. 9), 162–178; Campbell and Detweiler (n. 7), 3–4; McKenzie (n. 16), 496; Rallie Health Belt ad, *New Health* (November 1934) 9:32.

18. Ad for Kolon-Motor, AMA, box 867, folder 9; McKenzie (n. 15), 352–363; M. L. H. Snow, *Mechanical Vibration. Its Physiological Application in Therapeutics* (New York: Scientific Authors' Publishing, 1912), 1–43.

19. Gant (n. 12), 226, 274, 280; Snow (n. 18), 55–81, 419–427; a Veedee vibrator and advertisement are in the collection of St. Thomas's Operating Theatre Museum, London.

20. Snow (n. 18), 428–434.

21. Susan Ehlers, Currents. Electrotherapy in America in the Late Nineteenth Century. MA thesis, University of Washington, 1983; Margaret Rowbottom and Charles Susskind, *Electricity and Medicine. History of Their Interaction* (San Francisco: San Francisco Press, 1984), 1–200; Hector Colwell, *An Essay on the History of Electrotherapy and Diagnosis* (London: Heinemann, 1922).

22. Rowbottom and Susskind (n. 21), 17; Elkin Cumberbatch, *Essentials of Medical Electricity*, 6th ed. (St. Louis: Mosby, 1929), 349.

23. Cumberbatch (n. 22), 349; Gant (n. 12), 282, 295.

24. Gant (n. 12), 246–262.

25. R. H. Ferguson, *The Non-Surgical Treatment of Intestinal Stasis and Constipation* (New York: Squibb, 1916); Liquid petrolatum as a laxative. *Journal of the American Medical Association* (1919) 73:1612–1613, p. 1612; Nujol, *American Druggist and Pharmaceutical Record*, December 1916, 9; Hyginol, *American Druggist and Pharmaceutical Record*, December 1915, 6. A particularly impressive example of the zeal with which mineral oil was promoted to the public and the medical profession is the collection of advertisements for Angier's Emulsion, spanning the 1910s through the 1930s. In: Uncatalogued Pamphlets, Library of the College of Physicians of Philadelphia.

26. Liquid Petrolatum (n. 25), 1613; Harold Aaron, *Our Common Ailment. Constipation: Its Cause and Cure* (New York: Dodge, 1938), 118.

27. Walter Bastedo, Clinical experience with liquid paraffin. *Journal of the American Medical Association* (1915) 64:807–808, p. 808; The oil enema. *Journal of the American Medical Association* (1919) 73:1528–1529, p. 1528; Liquid Petrolatum Squibb, *American Druggist*, January 1921, 49; Stemmerman (n. 17), 161–162; Liquid Petrolatum (n. 25), 1613; F. Parkes Weber,

in discussion of Arthur Hurst, The uses and abuses of purgatives. *Transactions of the Medical Society of London* (1939) 62:127–143, p. 141.

28. Élie Metchnikoff, *The Prolongation of Life. Optimistic Studies*, P. Chalmers Mitchell, trans. (New York: Putnam, 1908), 156–157; Adolphe Combe, *Intestinal Auto-Intoxication*, William States, trans. (New York: Rebman, 1910), 396–403; H. Douglas Wilson, Discussion on alimentary toxaemia. *Proceedings of the Royal Society of Medicine* (1913) i:340–344, p. 344 (also see Walter Bastedo, Rambles in the field of gastro-intestinal therapeutics. *New York State Journal of Medicine* (1927) 27:1173–1184, p. 1176); Pancrobilin, Warshaw, box 37, file 20; Reed and Carnrick, *Gland Therapy* (New York: Equity, 1924), 4; Gant (n. 12), 210–213.

29. Edward Muller, Intestinal self-poisoning greatest single case [sic?] of ill-health. *Naturopath and Herald of Health* (1934) 33:59; J. H. Tilden, *Constipation. A New Reading on the Subject* (Denver: Author, 1923), 37; G. R. Clements, Deadly constipation. *Naturopath* (1923) 28:764, 766; Kneipp's Laxative Herbs, *Nature's Path* (1937) 42:241, and *Nature's Path* (1938) 43:121.

30. Eugene Christian, *Why Die?* (New York: Little and Ives, 1928), 263–271; ad for Eugene Christian, *The Naturopath and Herald of Health* (1912) 17:45; George Drews, Apyrotropher section. *The Naturopath and Herald of Health* (1912) 17:819–825; Cameron Woodworth, Raw food delights. *Tacoma Reporter*, August 20, 1998, 5; Arnold Ehret, *Prof. Arnold Ehret's Mucusless-Diet Healing System*, 11th ed. (Beaumont, CA: Author, 1953), 23, 126; Jess Stearn, *Edgar Cayce—The Sleeping Prophet* (New York: Doubleday, 1967). Harold Reilly and Ruth Brod, *The Edgar Cayce Handbook for Health Through Drugless Therapy* (Virginia Beach, VA: ARE Press, 1975), x–xix, 232, 236. Cayce readings can be examined at the Association for Research and Enlightenment in Virginia Beach, Viginia.

31. James Whorton, 'Physiologic optimism': Horace Fletcher and hygienic ideology in progressive America. *Bulletin of the History of Medicine* (1981) 55:59–87; Whorton, *Crusaders for Fitness. The History of American Health Reformers* (Princeton, NJ: Princeton University Press, 1982), 168–200; Harvey Green, *Fit For America. Health, Fitness, Sport, and American Society* (New York: Pantheon, 1986), 294–302.

32. Horace Fletcher, *Fletcherism. What It Is, Or How I Became Young at Sixty* (New York: Stokes, 1913), 5, 121. (Fletcher's analysis of dietetic error residing in the mouth since that is the only area where a person has control of his food was anticipated, incidentally, by the nineteenth-century health reformer Dioclesian Lewis. In: *Our Digestion; or, My Jolly Friend's Secret* (Philadelphia: McLean, 1872), 29–30.)

33. Horace Fletcher, *The New Glutton or Epicure* (New York: Stokes, 1903), 182, 188–190.

34. Fletcher (n. 32), 93–94.

35. Horace Fletcher, *The A.B.-Z. of Our Own Nutrition* (New York: Stokes, 1903), 11; Fletcher, *Happpiness, as Found in Forethought Minus Fearthought* (New York: Stokes, 1898), 187–189; Fletcher (n. 32), 203.

36. Finley Peter Dunne, *The World of Mr. Dooley* (New York: Collier, 1962), 75, 77; William Anderson, Observations on the results of tests for physical endurance at the Yale gymnasium. *New York Medical Journal* (1907) 86:1009–1013; James Crichton Browne, *Parcimony in Nutrition* (London: Funk and Wagnall, 1909), 73; Harold Holck, *Diet and Efficiency* (Chicago: University of Chicago Press, 1929), 70; Horace Fletcher, Possible progressive growth: In

muscular efficiency after fifty years of life without systematic physical exercise. *New York Medical Journal* (1907) 86:1005–1009, p. 1008.

    37. Horace Fletcher, *Menticulture, or the A-B-C of True Living* (Stone: Chicago, 1898).

    38. Whorton, *Crusaders* (n. 31), 191–200; Tim Armstrong, Disciplining the corpus. Henry James and Fletcherism. In: Tim Armstrong, ed., *American Bodies. Cultural Histories of the Physique* (New York: New York University Press, 1996), 101–119; *Punch* (1906) 130:189; Hillel Schwartz, *Never Satisfied. A Cultural History of Diets, Fantasies and Fat* (New York: Free Press, 1986), 126.

    39. The Radical Cure (n. 1), 1–2, 8, 11–13.

    40. The Radical Cure (n. 1), 8, 18.

    41. The Radical Cure (n. 1), 2, 13, 34–36, 49, 58–59.

    42. Correspondence between R. H. Bragdon and E. M. Crump, May and June 1912, AMA, box 113, folder 3; Alcinous Jamison, *Intestinal Ills* (New York: Tyrrell's Hygienic Institute, 1919), 76–77; Victor Pauchet and H. Gaehlinger, *Hygiène du Constipe* (Paris: Doin, 1932), 23; Benko's, *The Naturopath* (1923) 28:145; Nicky, *Herald of Health and Naturopath* (1919) 24:413; Pneumatic Dilator, *Herald of Health and Naturopath* (1918) 23:no page; Macfadden, *Constipation* (n. 11), 80–81, 244; Vestvold, *The Naturopath and Herald of Health* (1935), 191.

    43. Aaron (n. 26), 70–71; Gant (n. 12), 296; J. F. Montague, *I Know Just the Thing for That* (New York: John Day, 1934), 212–213.

CHAPTER 7

The chapter-opening quotations are from The spectator. *Outlook* (1902) 70:612–614, pp. 612–613; and John Harvey Kellogg, *The Itinerary of a Breakfast* (Battle Creek, MI: Modern Medicine, 1918), 25, 71.

    1. Ad for Kellogg's All-Bran, *Physical Culture*, May 1937, 65.

    2. Elmer McCollum, *A History of Nutrition* (Boston: Houghton Mifflin, 1957), 63, 115–156; James Whorton, Eating to win: Popular concepts of diet, strength, and energy in the early twentieth century. In: Kathryn Grover, ed., *Fitness in American Culture. Images of Health, Sport, and the Body, 1830–1940* (Amherst, MA: University of Massachusetts Press, 1989), 86–122.

    3. The facts about proprietary foods. *Hygeia* (1933) 11:682–683, p. 682.

    4. Elmer McCollum, Scientific nutrition and public health. *Hygeia* (1923) 1:233–236, pp. 234–235; Vegetables as life insurance. *Literary Digest*, April 5, 1924, 75–77; "Use More Milk" health poster, *Hygeia* (1924) 2:630; Eugene Christian, *Ten Little Lessons on Vitamins* (Westfield, MA: Vitamin Research Association, 1922), 8; Experiment succeeds in child health work. *New York Times*, September 24, 1927, p. 17. For additional surveys of eating habits and calls for dietary reform, see Lovell Langstroth, Relation of American dietary to degenerative disease. *Journal of the American Medical Association* (1929) 93:1607–1613; and Willard Stone, Dietary facts, fads and fancies. *Journal of the American Medical Association* (1930) 95:709–715; United States Department of Agriculture, *Food and Life* (Washington, DC: U.S. Government Printing Office, 1929), 128–129.

    5. Walter Alvarez, Opinions of 470 physicians in regard to the advantages of using bran and roughage. *Minnesota Medicine* (1931) 14:296–300, p. 300; Rima Apple, *Vitamania. Vitamins in American Culture* (New Brunswick, NJ: Rutgers University Press, 1996); Russell

Wilder, The significance of diet in treatment. *Journal of the American Medical Association* (1931) 97:435–436, p. 435.

6. *Literary Digest*, November 18, 1922, 55; William Stemmerman, *Intestinal Management for Longer, Happier Life* (Asheville, NC: Arden, 1928), 199; Carl Malmberg, *Diet and Die* (New York: Hillman, Curl, 1935), 12–14; Harvey Levenstein, *Revolution at the Table. The Transformation of the American Diet* (New York: Oxford University Press, 1988), 197–198.

7. Florence Brown, Mary Campbell, Neva Stoner and Icie Macey, A study of the therapeutic value of yeast. *Journal of the American Dietetic Association* (1934–5) 10:29–39, pp. 30, 38; John Murlin and Henry Mattill, The laxative action of yeast. *American Journal of Physiology* (1923) 64:75–96; Fleischmann's, *Literary Digest*, February 10, 1923, 67; March 10, 1923, 65; and October 6, 1928, 35.

8. *Literary Digest*, October 20, 1923, 79, 87.

9. *Literary Digest*, February 10, 1923, 71.

10. Olga Metchnikoff, *Life of Élie Metchnikoff* (Boston: Houghton Mifflin, 1921); Edwin Slosson, *Major Prophets of To-day* (Boston: Little, Brown, 1916), 147–189; R. B. Vaughan, The romantic rationalist. A study of Élie Metchnikoff. *Medical History* (1965) 9:201–215; and G. E. Trease, Élie Metchnikoff 1845–1916. *British Journal of Pharmaceutical Practice* (1981) 3:26–27.

11. Élie Metchnikoff, *The Nature of Man. Studies in Optimistic Philosophy*, P. Chalmers Mitchell, trans. (New York: Putnam, 1908), 253, 257.

12. Metchnikoff (n. 11), 69, 285, 300.

13. Metchnikoff (n. 11), 76, 252; Metchnikoff, *The Prolongation of Life. Optimistic Studies*, P. Chalmers Mitchell, trans. (New York: Putnam, 1908) (Metchnikoff also gave credit to alcoholism and syphilis as causes of premature senility).

14. Metchnikoff, *The Prolongation* (n. 13), 151; J. Ellis Barker, *Chronic Constipation, the Most Insidious and the Most Deadly of Diseases* (London: Murray, 1927), 29; autobiography of William Arbuthnot Lane, Wellcome Institute of the History of Medicine; Lane, Chronic intestinal stasis. *Surgery, Gynecology and Obstetrics* (1910) 11:495–500, p. 499.

15. Metchnikoff, *The Prolongation* (n. 13), 255–257.

16. Élie Metchnikoff, The utility of lactic microbes. *The Century Illustrated Monthly Magazine* (1909–10) 79:53–59, pp. 56, 58; Metchnikoff, *The Prolongation* (n. 13), 175.

17. Metchnikoff (n. 11), 262, 287–288, 299–300; Adolphe Combe, *Intestinal Auto-Intoxication*, William States, trans. (New York: Rebman, 1910), 247.

18. Olga Metchnikoff (n. 10), 232, 234; Vaughan (n. 10), 215.

19. Slosson (n. 10), 175; Metchnikoff, *The Prolongation* (n. 13), 178–181; Metchnikoff, The utility (n. 16), 56; Olga Metchnikoff (n. 10), 198.

20. Anstey Guthrie, The cult of the microbe. *Punch* (1908) 134:344–347, p. 344.

21. A. Brown, Some notes on 'Curdled Milk'. *Edinburgh Medical Journal* [n.s.] (1910) 4:49–60, p. 49; A modern elixir of life. *British Medical Journal* (1908) ii:847–849, p. 847; Metchnikoff and buttermilk. *Journal of the American Medical Association* (1916) 67:939; Vaughan Harley. In: discussion of George Herschell, The therapeutical value of the lactic-acid bacillus. *Proceedings of the Royal Society of Medicine*, 1909–10, Part III. Therapeutical and Pharmacological Section, 51–63, p. 57.

22. Combe (n. 17); D. Fraser Harris, Longevity and the milk diet of 'Old Parr'. *Lancet* (1908) ii:1399; Modern elixir (n. 21), 849; Harley (n. 21); Thomas Luke, The use of sour milk in the treatment of constipation. *Practitioner* (1910) 84:653–661, p. 661.

23. P. G. Heinemann and Mary Hefferan, A study of bacillus bulgaricus. *Journal of Infectious Diseases* (1909) 6:304–318; Leo Rettger and Harry Cheplin, *Soured Milk and Pure Cultures of Lactic Acid Bacilli* (New Haven, CT: Yale University Press, 1921), 181; Walter Alvarez, Intestinal autointoxication. *Physiological Reviews* (1924) 4:352–393, p. 372; Intesti-Fermin, AMA, box 115, folder 9; Combe (n. 17), 341–342; George Herschell, *Soured Milk and Pure Cultures of Lactic Acid Bacilli in the Treatment of Disease*, 2nd ed. (London: Glaisher, 1909), 29–41; Metchnikoff and buttermilk (n. 21).

24. Walter Bastedo, Rambles in the field of gastro-intestinal therapeutics. *New York State Journal of Medicine* (1927) 27:1173–1184, pp. 1173–1174; Leo Rettger and Harry Cheplin, *A Treatise on the Transformation of the Intestinal Flora* (New Haven, CT: Yale University Press, 1921), 1–10; Nicholas Kopeloff, *Lactobacillus Acidophilus* (Baltimore: Williams and Wilkins, 1926), 1–32, 39; ads for acidophilus products were prolific in both popular and pharmaceutical publications—for examples, see issues of *American Druggist*, December 1926, 8, and March 1931, 64; Lederle Bacillus Acidophilus Milk, *Hygeia* (November 1927) 5:38; Yog-a-Lax, *Nature's Path* (1942) 47:36; Insta'ghurt, *Nature's Path* (1947) 51:434.

25. Bastedo (n. 24), 1174.

26. Post's Bran Flakes, *Literary* Digest, March 31, 1928, 57; Alexander Walker, The effect of recent changes of food habits on bowel motility. *South African Medical Journal* (1947) 21:590–596, p. 591; Richard Cummings, *The American and His Food. A History of Food Habits in the United States*, 2nd ed. (Chicago: University of Chicago Press, 1941), 111–121; Robert Hutchison, *Food and the Principles of Dietetics*, 3rd ed. (New York: Wood, 1911), 560; Leonard Williams, *The Science and Art of Living* (London: Hodder and Stoughton, 1924), 210.

27. The national mania. *Hygeia* (1924) 2:53–54; Morris Fishbein, *Your Diet and Your Health* (New York: Whittlesey House, 1937), 36; F. C. M., Bran lemonade. *Hygeia* (1927) 5:269; Postum Cereal Company, *The Road to Wellville* (Battle Creek, MI: Postum Cereal Company, 1926), 43; Diet-minded laymen. *Journal of the American Dietetic Association* (1929–30) 5:49–51, p. 50.

28. Richard Schwarz, *John Harvey Kellogg, M.D.* (Nashville: Southern Pubblishing, 1970); James Whorton, *Crusaders For Fitness. The History of American Health Reformers* (Princeton, NJ: Princeton University Press, 1982), 201–238; Irving Fisher, *My Father, Irving Fisher* (New York: Comet, 1956), 109.

29. John Kellogg, Should the colon be sacrificed or may it be reformed? *Journal of the American Medical Association* (1917) 68:1957–1959, p. 1958; Kellogg, *Colon Hygiene*, 4th ed. (Battle Creek, MI: Good Health Publishing, 1917), 370–390; Kellogg, *The Itinerary of a Breakfast* (Battle Creek, MI: Modern Medicine Publishing, 1918), 87, 93, 99; Kellogg, *Plain Facts for Young and Old* (Burlington, IA: Segner and Condit, 1881), 202; Kellogg, *Ladies' Guide in Health and Disease* (Des Moines: Condit, 1884), 164.

30. Kellogg, *Colon Hygiene* (n. 29), 48, 123, 359; Kellogg, The crippled colon. How to help it. *Good Health* (1938) 73:294–295; Kellogg, *The Itinerary* (n. 29), 71, 90–91.

31. Kellogg, *The Itinerary* (n. 29), 33–35, 115; Kellogg, *Autointoxication; or, Intestinal Toxemia* (Battle Creek, MI: Modern Medicine Publishing, 1919), 95, 266.

32. Kellogg, *Autointoxication* (n. 31), 96, 271–272.

33. Kellogg, Should the colon be sacrificed? (n. 29), 1957–1958.

34. Kellogg, *Autointoxication* (n. 31), 254, 310; Kellogg, *The Itinerary* (n. 29), 143, 155, 163; Kellogg, *Colon Hygiene* (n. 29), 115, 123.

35. Kellogg, *Rational Hydrotherapy*, 2nd ed. (Philadelphia: Davis, 1902); Kellogg, *Colon Hygiene* (n. 29), 241–257, 272–290.

36. R. Tait McKenzie, *Exercise in Education and Medicine*, 3rd ed. (Philadelphia: Saunders, 1923), 353–354; Whorton (n. 28), 205; Kellogg, *The Itinerary* (n. 29), 88–89; Kellogg, Some diet fads and their dangers. *Literary Digest*, October 15, 1927, 70–72, p. 72; Kellogg, *Colon Hygiene* (n. 29), 89. Kellogg was not alone in blaming Fletcher's death on autointoxication. Metchnikoff did as well, charging that bradyfagy, as he (and some physicians) called the slow consumption of food, promoted extreme intestinal putrefaction, and resulted in a short duration of life (Fletcher died in 1919, at an even three score and ten; Metchnikoff lived to 71). See Metchnikoff, *The Prolongation* (n. 13), 159–160. Also see R. L. Alsaker, Was Horace Fletcher wrong? *Physical Culture*, June 1920, 40, 76.

37. Kellogg, *Autointoxication* (n. 31), 307–311.

38. Kellogg, Should the colon (n. 29), 1957; Kellogg, *Colon Hygiene* (n. 29), 85; Kellogg, *The Itinerary* (n. 29), 134–135, 163.

39. Leonard Williams, The spa treatment of chronic constipation. *Practitioner* (1910) 84:662–670, p. 662; Kellogg, *Colon Hygiene* (n. 29), 231–240; Kellogg, *The Itinerary* (n. 29), 105; Healthful living, 25–26, Warshaw, cereal collection, box 1, file 5.

40. Gerald Carson, *Cornflake Crusade* (New York: Rinehart, 1957), 93–210; Healthful Living (n. 39), 15.

41. Carson (n. 40), 146.

42. Quaker Oats, *Collier's Weekly*, April 7, 1906, 32; Shredded Wheat, *Collier's Weekly*, May 26, 1906, 32.

43. George Williams, A study of the laxative action of wheat bran. *American Journal of Physiology* (1927) 83:1–14, p. 1; All-Bran, Warshaw, cereal collection, box 1, file 20; Healthful living (n. 39), 8; A new way of life, Warshaw, cereal collection, box 1, file 22; Mealene, *Nature's Path* (1944) 48:427; Bran-O-Lax, AMA, box 113, folder 4; Harvey Levenstein, *Revolution at the Table. The Transformation of the American Diet* (New York: Oxford University Press, 1988), 189.

44. Fleischmann's Yeast, *Literary Digest*, July 8, 1922, 57.

45. Post's Bran Flakes, *Hygeia* (1931) 9:1078; The national mania (n. 27), 54.

46. Pillsbury Health Bran, *Literary Digest*, February 16, 1924, 52; Post Bran Flakes ads, *Saturday Evening Post*, July 3, 1926, 32, and November 6, 1926, 42.

47. Kellogg's All-Bran ads, n. 24 and *Saturday Evening Post*, October 9, 1926, 46.

48. Post Bran Flakes ads in *Hygeia* (February 1926) 4:15; (November 1926) 4:17; and (1932) 10:1152.

49. John Harvey Kellogg, Laxatives shorten body length as well as life length. *Good Health* (January 1939) 74:18; Pettijohn's Bran and Kellogg's All-Bran ads *Hygeia* (1931) 9:390, 592; LAXA Biscuits and Lacto-Dextrin ads, *Literary Digest*, January 12, 1929, 61 and April 6, 1929, 88; Charles LaWall, So psyllium is a new drug! *American Druggist*, June 1929, 107; ad for Paraffin Tablets, Kremers, C39 (k); KABA, *Good Health* (February 1934) 69:28–29; ads

for LD-LAX in *Good Health* (April 1940) 75:34; *Good Health* (June 1942) 77:87; *Good Health* (June 1951) 86:144.

50. Postum Cereal Company (n. 27), 41–42; Eating for efficiency, KRF, C 39(k); The simple life, KRF, C 39(k); Healthful living (n. 39), 43.

51. Malmberg (n. 6), 10; Luther Gulick, *The Efficient Life* (New York: Doubleday, Page, 1907), 50; R. Tait McKenzie, The quest for El Dorado. *American Physical Education Review* (1913) 18:295–303, p. 303; Whorton (n. 28), 166–167.

52. Fleischmann's Yeast, *Literary Digest*, June 9, 1923, 55.

CHAPTER 8

The chapter-opening quotations are from J. Ellis Barker, *Cancer. How it is Caused; How it Can be Prevented* (New York: Dutton, 1924), 220–221, 295, 427; and Arbuthnot Lane, *The Prevention of the Diseases Peculiar to Civilization* (London: Faber and Faber, 1929), 65.

1. Alfred Jordan, Stasis the destroyer. *Medical Journal and Record* (1925) 22:328–330, p. 330.

2. Jordan (n. 1), 330.

3. Autobiography of William Arbuthnot Lane, Wellcome Institute for the History of Medicine.

4. Lane (n. 3).

5. New health news. *New Health* (January 1928) 3:55; Lane (n. 3); *Harrogate Advertiser*, January 28, 1928, 3, 10; New health news. (July 1927) 2:32; *New Health* (August 1927) 2:35.

6. Are Waerland. In: *the Cauldron of Disease* (London: Nutt, 1934), 193; A school of dietetics. *New Health* (November 1932) 7:18–19.

7. Thomas Partington, Noise and inefficiency. *New Health* (February 1927) 2:24; W. Arbuthnot Lane, British spas. *New Health* (May 1932) 7:32–33; Lane, *New Health for Everyman* (London: Bles, 1932), 146–163, 177; Lane, pamphlets for Defence of Rights and Amusements Force, Wellcome Institute of the History of Medicine; Lane, *Blazing the Health Trail* (London: Faber and Faber, 1929), 53; *New Health* (November 1937) 12:7; *New Health* (January 1929) 4:54.

8. W. Arbuthnot Lane, The New Health Society. *New Health Society Bulletin* (January 1926) 1:5; Lane, *Blazing the Health Trail* (n. 7), 74.

9. Postum Cereal Company, The Road to Wellville (Battle Creek, MI: Postum Cereal Company, 1926), 49.

10. W. Arbuthnot Lane, Introduction. In: R. H. A. Plimmer and Violet Plimmer, *Vitamins: What We Should Eat and Why* (London: People's League of Health, 1924), 3–4, p. 3; Lane, *An Apple a Day* (London: Methuen, 1935), 89; Lane, *Every Woman's Book of Health and Beauty* (London: Thornton Butterworth, 1936), 28; Lane, *Blazing the Health Trail* (n. 7), 32. The phrase white man's burden to describe intestinal stasis was used by at least two writers in the 1920s and '30s. See J. Ellis Barker, More light upon cancer. *New Health* (May 1927) 2:56–60, p. 58; and F. A. Hornibrook, *The Culture of the Abdomen. The Cure of Obesity and Constipation* (Garden City, NY: Doubleday, Doran, 1934), 8.

11. Robert McCarrison, *The Work of Sir Robert McCarrison*, H. M. Sinclair, ed. (London: Faber and Faber, 1953); McCarrison, An address on faulty food in relation to gastrointestinal disorder. *Lancet* (1922) i:207–212, pp. 207–208.

12. McCarrison, *The Work of Sir Robert McCarrison* (n. 11), 279–281, 285–288; W. Arbuthnot Lane, *New Health for Everyman* (n. 7), 78–96.

13. Lane, *New Health for Everyman* (n. 7), 103–112; M. Cameron Blair, Freedom of Negro races from cancer. *British Medical Journal* (1923) ii:130–131; James Patterson, *The Dread Disease. Cancer and Modern Amerian Culture* (Cambridge, MA: Harvard University Press, 1987), 78–81; Frederick Hoffman, *The Mortality From Cancer Throughout the World* (Newark, NJ: Prudential Press, 1915), 146–147.

14. Lane, *The Prevention of the Diseases Peculiar to Civilization* (London: Faber and Faber, 1929), 55; Alfred Jordan, Stasis and the prevention of cancer. *British Medical Journal* (1920) ii:959–962; Leonard Williams, *Middle Age and Old Age* (London: Oxford University Press, 1925), 182–183; J. Ellis Barker, *Cancer. How it is Caused; How it Can be Prevented* (New York: Dutton, 1924).

15. Ernest Tipper, *The Cradle of the World and Cancer; A Disease of Civilization* (London: Murray, 1927), 10, 53, 137.

16. John Cope, *Cancer: Civilization: Degeneration*, (London: Lewis, 1932), 26, 116–117, 229.

17. Barker (n. 14), 180; review of Barker, *Journal of the American Medical Association* (1924) 83:785; Albert Ochsner, Cancer infection. *Surgery, Gynecology and Obstetrics* (1925) 40:336–342, 336; Thomas Horder, Diet and dietists. *The Lancet* (1927) ii:103–107, 106; Patterson (n. 13), 104.

18. Lane, *New Health for Everyman* (n. 7), 97–100; Cancer: The great darkness. *Fortune*, March 1937, 112–114, 162–179.

19. Lane, *Blazing the Health Trail* (n. 7), vii (Lane did not abandon intestinal kinking altogether, but it played a considerably less important role in his overall scheme; see *The Prevention of the Diseases Peculiar to Civilization* (n. 14), 75–76); Victor Pauchet and H. Gaehlinger, *Hygiène du Constipe* (Paris: Doin, 1932), 5; Hornibrook (n. 10), 75–76; Thomas Layton, *Sir William Arbuthnot Lane, Bt. An Enquiry into the Mind and Influence of a Surgeon* (London: Livingston, 1956), 102–103; Hygienic Lavatory Foot Rest ad, *New Health* (March 1929) 4:85; James Sawyer, *Coprostasis: Its Causes, Prevention and Treatment* (Birmingham, England: Cornish, 1912), 18. Also see William Stemmerman, *Intestinal Management for Longer, Happier Life* (Asheville, NC: Arden, 1928), 51–57.

20. Lane, *Every Woman's Book* (n. 10), 32–33; Lane, *Blazing the Health Trail* (n. 7), 73; Leonard Williams, *The Science and Art of Living* (London: Hodder and Stoughton, 1924), 88; Notes on books. *British Medical Journal* (1927) ii:791–792.

21. Leonard Williams, *Minor Maladies and Their Treatment* (New York: Wood, 1906), 102–103; Williams, The medical aspect of intestinal stasis. In: W. Arbuthnot Lane, *The Operative Treatment of Chronic intestinal stasis*, 4th ed. (London: Frowde, Hodder, and Stoughton, 1918), 250–263, p. 251.

22. Williams, *Minor Maladies* (n. 21), 102–103; Lane, *Every Woman's Book* (n. 10), 65–7; Lane, Physical training in our public schools. *New Health* (May 1927) 2:9–10, p. 9.

23. Michael O'Donnell, quoted by Lynn Payer, *Medicine and Culture* (New York: Holt, 1988), 118; Arbuthnot Lane, *The Prevention of the Diseases Peculiar to Civilization* (n. 14), 64, 93; Williams, *Minor Maladies* (n. 21), 103; Williams (n. 20), 90.

24. Lane, *New Health for Everyman* (n. 7), 113, 127; Lane, Talks to children. *New Health* (January 1929) 4:42; Lane, A visit to Allinson's. *New Health* (April 1928) 3:53; Lane, Presi-

dential address. *New Health* (February 1927) 2:35; Lane quoted in Against white bread. *Journal of the American Medical Association* (1924) 83:1179; A. Rendle Short, The causation of appendicitis. *British Journal of Surgery* (1920–1) 8:171–188, pp. 184, 187–188.

25. Barker, *Cancer* (n. 14), 316; McCarrison, An address on faulty food (n. 11), 208.

26. Lane, *New Health for Everyman* (n. 7), 120.

27. Arbuthnot Lane, *Blazing the Health Trail* (n. 7), 16–18; *New Health* (April 1927) 2:10; J. W. Scott, The Homecroft scheme of new health housing. *New Health* (March 1927) 2:21–24; *New Health* (April 1928) 3:29–31; Mark Weatherall, Bread and newspapers: The making of 'a revolution in the science of food'. *Clio Medica* (1995) 32:179–212.

28. Horder (n. 17), 106–107; Gladys Hartwell, Thomas Horder, S. G. Moore, V. H. Mottram, H. E. Roaf and T. B. Wood, Diet and dietists. *The Lancet* (1927) ii:201.

29. Millers' questionnaire on white flour. *Journal of the American Medical Association* (1927) 88:938; The bread controversy. *Journal of the American Medical Association* (1927) 88:1334; Brown versus white bread. *Journal of the American Medical Association* (1927) 89:893; Medical news. *British Medical Journal* (1927) i:267.

30. Morris Fishbein, *The New Medical Follies* (New York: Boni and Liveright, 1927), 132; Studies on cancer and diet. *Hygeia* (1927) 5:99; Alfred McCann, *The Science of Eating*, 2nd ed. (New York: Doran, 1919), vi, 162.

31. McCann (n. 30), 19, 24, 111–113, 118, 291; McCann, *Starving America* (New York: Doran, 1913), 65.

32. McCann nips another plot. *Journal of the American Medical Association* (1925) 84:1922; Prof. Paul C. Bragg. *Journal of the American Medical Association* (1931) 96:288–289; Paul Bragg, *Golden Keys to Internal Physical Fitness* (Desert Hot Springs, CA: Health Science, 1975).

33. Morris Fishbein (n. 30), 133; David Lewis, *The Public Image of Henry Ford. An American Folk Hero and His Company* (Detroit: Wayne State University Press, 1976), 229, 406.

34. James Whorton, Eating to win: Popular concepts of diet, strength, and energy in the early twentieth century. In: Kathryn Grover, ed., *Fitness in American Culture. Images of Health, Sport, and the Body, 1830–1940* (Amherst, MA: University of Massachusetts Press, 1989), 86–122; Walter Alvarez, The mechanics of digestion. *Journal of the American Dietetic Association* (1929–30) 5:180–183, p. 182.

35. Carl Malmberg, *Diet and Die* (New York: Hillman, Curl:, 1935), xx, 10; F. J. Schlink, *Eat, Drink and Be Wary* (New York: Covici, Friede, 1935), 56; T. Swann Harding, Spinach— for others. *North American Review*, November 1928, 557–565, p. 559; The wonders of diet. *Fortune*, May 1936, 86–91, p. 88. Also see Margaret Barnet, 'Every man his own physician': Dietetic fads, 1890–1914. *Clio Medica* (1995) 32:155–178.

36. Too much acid. *Journal of the American Dietetic Association* (1933–4) 9:498–502, p. 499; Kenneth Roberts, An inquiry into diets. *Saturday Evening Post*, October 15, 1932, 14–15, 75–78, p. 15; Keith Sward, *The Legend of Henry Ford* (New York: Rinehart, 1948), 108–109; Ionite ad, *New Health* (February 1928) 3:60; AMA, box 768, folder 13; Science and Sal Hepatica. *Journal of the American Medical Association* (1940) 114:1082–1083, p. 1082; Sal Hepatica—Not acceptable for A.D.R. *Journal of the American Dental Association* (1935) 22:854–856, 854; Whorton (n. 34), 114–117.

37. Roberts (n. 36), 15; Against white bread. *Journal of the American Medical Association* (1925) 84:688.

38. Whole grain wheat. *Journal of the American Medical Association* (1924) 83:1788; Whole grain wheat. *Journal of the American Medical Association* (1925) 84:1441–1443; Berhalter's booklet, Warshaw, cereal collection, box 1, file 7.

39. Thomas Hunt, Dr. Allinson and the wholemeal loaf. *World Medicine*, March 24, 1976, 58–59; the cited Allinson ads are in several issues of *New Health* (April 1927) 2:53; (May 1927) 2:48; (July 1927) 2:37; (April 1928) 3:53; (August 1930) 5:47; (May 1932) 7:43; (March 1935) 10:47.

40. All-Bran booklet, A New Way of Living, Warshaw, cereal collection, box 1, file 22; Grape Nuts, *New Health* (May 1932) 7:4; Colonator, *New Health* (April 1934) 9:37; Fleischmann, *Literary Digest*, June 10, 1922, 67; Post Bran Flakes, *Ladies' Home Journal*, August 1931 (I am indebted to Dale Smith for calling this advertisement to my attention).

41. W. Arbuthnot Lane, *Every Woman's Book* (n. 10), 128; F. D. Saner, Some impressions of Lane. *Guy's Hospital Gazette* (1956) 70:227–229, p. 227; personal communication from Barbara Clarkson; W. Arbuthnot Lane, Chronic constipation and self-poisoning—A sword of Damocles. *Heal Thyself* (1941) 76:49–51; Lane, The paramount importance of effective intestinal drainage in preventing ill health and disease. *American Medicine* [n.s.] (1926) 21:689–693, p. 692; Robert McCarrison, Food and physical efficiency. *New Health* (Autumn 1956) 31:8–14, p. 9; C. M. Kohan, Centenary. *New Health* (1956) 31:2.

CHAPTER 9

The chapter-opening quotation is from George Dupain, quoted by Frederick Hoffman, *Cancer and Diet* (Baltimore: Williams and Wilkins, 1937), 507.

1. J. Ellis Barker, *Cancer. How it is Caused; How it Can be Prevented* (New York: Dutton, 1924), 416–418.

2. Barker (n. 1), 418–422.

3. Barker (n. 1), 421.

4. 'Rough Stuff'—In the diet. *Good Health* (January 1925) 60:16. For examples of criticism of bran as irritating see James Gully, *The Water-Cure in Chronic Disease* (New York: Wiley and Putnam:, 1847), 260; and Arthur Hurst, *Constipation and Allied Intestinal Disorders*, 2nd ed. (London: Frowde, 1921), 335.

5. Walter Alvarez, Opinions of 470 physicians in regard to the advantages of using bran and roughage. *Minnesota Medicine* (1931) 14:296–300, p. 298; Alvarez, quoted by T. Swann Harding, Diet and common-sense. *Journal of the American Dietetic Association* (1930–1) 6:193–208, pp. 196–197.

6. Alvarez, Opinions (n. 5), 296–298; Walter Bastedo, Rambles in the field of gastro-intestinal therapeutics. *New York State Journal of Medicine* (1927) 27:1173–1184, p. 1177; Morris Fishbein, *Your Diet and Your Health* (New York: Whittlesey House, 1937), 34–37; J. F. Montague, *How to Overcome Nervous and Other Forms of Constipation*, 2nd ed. (Chicago: Nelson-Hall, 1956), 109–110; Murray Davis, Intestinal obstruction from eating bran. *Journal of the American Medical Association* (1931) 97:24–25; J. F. Montague, *I Know Just the Thing for That* (New York: John Day, 1934), 32.

7. The nutritional significance of bran. *Journal of the American Medical Association* (1936) 107:874–877, p. 877; R. A. McCance and E. M. Widdowson, *Breads White and Brown. Their*

Place in Thought and Social History (London: Pittman, 1956), 85–119; Hugh Trowell, Denis Burkitt, and Kenneth Heaton, eds., *Dietary Fibre, Fibre-Depleted Foods and Disease* (London: Academic Press, 1985), 4; The national loaf. *British Medical Journal* (1942) i:393; E. M. Dimock, The prevention of constipation. *British Medical Journal* (1937) i:906–909, p. 907; A visit to a Hovis factory. *New Health*, October 1927, 73–74, p. 74; ad for Heinz Rice Flakes, *Hygeia* (1930) 8:673; Robert Jackson, *How to Keep Well*, pamphlet, Warshaw, box 2, file "miscellaneous publications."

8.   Use and abuse of cathartics. *Journal of the American Medical Association* (1919) 73:1768–1769, p. 1768 (also see Arbuthnot Lane, *New Health for Everyman* (London: Bles, 1932), 129; George Everett, *Health Fragments or, Steps Toward a True Life* (New York: Somerby, 1875), 89; Erwin Nelson, The treatment of constipation. *International Medical Digest* (1943) 42:308–310; Mary Rose, Grace MacLeod, Ella Vahlteich, Esther Funnell and Catherine Newton, The influence of bran on the alimentary tract. *Journal of the American Dietetic Association* (1932–3) 8:133–156, p. 137; Victor Levine, Should whole wheat products displace the refined products? *Archives of Pediatrics* (1929) 46:281–296, p. 285.

9.   George Cowgill and William Anderson, Laxative effects of wheat bran and 'washed bran' in healthy men. *Journal of the American Medical Association* (1932) 98:1866–1875; Rose (n. 8).

10.   E. M. Dimock (n. 7); Alexander Walker, The effect of recent changes of food habits on bowel motility. *South African Medical Journal* (1947) 21:590–596, pp. 591, 594.

11.   T. L. Cleave, *The Saccharine Disease* (Bristol, England: Wright, 1974), 38–39; Cleave, Danger of purgatives. *British Medical Journal* (1962) i:191; Sylvester Graham, *Lectures on the Science of Human Life* (Boston: Marsh, Capen, Lyon, and Webb, 1839), Vol. 2, 435.

12.   F. Parkes Weber, Prepared bran in the prevention of constipation. *British Medical Journal* (1941) i:252–253; M. E. Lampard, Bran in the prevention of constipation. *British Medical Journal* (1941) i:390; T. L. Cleave, Natural bran in the treatment of constipation. *British Medical Journal* (1941) i:461.

13.   T. L. Cleave, The neglect of natural principles in current medical practice. *Journal of the Royal Naval Medical Service* (1956) 42:55–83, pp. 55, 69–70.

14.   Cleave (n. 13), 58, 63, 64.

15.   Cleave (n. 13), 69, 72.

16.   T. L. Cleave, *Fat Consumption and Coronary Disease* (Bristol, England: Wright, 1957); Cleave, *On the Causation of Varicose Veins* (Bristol, England: Wright, 1960); Cleave, *Peptic Ulcer. A New Approach to its Causation, Prevention, and Arrest, Based on Human Evolution* (Bristol, England: Wright 1962), 126–129; T. L. Cleave and G. D. Campbell, *Diabetes, Coronary Thrombosis, and the Saccharine Disease* (Bristol, England: Wright, 1966); Brian Kellock, *The Fiber Man. The Life Story of Dr. Denis Burkitt* (Belleville, MI: Lion, 1985), 126.

17.   Cleave and Campbell (n. 16), iv.

18.   Cleave and Campbell (n. 16), 35–38, 75; Arbuthnot Lane, *The New Health Guide*, (London: Bles, 1935), 16; T. L. Cleave, *The Saccharine Disease* (Bristol, England: Wright, 1974), 185–186; Montague (n. 6), 130.

19.   Cleave and Campbell (n. 16), 6, 8, 75–76, 126, 137–138; Cleave, *Peptic Ulcer* (n. 16), 128; Cleave, *The Saccharine Disease* (n. 18), 40.

20. Derrick Dunlop, The saccharine disease. *British Medical Journal* (1966) ii:163; Cleave, *The Saccharine Disease* (n. 18), 185; Denis Burkitt, *Journal of the Royal Naval Medical Service* (1984) 70:51–52; Kenneth Vickery, *Journal of the Royal Naval Medical Service* (1984) 70:52; personal communication, Denis Burkitt.

21. G. J. Milton-Thompson, *Journal of the Royal Naval Medical Service* (1984) 70:51; Burkitt (n. 20), 51; Denis Burkitt, *Don't Forget Fiber in Your Diet*, 2nd ed. (New York: Arco, 1984), 44; News and notes. *British Medical Journal* (1978) i:54. A good outline of the development of the dietary fiber hypothesis, though a journalistic account, is Lawrence Galton, *The Truth About Fiber in Your Diet* (New York: Crown, 1976).

22. Personal communication, Denis Burkitt; Denis Burkitt. *The Times* (London), March 27, 1993, 17; Letter, *British Medical Journal* (1972) ii:645.

23. Bernard Glemser, *Mr. Burkitt and Africa* (New York: World, 1970); Kellock (n. 16); Denis Burkitt and D. H. Wright, *Burkitt's Lymphoma* (Edinburgh: Livingstone, 1970); Kenneth Heaton, Denis Burkitt. *The Lancet* (1993) 342:951–952, p. 951.

24. Personal communication, Denis Burkitt; Burkitt, Related disease—Related cause. *The Lancet* (1969) ii:1229–1231.

25. Burkitt, *Don't Forget Fiber* (n. 21), 24; Burkitt, Related disease—Related cause (n. 24).

26. Burkitt, Related disease—Related cause (n. 24).

27. Denis Burkitt, Relationship as a clue to causation. *The Lancet* (1970) ii:1237–1240; Burkitt, Some diseases characteristic of modern Western civilization. *British Medical Journal* (1973) i:274–278, p. 275.

28. Denis Burkitt, Alexander Walker, and N. S. Painter, Effect of dietary fibre on stools. *The Lancet* (1972) ii:1408–1412, p. 1408; Burkitt, Possible relationships between bowel cancer and dietary habits. *Proceedings of the Royal Society of Medicine* (1971) 64:964–965; E. M. Dimock, The Treatment of Habitual Constipation by the Bran Method. MD Thesis, University of Cambridge, 1936 (I have been unable to locate this thesis at Cambridge, but it is discussed in Galton, n. 21, p. 27); Walker, The effect (n. 10), 595; Walker, Diet, bowel motility, faeces composition and colonic cancer. *South African Medical Journal* (1971) 45:377–379, p. 378; Walker, Plumbing and bowel habit. *The Lancet* (1975) ii:456.

29. Personal communication, Denis Burkitt; Burkitt, Walker, and Painter (n. 28); M. M. Schuster. In: Richard Reilly and Joseph Kirshner, eds., *Fiber Deficiency and Colonic Disorders* (New York: Plenum, 1975), 85.

30. Personal communication, Denis Burkitt; Kellock (n. 16), 183–184.

31. Burkitt, Possible relationships (n. 28); Burkitt, Epidemiology of cancer of the colon and rectum. *Cancer* (1971) 28:3–13; Burkitt, Large-bowel cancer: An epidemiologic jigsaw puzzle. *Journal of the National Cancer Institute* (1975) 54:3–6, p. 4.

32. Burkitt, Epidemiology (n. 31), 7, 11.

33. Denis Burkitt and Hugh Trowell, eds., *Refined Carbohydrate Foods and Disease. Some Implications of Dietary Fibre* (London: Academic Press, 1975), 153–154, 189; personal communication, Denis Burkitt.

34. Walker, Diet (n. 28); Walker and Denis Burkitt, Colon cancer: Epidemiology. *Seminars in Oncology* (1976) 3:341–350; Walker and Burkitt, Colonic cancer—Hypotheses of causation, dietary prophylaxis, and future research. *American Journal of Digestive Diseases*

(1976) 21:910–917; Trowell et al., *Dietary Fibre* (n. 7), 13; Trowell, *Non-Infective Disease in Africa* (London: Arnold, 1960), 217–222.

35. Personal communication, Denis Burkitt; Denis Burkitt and Hugh Trowell, eds., *Western Diseases: Their Emergence and Prevention* (Cambridge, MA: Harvard University Press, 1981), xiv, 427.

36. Burkitt and Trowell (n. 33), vii–viii, 343; Burkitt, *Don't Forget* (n. 25), 49–84.

37. Cleave, *Diabetes* (n. 16), 106–110; Burkitt, *Don't Forget Fiber* (n. 21), 67, 72.

38. Personal communications, Denis Burkitt, Albert Jonsen; Michael O'Donnell, One man's burden. *British Medical Journal* (1983) 287:368; Heaton, Denis Burkitt (n. 23), 952; Alex Shulman, For health, don't go against the grain. *Los Angeles Times*, August 27, 1972, H8; David Kritchevsky, Charles Bonfield, and James Anderson, eds., *Dietary Fiber. Chemistry, Physiology, and Health Effects* (New York: Plenum, 1990); Gene Spiller, ed., *CRC Handbook of Dietary Fiber in Human Nutrition* (Boca Raton, FL: CRC Press, 1986), preface (no pagination).

39. O'Donnell (n. 38); Heaton, Denis Burkitt (n. 23), 952.

CHAPTER 10

The chapter-opening quotations are from J. F. Montague, *How to Overcome Nervous and Other Forms of Constipation*, 2nd ed. (Chicago: Nelson-Hall, 1956), 15; and Bernard Jensen and Sylvia Bell, *Tissue Cleansing Through Bowel Management* (Escondido, CA: Author, 1981), 3.

1. Nicholas LaRusso and Douglas McGill, Surreptitious laxative ingestion. Delayed recognition of a serious condition: A case report. *Mayo Clinic Proceedings* (1975) 50:706–708, pp. 706–707.

2. LaRusso and McGill (n. 1), 707.

3. F. Avery Jones, J. W. P. Gummer, and J. E. Lennard-Jones, *Clinical Gastroenterology*, 2nd ed. (Oxford: Blackwell Scientific Publications, 1968), 49, 57; Dangers of purgatives. *British Medical Journal* (1961) ii:1694–1695, p. 1694; John Cummings, Laxative abuse. *Gut* (1974) 15:758–766; Gail Sekas, The use and abuse of laxatives. *Practical Gastroenterology* (1987) 11:33–39; LaRusso and McGill (n. 1), 707.

4. Value judgment: The straight poop on laxatives. *Moneysworth*, August 9, 1971, in AMA, box 113, folder 4; J. F. Montague, *How to Overcome Nervous and Other Forms of Constipation*, 2nd ed. (Chicago: Nelson-Hall, 1956), 25; Purgatives and the colon. *British Medical Journal* (1968) 3:74.

5. Melva Weber, Laxatives: Overused and undersafe. *Vogue* (June 1975), 60; Leslie Wright, *Bowel Function in Hospital Patients*, The Study of Nursing Care Project Reports, No. 4 (London: Royal College of Nursing, 1974), 27–28; J. T. Boyd and R. Doll, Gastrointestinal cancer and the use of liquid paraffin. *British Journal of Cancer* (1954) 8:231–237, p. 232; R. D. G. Creery, Magnesia and alkaline carminatives in infancy. *British Medical Journal* (1955) ii:178–179; Austin Smith, *The Drugs We Use* (New York: Revere, 1948), 68; Teething powders. *British Medical Journal* (1954) ii:265; J. J. A. Reid, Regular use of laxatives by schoolchildren. *British Medical Journal* (1956) ii:25–27, p. 26; The treatment of constipation. *The Lancet* (1962) i:1010–1011, p. 1010; Horace Davenport, *Physiology of the Digestive Tract*, 3rd ed. (Chicago: Year Book Medical Publishers, 1971), 216; Denis Burkitt, *Don't Forget Fibre in Your Diet*, 2nd ed. (New York: Arco, 1984), 42–44; Bill Rados and Harold Hopkins, Laxa-

tives overused in the quest for regularity. *FDA Consumer*, May 1985, 12–15; Sheryl Stolberg, FDA statement prompts Ex-Lax to pull products from the shelves. *Tacoma News Tribune*, August 30, 1997, A1, 49.

6. T. L. Hardy, Order and disorder in the large intestine. *The Lancet* (1945) i:519–524, 553–559, p. 523; J. Ned Smith and Kyo Lee, *Essentials of Gastroenterology* (St. Louis: Mosby, 1969) (also see Jones et al., n. 3, 47); Investigating constipation. *British Medical Journal* (1980) 280:669–670, p. 669; Marvin Shuster, What is constipation. (Washington, DC: National Institutes of Health Publication #86–2754, 1986) (also see Robert Pietrusko, Use and abuse of laxatives. *American Journal of Hospital Pharmacy* (1977) 34:291–300, p. 291).

7. William Glafke, Treat your colon kindly. *Readers Digest*, October 1949, 64; The Advertising Association, Advertising of laxatives. London, 1962; Smith (n. 5), 169; James Harvey Young, *The Medical Messiahs. A Social History of Health Quackery in Twentieth-Century America* (Princeton, NJ: Princeton University Press, 1967), 151.

8. Nature's remedy. *Life*, March 6, 1950, 108; Dr. Edward's Olive Tablets. *Collier's*, February 10, 1951, 71; Feen-a-mint, *Collier's*, March 17, 1952, 80; Carter's, *Collier's*, February 17, 1951, 62; Serutan, *Life*, March 5, 1951, 134; Adolphe Abrahams, Chronic constipation. *The Practitioner* (1953) 170:266–272, p. 268; Rados and Hopkins (n. 5), 12.

9. Charles Beek, Laxatives: What does regular mean? *FDA Consumer*, May 1975, 16–21, pp. 16, 19; Ex-Lax, *Good Housekeeping*, August 1984, 72; Rados and Hopkins (n. 5), 12.

10. Catalog for Your Health Inc., Puyallup, WA, 1996, p. 6; pamphlet from The Herbalist, Seattle, early 1990s; Bernard Jensen and Sylvia Bell, *Tissue Cleansing Through Bowel Management* (Escondido, CA: Author, 1981) (this volume is a prime example of New Age detoxification theory, indiscriminately mixing together diet, enema treatments, iridology, and other elements of hygiene and medicine).

11. James Thomson, *Constipation and Our Civilisation* (Lewes, England: Lewes Press, 1944), 153; Charles Hunt, Constipation! Auto intoxication! Self poisoning! *Nature's Path* (1937) 42:290, 303; R. A. Riggs, Constipation. Civilization's curse. *Nature's Path* (1946) 50:632, 658–660; Alice Everett, Constipation. The greatest menace to beauty. *Nature's Path* (1940) 45:124, 135–137; Patrick Lackey, Eliminate constipation for all time. *Nature's Path* (1940) 45:46–48; Edwin Ross, Constipation. *Nature's Path* (1944) 48:48, 55.

12. Patrick Donovan, Bowel toxemia, permeability and disease: New information to suppport an old concept. In: Joseph Pizzorno and Michael Murray, eds., *A Textbook of Natural Medicine* (Seattle: Bastyr University Publications, 1993), Vol. 1, no pagination.

13. Jack LaLanne, *The Jack LaLanne Way to Vibrant Good Health* (Englewood Cliffs, NJ: Prentice Hall:, 1960), 80–81, 184; Personalities this month. Paul C. Bragg. *Nature's Path* (1947) 51:17, 24, 31, 55; Paul Bragg, Don't live in an unclean body. *Nature's Path* (1948) 52:70, 110; C. Leslie Thomson, *Intestinal Fitness* (London: Thorsons:, 1961), 135–144.

14. Lust's Pills, *Nature's Path* (1940) 45:441; Gastro-Intestinal Cleanser. *Nature's Path* (1946) 50:432; Structor. *Nature's Path* (1943) 47:400.

15. Eugene Wimmershoff, Colonic irrigation in relation to good health. *Nature's Path* (1942) 47:472; Clark Internal Baths, *Nature's Path* (1942) 47:429; *Nature's Path* (1946) 50:482; Thermaire, *Nature's Path* (1941) 46:226.

16. Drew Collins, Colon therapy. In: Joseph Pizzorno and Michael Murray, eds., *A Textbook of Natural Medicine* (Seattle: Bastyr University Publications, 1993), Vol. 1, no pagi-

nation; *Colonic Therapy. A Modern Road to Health*, AMA, box 156, file 15; Norman Walker, *Colon Health: The Key to a Vibrant Life* (Phoenix: O'Sullivan Wodoside, 1979), 5, 173; *Cleansing the Body and Colon for a Happier and Healthier You*, free book advertised in leaflet placed under windshield wiper (no author identified).

17. William Tiller, *Are You a Toxic Waste Site?* (San Antonio: Author, 1996), 5, 7, 22; Jan Alexander, High colonics: The return of the purge. *Ms* (July 1983), 78–80; Mark Baker, *Colon Irrigation: A Forgotten Key to Health* (St. Louis: Baker, 1989); James Strohecker, ed., *Alternative Medicine. The Definitive Guide* (Puyallup, WA: Future Medicine Publishing, 1994), 145.

18. Arlis Loe, Colonic irrigation. *Journal of the American Medical Association* (1981) 246:1869; Thomas Merar, Colonic irrigations. *Journal of the American Medical Association* (1961) 175:642; Use of enemas is limited. *FDA Consumer*, June 1984, 33; Gregory Istre, Kathleen Kreiss, Richard Hopkins, George Healy, Michael Benzinger, Thomas Canfield, Patricia Dickinson, Timothy Englert, Roy Compton, Henry Mathews and Robert Simmons, An outbreak of amebiasis spread by colonic irrigation at a chiropractic clinic. *New England Journal of Medicine* (1982) 307:339–442; John Eisele and Donald Reay, Deaths related to coffee enemas. *Journal of the American Medical Association* (1980) 244:1608–1609; Congress of the United States, Office of Technology Assessment, *Unconventional Cancer Treatments* (Washington, DC: U.S. Government Printing Office, 1990), 51; Medicolegal abstracts. *Journal of the American Medical Association* (1947) 135:307–308.

19. Lynn Barber, Nobody's business but theirs. *The Independent* [London], December 1, 1991, 25.

20. Abrahams (n. 8), 267; Lawrence Galton, Is a vital ingredient missing from your diet? *Readers Digest*, December 1974, 105–109; Carl Flath, *The Miracle Nutrient. How Dietary Fiber Can Save Your Life* (New York: Evans, 1975), 49; Burkitt (n. 5): *Don't Forget Fibre in Your Diet* was initially published in the United States as *Eat Right—To Keep Healthy and Enjoy Life More*, a title the author strongly disliked (personal communication).

21. S. Boyd Eaton, Marjorie Shostak, and Melvin Konner, *The Paleolithic Prescription. A Program of Diet and Exercise and a Design For Living* (New York: Harper and Row, 1988), 8, 46, 67–68, 93, 133, 136, back of dust jacket. Also see S. Boyd Eaton and Melvin Konner, Paleolithic nutrition. A consideration of its nature and current implications. *New England Journal of Medicine* (1985) 312:283–289.

22. Jerome Rodale, *The Health Finder* (Emmaus, PA: Rodale, 1956), 278; Bill Gottlieb, The power in yogurt. *Prevention*, May 1978, 119; Robert Rodale, Stories your bowels can tell. *Prevention*, January 1973, 35–47. The constipation-avoidance points made in *Prevention*'s articles were reiterated by Rodale in books. Jerome Rodale, *J. I. Rodale's Health Treasury* (Emmaus, PA: Rodale, 1962), 265–270, presented Cleave's ideas as early as 1962 as one of the Health Secrets of Famous Doctors; also see Rodale, ed., *The Encyclopedia for Healthful Living* (Emmaus, PA: Rodale, 1974), 222–240.

23. Bran, a blessing for the lower you. *Prevention*, February 1977, 98; Mark Bricklin, Bran for what probably ails you. *Prevention*, August 1974, 85–92; Bricklin, Bathroom death, and how to prevent it. *Prevention*, July 1974, 71–79.

24. Hugh Trowell, Denis Burkitt, and Kenneth Heaton, eds., *Dietary Fibre, Fibre-Depleted Foods and Disease* (London: Academic Press, 1985), xiii; U.S. Department of Health,

Education, and Welfare, *Healthy People. The Surgeon General's Report on Health Promotion and Disease Prevention* (Washington, DC: U.S. Government Printing Office, 1979), 66; U.S. Department of Health and Human Services, *Cancer Prevention* (Washington, DC: U.S. Government Printing Office, 1982), 21; Eliot Marshall, Diet advice, with a grain of salt and a large helping of pepper. *Science* (1986) 231:537–539; U.S. Department of Health and Human Services, *The Surgeon General's Report on Nutrition and Health* (Washington, DC: U.S. Government Printing Office, 1988), 12; Updates, *FDA Consumer*, April 1990, 2; Charles Fuchs, Edward Giovannucci, Graham Colditz, David Hunter, Meir Stampfer, Bernard Rosner, Frank Speizer and Walter Willett, Dietary fiber and the risk of colorectal cancer and adenoma in women. *New England Journal of Medicine* (1999) 340:169–176, p. 169; John Potter, Fiber and Colorectal Cancer—Where to Now? *New England Journal of Medicine* (1999), 340:223–224, p. 224. For a statement of the medical profession's reservations about the fiber hypothesis see Rodney Taylor, Bran yesterday . . . Bran tomorrow? *British Medical Journal* (1984) 288:69–70.

25. Surgery . . . or bran? *Prevention*, December 1974, 143; Judith Stern, Eat rough: It may save your life. *Vogue*, July 1976, 22; Margot Gilman, Fiber mania. *Psychology Today*, December 1989, 33; The Proprietary Association, *Health Care Practices and Perceptions. A Consumer Survey of Self-Medication* (no city: Proprietary Association, 1984), 97; Cory Servaas, Time for a bran new diet. *Saturday Evening Post*, March 1977, 74; Audrey Eyton, *The F-Plan Diet* (Harmondsworth, England: Penguin, 1982); M. A. Eastwood and R. Passmore, Dietary fibre. *The Lancet* (1983) ii:202–206, p. 202; Lynn Langway, F is a five-letter word. *Newsweek*, February 7, 1983, 70; Rosalind Coward, *The Whole Truth: The Myth of Alternative Health* (Boston: Faber and Faber, 1989), 145; Ducks use their loaf. *The People* [London, December 31, 1989, 5; Oat-bran heartburn. *Newsweek*, January 29, 1990, 50–51; Tapping into the oat bran market. *Newsweek*, November 13, 1989, 65; William Connor, Dietary fiber—Nostrum or critical nutrient. *New England Journal of Medicine* (1990) 322:193–195.

26. Thomas Moore, Dietary fibre: Food or fetish? *The Lancet* (1986) i:1040; cartoon, *New Yorker*, November 2, 1987, 43; Wizard of Id. *Seattle Times*, July 22, 1986.

27. George Vahouny and David Kritchevsky, eds., *Dietary Fiber in Health and Disease* (New York: Plenum, 1982), ix; Andrew Ferguson, D. P. Burkitt, *British Medical Journal* (1993) 306:996; All-Bran, *Life*, June 23, 1961, 71, and *National Geographic*, January 1992, back cover.

28. Marshall (n. 24), 537.

29. David Kessler, The federal regulation of food labeling. *New England Journal of Medicine* (1989) 321:717–725; Joanne Silberner, Untangling the fiber story. *U S News and World Report*, November 30, 1987, 71; Stephen McNamara, Health claims for foods—What are the rules. *Food Drug Cosmetic Law Journal* (1985) 40:1–12; Peter Hutt, Government regulation of health claims in food labeling and advertising. *Food Drug Cosmetic Law Journal* (1986) 41:3–73; Sarah Taylor, Health claims for foods: Present law, future policy. *Food Drug Cosmetic Law Journal* (1988) 43:603–635. A good presentation of the state of knowledge of fiber and cancer at the time of the Kellogg ads is Bandaru Reddy, Dietary fiber and colon carcinogenesis. In: George Vahouny and David Kritchvesky, *Dietary Fiber in Health and Disease* (New York: Plenum, 1982), 265–285.

30. Kim Foltz, Policing the health ads. *Newsweek*, November 26, 1984, 75; *Seattle Times*, August 8, 1986, D3; Kenmei ad, *Newsweek*, November 12, 1990, advertising section; Selling high-fiber cereals. *FDA Consumer* (September 1987) 21:6; Laura Shapiro, Labels we can live

by. *Newsweek*, November 18, 1991, 90; Ruth Papazian, Bulking up fiber's healthful reputation. *FDA Consumer* (July–August 1997) 31:22–27, p. 24.

31. Dave Barry, Flush your tax relief down the space toilet. *Seattle Times*, March 8, 1993, A6; Martin Amis, *London Fields* (New York: Harmony, 1989), 212.

32. Saraka, AMA, Box 113, folder 14.

33. Saraka (n. 32).

34. Victor Lindlahr, *The Truth About Constipation* (no publication data given), 25–26; Peter Morell, *Poisons, Potions, and Profits. The Antidote to Radio Advertising* (New York: Knight, 1937), 201; Jason Winters ad in *Health Newsline* (1996) 9(2):54; ads for Perdiem and FibreSonic in personal collection.

35. Metamucil, *Good Housekeeping*, August 1984, 204, and *Newsweek*, June 27, 1988, 49; Naomi Freundlich, The experiment that could clobber Ex-Lax. *Business Week*, June 30, 1997, 93–94; The phenolphthalein fiasco. *Drug Store News*, May 25, 1998, CP37B; Karyn Snyder, Laxative-cancer scare sowing confusion in market. *Drug Topics*, July 7, 1997, 62; Paul Recer, Study finds laxative ingredient causes cancer in rats. *Tacoma News Tribune*, May 1, 1997, A8; Stolberg (n.5); Year book and price list. *American Druggist* (1930) 81:3.

36. D. M. Preston, Arbuthnot Lane's disease: Chronic intestinal stasis. *British Journal of Surgery* (September 1985) 72(Suppl):S8–S10; D. M. Preston and J. E. Lennard-Jones, Severe chronic constipation of young women: 'Idiopathic slow transit constipation'. *Gut* (1986) 27:41–48; D. M. Preston, J. M. Pfeffer, and J. E. Lennard-Jones, Psychiatric assessment of patients with severe constipation. *Gut* (1984) 25:A582–583.

37. Preston and Lennard-Jones (n. 36), 41, 45–47.

38. D. M. Preston, P. R. Hawley, J. E. Lennard-Jones and I. P. Todd, Results of colectomy for severe idiopathic constipation in women (Arbuthnot Lane's disease). *British Journal of Surgery* (1984) 71:547–552, p. 551.

39. Preston (n. 36), S10; Sidney Winawer, ed., *Management of Gastrointestinal Diseases* (New York: Gower, 1992), Vol. 2, 33.20; M. A. Kamm, P. R. Hawley, and J. E. Lennard-Jones, Outcome of colectomy for severe idiopathic constipation. *Gut* (1988) 29:969–973, p. 973; Norman Williams and N. R. Womack, Surgical therapy of constipation and incontinence. In: Sidney Phillips, John Pemberton, and Roy Shorter, eds., *The Large Intestine. Physiology, Pathophysiology, and Disease* (New York: Raven, 1991), 757–773, p. 757; Edgar Achkar, Richard Farmer, and Bertram Fleshler, eds., *Clinical Gastroenterology*, 2nd ed. (Philadelphia: Lea and Febiger, 1992), 79.

40. H. L. Mencken, A *Mencken Chrestomathy* (New York: Knopf, 1949), 444.

41. Mencken (n. 40), 445.

42. John Collins Warren, *Physical Education and the Preservation of Health*, 2nd ed. (Boston: Ticknor, 1846), 5.

43. Tom Morgenthau, Chasing the Unabomer. *Newsweek*, July 10, 1995, 41; William Alcott, Habitual constipation. *Library of Health and Teacher on the Human Constitution* (1842) 6:92–94; Alcott, Intestinal gases, *Teacher of Health and the Laws of the Human Constitution* (1843) 1:250–254, p. 253.

44. Eaton et al. (n. 21), 285.

45. Newsclips from the University of Virginia Office of University Relations, January 15, 1993; personal communication, Daniel Cox; Daniel Cox, James Sutphen, Stephen

Borowitz, Margie Dickens, Janice Singles and William Whitehead, Simple electromyographic biofeedback treatment for chronic pediatric constipation/encopresis: Preliminary report. *Biofeedback and Self-Regulation* (1994) 19:41–50; *The New Yorker*, March 8, 1993, 78.

46. Rene Dubos, *Man Adapting* (New Haven, CT: Yale University Press, 1965), 362; Reed and Carnrick, *Gland Therapy* (New York: Equity Press, 1924), 23. Also see Scott Podolsky, Cultural divergence: Elie Metchnikoff's *Bacillus bulgaricus* therapy and his underlying concept of health. *Bulletin of the History of Medicine* (1998) 72:1–27; and Charles Rosenberg, Pathologies of progress: The idea of civilization as risk. *Bulletin of the History of Medicine* (1998) 72:714–730.

47. H. L. Mencken, *Prejudices. Third Series* (New York: Knopf, 1922), 269; Ellen Goodman, Nouvelle nutrition isn't good for mind. *Seattle Times*, May 24, 1989, C1; News and notes. *British Medical Journal* (1978) i:54. Also see Arthur Barsky, *Worried Sick. Our Troubled Quest for Wellness* (Boston: Little, Brown, 1988), 136–137.

48. Paul Donohue, Longtime laxative user will be able to break habit. *Tacoma News Tribune*, September 2, 1997.

49. Astley Cooper, *The Lectures of Sir Astley Cooper*, 3rd American ed. (Boston: Lilly and Wait, 1831), 56.

INDEX